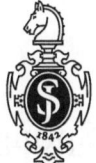

Springer-Verlag Berlin Heidelberg GmbH

33rd Hemophilia Symposium

Hamburg 2002

Editors: I. Scharrer, W. Schramm

Presentation:

Epidemiology
New Findings and Possibilities in the Therapy of Antibodies
Hemophilia: Therapeutic Exercise and Sport
Laboratory Diagnostics
Pediatric Hemostaseology
Free Lectures

Scientific Board:
I. Scharrer, Frankfurt/Main
W. Schramm, Munich

Chairmen:
G. Auerswald (Bremen); H.-H. Brackmann (Bonn); U. Budde (Hamburg);
M. von Depka Prondzinski (Hanover); L. Gürtler (Greifswald);
A. Kurth (Frankfurt/Main); I. Scharrer (Frankfurt/Main);
W. Schramm (Munich); R. Seitz (Langen); M. Spannagl (Munich);
A. H. Sutor (Freiburg); R. Zimmermann (Heidelberg)

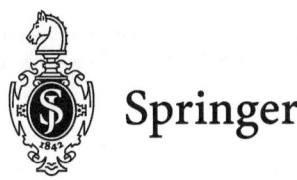 Springer

Professor Dr. med. INGE SCHARRER
Hemophilia Center, Dept. of Internal Medicine
University Hospital
Theodor-Stern-Kai 7
D-60590 Frankfurt am Main
Germany

Professor Dr. med. WOLFGANG SCHRAMM
Dept. of Hemostaseology
University Hospital
Ziemssenstr. 1a
D-80336 München
Germany

With 171 Figures

ISBN 978-3-540-00902-3

Library of Congress Cataloging-in-Publication Data

Hemophilia-Symposium (33rd : 2002 : Hamburg, Germany)
    33rd Hemophilia Symposium : Hamburg, 2002 / editors, I. Scharrer, W. Schramm ;
    chairman, G. Auerswald ... [et al.].
      p. ; cm.
    Includes bibliographical references and index.
     ISBN 978-3-540-00902-3   ISBN 978-3-642-18260-0 (eBook)
     DOI 10.1007/978-3-642-18260-0
     1. Hemophilia-Congresses. I. Title: Thirty-third Hemophilia Symposium. II. Scharrer,
    I. III. Schramm, W., 1943- IV. Title.
      [DNLM: 1. Hemophilia A--diagnosis--Congresses. 2. Hemophilia
    A--epidemiology---Congresses. 3. Hemophilia A--therapy--Congresses. WH 325 H228z 2004]
    RC642.H355 2002
    616.1'572--dc22   2003059113

http://www.springer.de/medizin

© Springer-Verlag Berlin Heidelberg 2004
Originally published by Springer Verlag Berlin Heidelberg New York in 2004

Typesetting: cicero Lasersatz, Dinkelscherben
Print: Saladruck, Berlin

Printed on acid-free paper   SPIN 10922170   21/3130   5 4 3 2 1 0

Contents

III. Hemophilia: Therapeutic Exercise and Sport

IV. Laboratory Diagnostics

V. Pediatric Hemostaseoloy

VI. Free Lectures

VII. Poster

a) Clinic and Casuistic

List of Participants

ANDRITSCHKE, K., Frau
Kinderklinik, Hämophilie-Ambulanz, J.-W.-Goethe-Universität,
D-Frankfurt/Main

ARENDS, P., Dr.
Arzt für Kinderheilkunde, A-Güssing

ASBECK, F., Prof. Dr.
Facharzt f. Innere Medizin, I. Medizinische Klinik, Städt. Krankenhaus, D-Kiel

ASPÖCK, G., Prim. Dr.
Labor I, Allgem. Österr. Krankenhaus der Barmherzigen Schwestern vom
heiligen Kreuz, A-Wels

AUERSWALD, G., Dr.
Professor-Hess-Kinderklinik, Zentralkrankenhaus, D-Bremen

AUMANN, V., Dr.
Klinik für Pädiatrische Hämatologie und Onkologie,
Otto-von-Guericke-Universität, D-Magdeburg

AYGÖREN-PÜRSÜN, E., Frau Dr.
Kinderklinik III, Abt. Hämatologie/Onkologie, Gerinnung,
J.-W.-Goethe-Universität, D-Frankfurt/Main

BALLEISEN, L., Prof. Dr.
Abt. Hämatologie und Onkologie, Innere Medizin, Evangelisches Krankenhaus,
D-Hamm

BARTHELS, M., Frau Prof. Dr.
Hannover

BASSEN, B., Frau Dr.
Praxis Dr. Pollmann, Praxis für Diagnose und Therapie für
Blutgerinnungsstörungen, D-Münster

BATOROVA, A., Frau M. D., Ph. D.
National Hemophilia Center, Institute of Hematology, Bratislava, Slovakia

BAUMGARTNER, CH., Dr.
Facharzt für Kinder und Jugendliche, spez. Hämatologie, CH-Gossau

BECK, CH., Frau Dr.
Ärztin für Kinderheilkunde, D-Berlin

BECK, K., Dr.
Med. Dienst der Krankenkassen, D-Lahr

BECKER, T., Dr.
Interessengemeinschaft Hämophiler (IGH), D-Bonn

BEESER, H., Prof. Dr.
Institute for Quality Management and Standardization in Transfusion Medicine
and Hemostaseology, D-Teningen

BEHA, L., Frau
D-Oberursel

BEILKEN, A., Dr.
Kinderklinik, Med. Hochschule Hannover, D-Hannover

BENEKE, H., Dr.
Sektion Hämostaseologie, Abteilung Innere Medizin III,
Medizinische Universitätsklinik, D-Ulm

BEREUTER, L., Dr.
Abteilung Pädiatrie, Landeskrankenhaus Feldkirch, A-Feldkirch

BEUTEL, K., Frau Dr.
Pädiatrische Hämatologie/Onkologie, Universitäts-Kinderklinik, D-Hamburg

BIDLINGMAIER, CH., Dr.
Abt. Hämostaseologie, Dr. von Haunersches Kinderspital, D-München

BLAZEK, B., Dr.
FNsP Ostrava, Childrens Dept. – Hematology, CZ-Ostrava – Poruba

BLICKHEUSER, R., Dr.
DRK-Kinderklinik, D-Siegen

BLUMENTRITT, H., Dr.
Paul-Ehrlich-Institut, D-Langen

BOBROWSKA, H., Dr.
Department of Hematology, Voievodship Children's Hospital,
PL-Poznan

BÖHM, M., Frau Dipl.-Biol.
Hämophilie-Ambulanz, J.-W.-Goethe-Universität,
D-Frankfurt/Main

BORCHERS, H., Frau
Abt. für Transfusionsmedizin, Medizinische Einrichtungen der
Heinrich-Heine-Universität, D-Düsseldorf

BOSSE, Z., Frau
Hämophilie-Zentrum, Med. Hochschule Hannover,
D-Hannover

BRACKMANN, H.-H., Dr.
Institut für Experimentelle Hämatologie und Transfusionsmedizin
der Universität, D-Bonn

BRACKMANN, CH., Frau
Institut für Experimentelle Hämatologie und Transfusionsmedizin
der Universität, D-Bonn

BRAND, B., Frau Dr.
Blutspendedienst SRK, Kantonsspital Chur, CH-Chur

BRAUN, U., Frau Dr.
CH-Zurzach

BROCKHAUS, W., Dr.
Abteilung für Hämostaseologie, Hämatologie und Angiologie, D-Nürnberg

BUDDE, U., Prof. Dr.
Gemeinschaftslabor Dr. Keeser und Prof. Arndt, D-Hamburg

CALATZIS, A., Dr.
Abteilung Hämostaseologie, Medizinische Klinik Innenstadt der
Ludwig-Maximilians-Universität, D-München

CARLSSON, L., Frau
Abt. Transfusionsmedizin, D-Greifswald

CASTER, CH., Frau
Abt. Hämostaseologie/Transfusionsmedizin, Universitäts-Kinderklinik,
D-Homburg/Saar

CVIRN, G., Mag.
Univ. Klinik für Kinder- und Jugendheilkunde,
Allgem. Österr. Landeskrankenhaus Graz, A-Graz

DEML, M., Frau Dr.
Dr. von Haunersches Kinderspital, D-München

DINGER, J., Dr.
Kinderklinik der Med. Fakultät der TU Dresden, D-Dresden

DITTMER, R., Frau Dr.
Gemeinschaftslabor Dr. Keeser und Prof. Arndt, D-Hamburg

DOCKTER, G., Prof. Dr.
Kinderklinik, Universitätskliniken des Saarlandes, D-Homburg

DOMSCH, CH., Dr.
Abteilung Hämostaseologie, Medizinische Klinik Innenstadt der
Ludwig-Maximilians-Universität, D-München

EBER, ST., Prof. Dr.
Abteilung Hämatologie, Kinderspital Zürich, CH-Zürich

EBERL, W., Dr.
Kinderklinik, Städtisches Klinikum Holwedestraße, D-Braunschweig

EFFENBERGER, W., Dr.
Institut für Exp. Hämatologie und Transfusionsmedizin der Universität, D-Bonn

EICKHOFF, H. H., Dr.
Orthopädische Klinik, St.-Josef-Hospital, D-Troisdorf

EIFRIG, B., Frau Dr.
Abteilung Onkologie/Hämostaseologie, Medizinische Klinik
Universitätskrankenhaus Eppendorf, D-Hamburg

EL-MAARRI, O., Dr.
Institut für Experimentelle Hämatologie und Transfusionsmed.,
Universitätsklinik, D-Bonn

ELANJIKAL, Z.
Zentrum für Kinderheilkunde, Klinikum der J.-W-.Goethe-Universität,
D-Frankfurt/Main

ESCURIOLA-ETTINGSHAUSEN, C., Frau Dr.
Zentrum der Kinderheilkunde, Klinikum der J.-W.-Goethe-Universität,
D-Frankfurt/Main

FÄSSLER, H., Dr.
FMH Medicina interna, CH-Chiasso

FENGLER, V., Frau
Kinder- u. Jugendmedizin KK3, Klinikum Frankfurt/O., D-Frankfurt/Oder

FISCHER, B., Frau
Kinderklinik, Hämatol./Onkol. Ambulanz, Universitätsklinikum Eppendorf,
D-Hamburg

FÖRSTER, T., Frau Dipl.-Biol.
Institut für Humangenetik, Biozentrum, D-Würzburg

FRANKE, D., PD Dr.
Schwerpunktpraxis für Gerinnungsstörungen und Gefäßkrankheiten,
D-Magdeburg

FREWERT, B., Frau Dr.
Inst. für Exp. Hämatologie und Transfusionsmedizin der Universität,
D-Bonn

FUNK, M., Dr.
Kinderklinik, Klinikum der J.-W.-Goethe-Universität, D-Frankfurt/Main

GABOR, K., Frau Dr.
Universitätsklinik Düsseldorf, D-Düsseldorf

GALLISTL, S., Prof. Dr.
Univ. Klinik für Kinder- und Jugendheilkunde, Allgem. Österr.
Landeskrankenhaus Graz, A-Graz

GEHRICH, S., Dr.
Klinikum der Carl-Gustav-Carus-Universität, D-Dresden

GEIB, R., Frau Dr.
Klinik für Kinder- u. Jugendmedizin, Klinikum Saarbrücken gGmbH,
D-Saarbrücken

GEISHOFER, G., Dr.
Universitäts-Kinderklinik, A-Graz

GNAD, Dr.
Abteilung Hämatologie, Universitätsklinik Regensburg, D-Regensburg

GÖHAUSEN, M., Frau Dr.
Praxis für Diagnostik und Therapie von Blutgerinnungsstörungen,
Ambulanzzentrum der Raphaelsklinik, D-Münster

GOTTSTEIN, S., Frau Dr.
Abt. Klin. Hämostaseologie, Hämophilie-Zentrum, Krankenhaus im Friedrichshain, D-Berlin

GRANDHAMME, B., Frau
D-Homburg

GROSS, J., Dr.
D-Homburg/Saar

GRÜNINGER, M., Dr.
Krankenhaus Dornbirn, A-Dornbirn

GÜLDENRING, H., Dipl.-Med.
Kinderklinik, Städt. Krankenhaus Dresden-Neustadt, D-Dresden

GÜRTLER, L., Prof. Dr.
Institut für Mikrobiologie, Ernst-Moritz-Arndt-Universität, D-Greifswald

GUTENSOHN, K., PD Dr.
Institut für Bioscientia und Laboruntersuchungen, D-Ingelheim

HABERLAND, H., Dr.
Kinderklinik Lindenhof, Krankenhaus Lichtenberg, D-Berlin

HÄDRICH, H., Frau
Internistische Funktionsabt., Asklepias Fachklinik, D-Stadtroda

HALBMAYER, M., Dr.
Zentrallaboratorium, Krankenhaus der Stadt Wien-Lainz, A-Wien

HAMMANN, M., Frau
Paul-Ehrlich-Institut, D-Langen

HAMPEL, H., Frau Dr.
Kurpfalz-Krankenhaus, D-Heidelberg

HANFLAND, P., Prof. Dr.
Institut für Exp. Hämatologie und Transfusionsmedizin der Universität, D-Bonn

HARTMANN, S., Frau Dr.
Ärztin für Hämatologie u. Onkologie, CH-Chur

HASSENPFLUG, W., Dr.
Kinderklinik, Universitätsklinik Eppendorf, D-Hamburg

HAUSHOFER, A., Dr.
Zentrallabor Allgem. Österr. Krankenhaus der Landeshauptstadt St. Pölten,
A-St. Pölten

HEIDE, D., Frau
Kinderklinik K4 Ambulanz, Universitätskliniken Heinrich-Heine, D-Düsseldorf

HEINRICHS, CH., Frau Doz. Dr.
D-Berlin

HELLSTERN, P., Prof. Dr.
Institut für Transfusionsmedizin und Immunhämatologie, Klinikum der
Stadt Ludwigshafen, D-Ludwigshafen

HEMPELMANN, L., Dr.
D-Berlin

HENSELER, D., Frau
Molekulare Hämostaselologie, Universitätsklinik Bonn, D-Bonn

HERBINIAUX, U., Frau
Molekulare Hämostaseologie, Universitätsklinik Bonn, D-Bonn

HERRMANN, F., Prof. Dr. Dr.
Institut für Humangenetik, Medizinische Fakultät der
Ernst-Moritz-Arndt-Universität, D-Greifswald

HESPE-JUNGESBLUT, K., Frau
Zentrum für Gesundheitsethik, D-Hannover

HILBERG, T., Dr.
Lehrstuhl für Sportmedizin, Friedrich-Schiller-Universität, D-Jena

HOFMANN, H., Dr.
Facharzt für Transfusionsmedizin, DRK-Blutspendedienst, D-Potsdam

HOHMANN, D.
Interessengemeinschaft Hämophiler (IGH), D-Bonn

HOLECKOVA, M., Frau Dr.
Abteilung Hämatologie, Fakultäts-Krankenhaus, CZ-Ceské Budejovice

HOLZHÜTER, H., Prof. Dr.
Hämophilie-Zentrum Nordwest, D-Bremen

HORNEFF, S., Frau Dr.
Klinik für Kinderheilkunde der Martin-Luther-Universität Halle-Wittenberg,
D-Halle

HOVY, L., Prof. Dr.
Orthopädische Abt., Städtische Kliniken Frankfurt/M.-Höchst,
D-Frankfurt/Main

HUTH-KÜHNE, A., Frau Dr.
Kurpfalzkrankenhaus Heidelberg und Hämophiliezentrum gGmbH,
D-Heidelberg

IMAHORN, P., Dr.
Kinderspital Luzern, CH-Luzern

JULEN, E., Dr.
FMH Allgemeine Medizin, CH-Zermatt

KALNINS, W., Dr.
Deutsche Hämophilie-Gesellschaft (DHG), D-Marmagen

KÄSE, M., Frau
Päd. Hämostaseologie/Onkologie, Universitätsklinik Münster, D-Münster

KEHREL, B., Frau Prof. Dr.
Klinik und Poliklinik f. Anästhesie und Intensivmedizin, D-Münster

KEMKES-MATTHES, B., Frau Prof. Dr.
Zentrum für Innere Medizin, Klinikum der Justus-Liebig-Universität,
D-Gießen

KIESEWETTER, H., Prof. Dr. Dr.
Inst. f. Transfusionsmedizin u. Immunhämatologie, Campus Charité Mitte,
D-Berlin

Kilgert, K., Frau
Hämostaseologie, Med. Klinik Innenstadt, D-München

KIM, S., Frau Dr.
Abt. f. päd. Hämatologie/Onkologie, Universitäsklinik Hamburg, D-Hamburg

KLAMROTH, R., Dr.
Abt. Klinische Hämostaseologie, Hämophilie-Zentrum, Krankenhaus
im Friedrichshain, D-Berlin

KLARE, M., Dr.
II. Innere Klinik, Klinikum Berlin-Buch, D-Berlin

KLARMANN, D., Dr.
Kinderklinik der J.-W.-Goethe-Universität, D-Frankfurt/Main

KLIER, H., Dr.
Steiermärkische Gebietskrankenkasse, A-Graz

KNÖBL, P., Prof. Dr.
Abteilung für Hämatologie und Hämostaseologie, Allgem. Krankenhaus
der Stadt Wien, A-Wien

KNÖFLER, R., Dr.
Klinik und Poliklinik für Kinderheilkunde, Carl-Gustav-Carus-Universität,
D-Dresden

KOBELT, R., Dr.
FMH Kinder- und Jugendmedizin im Wabern-Zentrum, CH-Wabern

KÖHLER-VAJTA, K., Frau Dr.
Ärztin für Kinderheilkunde, D-Grünwald

KÖNIGS, CH.
Zentrum für Kinderheilkunde, J.-W.-Goethe-Universität, D-Frankfurt/Main

KOSCIELNY, J., Dr.
Institut für Transfusionsmedizin und Immunhämatologie,
Campus Charité Mitte, D-Berlin

KÖSTENBERGER, M., Dr.
A-Graz

KÖSTERING, H., Prof. Dr.
D-Lemgo

KRAUSE, M., Frau
Hämophilie-Ambulanz, Klinikum der J.-W.-Goethe-Universität,
D-Frankfurt/Main

KREBS, H., Dr.
Abteilung Hämostaseologie, Medizinische Klinik Innenstadt der
Ludwig-Maximilians-Universität, D-München

KREUZ, W., PD Dr.
Zentrum der Kinderheilkunde, Klinikum der J.-W.-Goethe-Universität,
D-Frankfurt/Main

KURME, A., Dr.
D-Hamburg

KURNIK, K., Frau Dr.
Kinderklinik im Dr. von Hauner'schen Kinderspital,
Ludwig-Maximilians-Universität, D-München

KURTH, A., PD Dr.
Orthopädische Universitätsklinik, D-Frankfurt/Main

LAHAYE, L.
D-Bonn

LAJOS, I., Prof. Dr.
Bluttransfusionsdienst, H-Szombathely

LEHMANN, I., Frau
Med. Klinik und Poliklinik I, Hämophiliezentrum, Universität Leipzig,
D-Leipzig

LENK, H., PD Dr.
Univ.-Klinik und Poliklinik für Kinder und Jugendliche, Universität Leipzig,
D-Leipzig

HEIKO-GUNDMAR L., Prof. Dr.
Institut für Labormedizin, Klinikum Schwerin, D-Schwerin

LIESE, Frau
Ltd. MTA – Labor, Medizinische Hochschule Hannover, D-Hannover

LIGHEZAN. D., Dr.
Clinica Medicina Interna II, Universitatea de Medicina si Farmacie Timisoara,
Spital Municipal, R-Timisoara

LORETH, R., Dr.
Gerinnungslabor, Westpfalz-Klinikum, D-Kaiserslautern

LOSONCZY, H., Doz. Dr.
1. Medizinische Klinik, Medizinische Universität, H-Pécs

LUBENOW, N., Dr.
Abt. Transfusionsmedizin, Universitätsklinik Greifswald, D-Greifswald

LUFT, B., Dr.
Kinderklinik, Hämophilie-Ambulanz 31–1,
Klinikum der J.-W.-Goethe-Universität, D-Frankfurt/Main

LÜHR, C., Frau
Abt. Hämophilie/Med. Poliklinik, Medizinische Hochschule Hannover,
D-Hannover

LUTZ, W., Dr.
Gerinnungslabor D-LAB 28, Universitätsspital, CH-Zürich

LUTZE, G., Prof. Dr.
Institut für Klinische Chemie und Pathobiochemie,
Otto-von-Guericke-Universität, D-Magdeburg

MAAK, B., Prof. Dr.
Thüringen-Klinik Georgius Agricola Saalfeld, D-Saalfeld

MAGENS, Mirko
Abt. Transfusionsmedizin, Transplantationsimmunologie,
Universitätskrankenhaus Eppendorf, D-Hamburg

MALE, CH., Dr.
Universitätsklinik für Kinderheilkunde, A-Wien

MANNHALTER, CH., Frau Prof. Dr.
Allgem. Krankenhaus der Stadt Wien, Klinisches Institut für Med. und
Chem. Labordiagnostik, A-Wien

MAREK, R., Dr.
Wiener Gebietskrankenkasse, A-Wien

MARTINEZ, I., Frau
Zentrum der Kinderheilkunde, Klinikum der J.-W.-Goethe-Universität,
D-Frankfurt/Main

MARTINKOVÁ, I., Frau Prim. Dr.
odd. Hematologie, Fakultni nemocnice v Plzni, CZ-Plzen-Bory

MATYSKOVA, M., Frau Dr.
Department of Hematology, II. Interni Klinika, CZ-Brno

MAURER, M., Prof. Dr.
D-Bernau/Chiemsee

MEILI, E., Frau Dr.
Gerinnungslabor, Universitätsspital, CH-Zürich

METZEN, E., Frau Dr.
Institut für Hämostaseologie und Transfusionsmedizin,
Universitätskliniken Heinrich-Heine, D-Düsseldorf

MIESBACH, W., Dr.
Innere Med., Hämophilie-Ambulanz, Klinikum der J.-W.-Goethe-Universität,
D-Frankfurt/Main

MIHAILOV, M., Frau Dr.
University of Medicine, Clinica I-a Pediatrie, R-Timisoara

MÖBIUS, D., Frau Dr.
Kinderklinik und Kinderpoliklinik, Carl-Thiem-Klinikum, D-Cottbus

MÖSSELER, J., Dr.
Arzt für Kinderheilkunde, D-Dillingen

MÜHLE, CH., Frau
Universität Erlangen-Nürnberg, Klinik für Kinder und Jugendliche,
D-Erlangen

MUNTEAN, E., Prof. Dr.
Univ.-Klinik für Kinder- und Jugendheilkunde,
Allgem. Österr. Landeskrankenhaus Graz, A-Graz

MUSS, N., Dr.
Salzburger Gebietskrankenkasse, A-Salzburg

NIEKRENS, C., Frau Dr.
Pädiatrie, Städt. Klinik Delmenhorst, D-Delmenhorst

NIMTZ-TALASKA, A., Frau Dr.
Klinik für Kinder- und Jugendmedizin, Klinikum Frankfurt/O.,
D-Frankfurt/Oder

OBERGSELL, A., Dr.
Inst. f. Biochemie/Pathobiochemie, Zentrallabor, Med. Universitätsklinik,
D-Würzburg

OBERNDORFER, M., Frau
Universitätsklinik für Innere Med., A-Wien

OLDENBURG, J., Dr.
Blutspendedienst Frankfurt/M., D-Frankfurt/Main

PABINGER, I., Frau Prof. Dr.
Universitätsklinik für Innere Medizin I, A-Wien

PETRESCU, C., Frau Dr.
Spitalul Clinic de copii, Louis Turcanu/Clin. Pediatrie III,
Compartimentul de Onco-Hematologie, R-Timisoara

PODEHL-KLOSE, J., Dr.
Orthopädisches Fachkrankenhaus, Annastift, D-Hannover

POEK, K.
Deutsche Hämophiliegesellschaft (DHG), D-Berlin

POEK, B., Frau
D-Berlin

PTOSZKOVA, H., Frau Dr.
Hämatologie, CZ-Ostrava-Zabreh

RABENSTEIN, C., Frau
Zentrum der Inneren Medizin, Hämophilie-Ambulanz,
Klinikum der J.-W.-Goethe-Universität, D-Frankfurt/M.

RAGER, K., PD Dr.
Kinderklinik, Caritas-Krankenhaus, D-Bad Mergentheim

RAMSCHAK, H., Dr.
I. Medizinische Universitätsklinik,
Allgem. Österr. Landeskrankenhaus Graz, A-Graz

RANK, A., Dr.
Med. Klinik III, Klinikum Großhadern, D-München

REHAK, T., Dr.
Universitätsklink, A-Graz

REHBERGER, G., Dr.
Ordination, A-Frastanz

REININGER, A., PD Dr.
Abt. Transfusionsmedizin, Universitätsklinik München, D-München

REITER, W., Dr.
Facharzt für Innere Medizin, Hämatologie/Intern. Onkologie, D-Viersen

RIES, M., PD Dr.
Klinik für Kinderheilkunde und Jugendmedizin, Klinikum Memmingen,
D-Memmingen

RINGKAMP, H., Frau
Praxis für Diagnostik und Therapie von Blutgerinnungsstörungen,
Ambulanzzentrum der Raphaelsklinik, D-Münster

ROOSENDAAL, G., Dr.
Van Creveld Clinic, NL-BN Utrecht

ROSCHITZ, B, Frau Dr.
Allgem. Österr. Landeskrankenhaus Graz, Univ.-Klinik für Kinder-
und Jugendheilkunde, A-Graz

Rost, S., Frau Dipl.-Biol.
Institut für Humangenetik, Biozentrum, D-Würzburg

Rützler, L., Dr.
CH-Altstätten

Schambeck, Ch., Dr.
Inst. f. klin. Biochemie u. Pathobiochemie/Zentrallabor,
Universitätsklinikum/Med. Klinik, D-Würzburg

Scharrer, I., Frau Prof. Dr.
Zentrum der Inneren Medizin, Hämophilie-Ambulanz,
Klinikum der J.-W.-Goethe-Universität, D-Frankfurt/Main

Scheel, H., Dr.
D-Leipzig

Schelle, G.
Interessengemeinschaft Hämophiler (IGH)
D-Bonn

Schimpf, K., Prof. Dr.
D-Heidelberg

Schleef, M., Dr.
Hämostaseologie, Medizinische Klinik, D-München

Schlenkrich, U., Dr.
D-Großlehna

Schmidt, O., Dr.
Praxis für Gefäßkrankheiten, D-Magdeburg

Schneppenheim, R., Prof. Dr.
Abt. Hämatologie/Onkologie, Kinderklinik Universitätsklinik Eppendorf,
D-Hamburg

Schön, A., Frau cand. med.
Abt. für Transfusionsmedizin und Transplantationsimmunologie,
Universitätsklinikum Eppendorf, D-Hamburg

Schramm, W., Prof. Dr.
Abteilung Hämostaseologie, Medizinische Klinik Innenstadt der
Ludwig-Maximilians-Universität, D-München

Schramm, B.
D-München

SCHRÖDER, W., Dr.
Institut für Humangenetik, Ernst-Moritz-Arndt-Universität, D-Greifswald

SCHUBERT, CH., Dr.
Medizinische Klinik, Klinikum Erfurt GmbH, D-Erfurt

SCHULTE-OVERBERG, U., Dr.
Kinderklinik, Campus Virchow Klinikum, D-Berlin

SCHULZ, M., Frau Dr.
Abteilung Blutspende- und Transfusionsmedizin der
Ernst-Moritz-Arndt-Universität, D-Greifswald

SCHUMACHER, R., Dipl.-Med.
Kinderklinik/Station A 2, Klinikum Schwerin, D-Schwerin

SCHWAAB, R., Dr.
Institut für Exp. Hämatologie u. Transfusionsmedizin der Universität,
D-Bonn

SEDLAK, M., Dr.
Interne II, Allgem. Krankenhaus der Stadt Linz, A-Linz

SEITZ, R., Prof. Dr.
Abteilung Hämatologie und Transfusionsmedizin, Paul-Ehrlich-Institut,
D-Langen

SELKE, K., Dr.
Nephrologisches Labor, Universitäts-Kinderklinik, D-Freiburg

SEPIC, A., Dr.
Ospedale Beata Vergine, CH-Mendrisio

SERBAN, M., Frau Prof. Dr.
IIIrd Paediatric Clinic, University of Medicine, R-Timisoara

SEUSER, A., Dr.
Kaiser-Karl-Klinik, Fachklinik für Orthopädie, D-Bonn

SEYFERT, U., Prof. Dr.
Abt. Klinische Hämostaseologie und Transfusionsmedizin,
Universitätskliniken d. Saarlandes, D-Homburg

SIEGEMUND, A., Frau Dr.
Institut für Klinische Chemie, Gerinnungslabor Innere Medizin,
Universität Leipzig, D-Leipzig

SIEGMUND, B.
  Praxis Dr. Pollmann, Praxis für Diagnostik und Therapie von
  Blutgerinnungsstörungen, D-Münster

SIEMENS, H. J., PD Dr.
  Gemeinschaftslabor und Gerinnungsambulanz, D-Plön

SIEMENSEN, M., Frau
  II. Med. Abt. Endokrinologie, Allgem. Krankenhaus Barmbek, D-Hamburg

SILLER, M.
  Deutsche Hämophiliegesellschaft (DHG), D-Berlin

SINGER, H.
  Institut für exp. Hämatologie und Transfusionsmedizin,
  Universitätsklinik Bonn, D-Bonn

SPANNAGL, M., Dr.
  Abt. Hämostaseologie, Med. Klinik Innenstadt der L. Maximilians-Universität,
  D-München

STOLL, H., Frau
  Kinderklinik, Klinikum der J.-W.-Goethe-Universität, D-Frankfurt/Main

STUMPE, CH., Frau
  Abt. f. Klinische Hämostaseologie, Krankenhaus Friedrichshain, D-Berlin

SUBERT, R., Frau Dr.
  Abt. für Hämatologie und Onkologie, Klinik für Innere Medizin II,
  Klinikum Schwerin, D-Schwerin

SULOVSKA, I., Frau Dr.
  Hämatologische Klinik, Fakultäts-Krankenhaus, CZ-Olomouc

SUTOR, H., Prof. Dr.
  Abt. Hämatologie und Hämostaseologie, Kinderklinik/Klinikum der
  Albert-Ludwigs-Universität, D-Freiburg

SUTTORP, M., Prof. Dr.
  Hämatologie/Onkologie, Klinik u. Poliklinik für Kinderheilkunde,
  Carl-Gustav-Carus Universität, D-Dresden

SYKORA, K.-W. PD Dr.
  Zentrum Kinderheilkunde, Medizinische Hochschule Hannover, D-Hannover

THEDIECK, S., Frau
D-Münster

TIEDE, A., Dr.
Hannover

TRUNZ-CARLISI, E.
Institut für Prävention und Nachsorge GmbH, D-Köln

TÜRK-KRAETZER, B., Frau Dr.
Ärztin für Kinderheilkunde, D-Oldenburg

UNKRIG, CH., Dr.
D-St. Augustin

VANDENDRIESSCHE, T., Prof. Dr.
Center for Transgene Technology and Gene Therapy, B-Leuven

VARVENNE, M., Dr.
Abt. Hämophilie/Med. Poliklinik, Medizinische Hochschule Hannover,
D-Hannover

VERMÖHLEN, K.
Orthopädie, Eifelhöhen-Klinik, D-Netternheim-Marmagen

VIGH, T., Dipl.-Biochemiker
Zentum der Inneren Med., Hämophilie-Ambulanz,
Klinikum der J.-W.-Goethe-Universität, D-Frankfurt/Main

VOERKEL, W., Dr.
Gemeinschaftspraxis für Labormedizin, Mikrobiologie,
Transfusionsmedizin, D-Leipzig

VOGEL, G., Prof. Dr.
D-Erfurt

VOGT, B., Frau
Abt. Hämatologie, Universitäts-Kinderklinik, D-Leipzig

VON AUER, CH., Frau Dr.
Zentrum der Inneren Med., Hämophilie-Ambulanz,
Klinikum der J.-W.-Goethe-Universität, D-Frankfurt/Main

VON DEPKA PRONDZINSKI, M., Dr.
Abt. Hämophilie/Med. Poliklinik, Medizinische Hochschule Hannover,
D-Hannover

VON DER WEID, N., Dr.
Medizinische Kinderklinik, Inselspital, CH-Bern

VORLOVA, Z., Frau Dr.
Institut für Hämatologie und Bluttransfusion, CZ-Praha 2

WALLNY, T., PD Dr.
Orthopädische Klinik, Med. Einrichtungen der Rheinischen
Friedrich-Wilhelms-Universität, D-Bonn

WANK, J., Dr.
St.-Anna-Kinderspital, A-Wien

WEISS, Josef
Österr. Hämophiliegesellschaft, A-Wien

WEISSER, J., Dr.
Kinderarzt/Rehabilitation, Fachkrankenhaus Neckargemünd gGmbH,
D-Neckargemünd

WENDISCH, E., Frau Dr.
Ärztin für Allgemeinmedizin, D-Dresden

WENZEL, E., Prof. Dr.
Abt. Klinische Hämostaseologie und Transfusionsmedizin,
Universitätskliniken d. Saarlandes, D-Homburg/Saar

WERMES, C., Frau Dr.
Abt. Hämophilie/Med. Poliklinik, Medizinische Hochschule Hannover,
D-Hannover

WIEDING, J., Dr.
D-Göttingen

WIEN, F., Dr.
Zentrum für Kinderheilkunde, Otto-von-Guericke-Universität, D-Magdeburg

WINTERSTEIN, E., Frau Dr.
D-Zimmernsupra

WOLF, H.-H., Dr.
Klinik u. Polikl. f. Innere Med. IV, Medizinische Fakultät,
M.-Luther-Universität Halle-Wittenberg, D-Halle

WULFF, K., Frau Dr.
Institut für Humangenetik, Ernst-Moritz-Arndt-Universität, D-Greifswald

ZANIER, U., Frau
  Krankenhaus, A-Dornbirn

ZELLHOFER, J.
  Personalvertretung, Allgem. Krankenhaus der Stadt Wien, A-Wien

ZIEGER, B., Frau PD Dr.
  Kinderklinik, Klinikum der Albert-Ludwigs-Universität, D-Freiburg

ZIMMERMANN, R., Prof. Dr.
  Kurpfalzkrankenhaus Heidelberg und Hämophiliezentrum gGmbH,
  D-Heidelberg

ZUPANCIC-SALEK, S., Frau Dr.
  Lug Samoborski, Croatia

ZYSCHKA, A., Frau
  Kinderklinik III, Abt. Hämatologie/Onkologie,
  Klinikum der J.-W.-Goethe-Universität, D-Frankfurt/Main

Johann Lukas Schoenlein Award 2002

I. Scharrer

The Johann Lukas Schoenlein Prize was first awarded in 1977, sponsored originally by Immuno company, now Baxter, to commemorate J. L. Schoenlein, who gave the name to hemophilia.

The objectives of the Prize are laid down in the statutes as follows:

The Prize serves to advance clinical research in the area of chronic blood diseases, particularly hemophilia and related congenital diseases of blood clotting. This is an exclusively charitable foundation and achieves the objective by the award of the J. L. Schoenlein Prize for exceptional scientific works.

The recipient of the award is decided by a curatorium consisting of seven scientists and one representative of the foundation

The criteria on which the committee bases its decision include scientific value, clinical relevance, innovation, originality, effectiveness and presentation.

This year we had 9 candidates for the award. We have had more female candidates this time than in the past. The median age of the candidates was 36 years old which was younger than before.

After very careful consideration, Prof. VandenDriessche was selected for his investigations of gene therapy of hemophilia A.

He submitted four publications which presented three different successful models of gene therapy.

The aims of gene therapy are to achieve high and long-lasting levels of FVIII. This goal can be achieved by vectors, which lead the gene into the target cell.

The vectors are the Achilles heel of the gene therapy.

Prof. VandenDriessche published 3 models, f.i. *the retroviral FVIII gene transfer*:

Using this model he could achieve therapeutical transient levels of FVIII in mice after transplantation of bone marrow cells which contained retroviral vectors with FVIII genes.

Prof. VandenDriessche was invited to present his work as a State of the Art Lecture during ISTH in Birmingham in July 2003.

He achieved persistent elevated levels of FVIII in neonatal hemophilic mice by a gene transfer into the liver.

By *lentiviral gene transfers* he achieved therapeutical levels of FIX in liver cells of adult mice, without need of a hepatectomy.

The new *HC-adenoviral vectors* give us a glimmer of hope. By using these he could achieve the highest long-lasting levels of FVIII in hemophilic mice and dogs.

Furthermore the HC-adenoviral vectors proved to be safe. They caused neither hepatoxicity nor blood cell damage.

Prof. VandenDriessche was also able to achieve therapeutical FVIII levels in a hemophilia A – dog model with the homologous dogs FVIII-gene.

As a result of the work of Prof. VandenDriessche we hope that our patients will soon profit from these positive results in mice and dogs.

It will no longer be necessary to rely on »Rasputin-therapy« needed by the Russian tsarevitch Alexis.

The J. W. Schoenlein Prize was awarded on November 08, 2002 for the 15th time to:

Prof. Thierry VandenDriessche.

He was born in 1965 in Ostende (Belgium).

He is working in the Center of Transgene Technology and Gene Therapy of the University of Leuven and he is a visiting professor at the Free University in Brussels.

He published 61 publications in well known peer-reviewed journals during the period of 1989–2002.

His research projects include methods of gene transfer and the gene therapy of hemophilia.

As he describes his wife as his best coworker, a part of the this year's Prize is awarded to her.

We congratulate Prof. VandenDriessche in his own words:

Van Harte Proficiat!

I. *Epidemiology*

Chairmen:

R. SEITZ (Langen)
L. GÜRTLER (Greifswald)

HIV Infection and Causes of Death in Patients with Hemophilia in Germany (Year 2001/2002 Survey)

W. SCHRAMM and H. KREBS, on behalf of the participating German hemophilia centers

Basic Facts on the Surveys

The annually survey »HIV Infection and Causes of Death in Patients with Hemophilia in Germany« goes along with a fine tradition. Already in the late 1970s Professor Landbeck began to survey annually hemophiliacs living at that time in West Germany for causes of death and the prevalence of diseases. This was carried on till today, so that our actual insights rest upon a broad database. However data quality could be much more improved in future. Especially incomplete and inconsistent filled in forms always weaken the statistical strength of our findings. Hence it is planned to complete the missing information by inquiring the according centers.

Participating Centers

Since the first survey the number of participating centers has increased every year with a particularly rise in 1991 when the hemophilia treatment centers of the former East Germany joined in. Today these centers contribute a significant portion of the overall data (Fig. 1). In this year's survey the number of reporting hemophilia centers slightly increased from 72 centers last year to 75 centers this year (Table. 1 and Fig. 1). Thereby the total number of patients (including patients with von-Willebrand disease) reported from all centers remained relatively constant and added up to 7759 patients compared to 8055 patients in last year's survey (Table. 2).

Table 1. Numbers of participating hemophilia centers

	1991	1992	1993	1994	1995	1996	1997	1998	1999	2000	2001	2002
East	47	62	79									
West	18	18	24									
Total	65	80	103	111	119	119	71	75	93	87	72	75

I. Scharrer/W. Schramm (Ed.)
33rd Hemophilia Symposium Hamburg 2002
© Springer-Verlag Berlin Heidelberg 2004

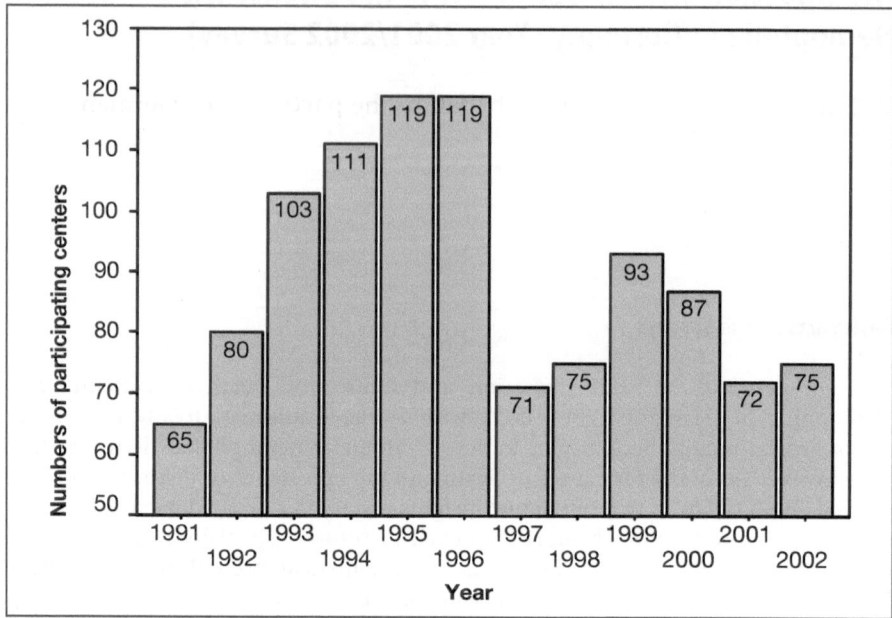

Fig. 1. Numbers of participating hemophilia centers

Patients

In the 2001/2002 survey, a total number of 7759 patients (including possible double registrations) have been reported from the participating centers. The distribution of patients with hemophilia A (51,79%), B (9,09%) and patients with von-

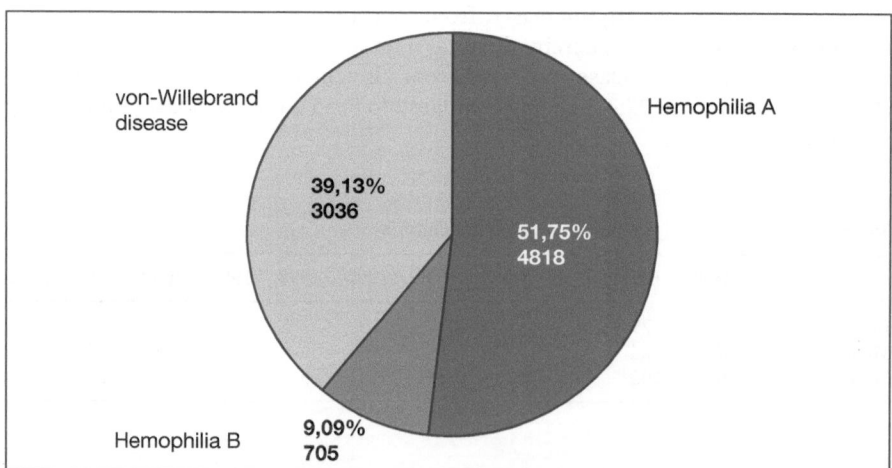

Fig. 2. Overall distribution of diseases

Willebrand disease (39,13%) is given in Fig. 2. Compared to the data of the previous surveys these are relative consistent findings.

When severity of disease is analyzed with a cut-off of 2% factor activity, the distribution between the two subgroups, i.e. below 2% and above 2%, is almost similar in patients with hemophilia A and B as shown in Fig. 3.

In 3,51% of the patients with hemophilia A and in 2,83% of the patients with hemophilia B, an inhibitor was found (see Fig. 4 and Tab. 2). 28% of patients with von-Willebrand disease showed ristocetin Cofactor levels below 30% as demonstrated in Fig. 5 and Table 2.

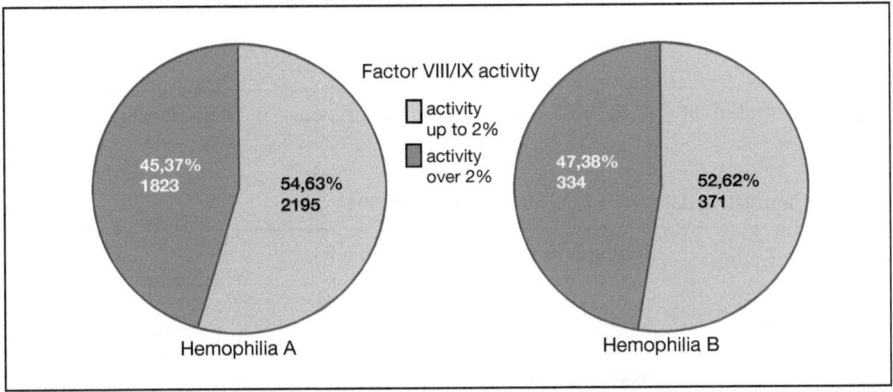

Fig. 3. Distribution of factor VIII/IX activity in patients with hemophilia A and B

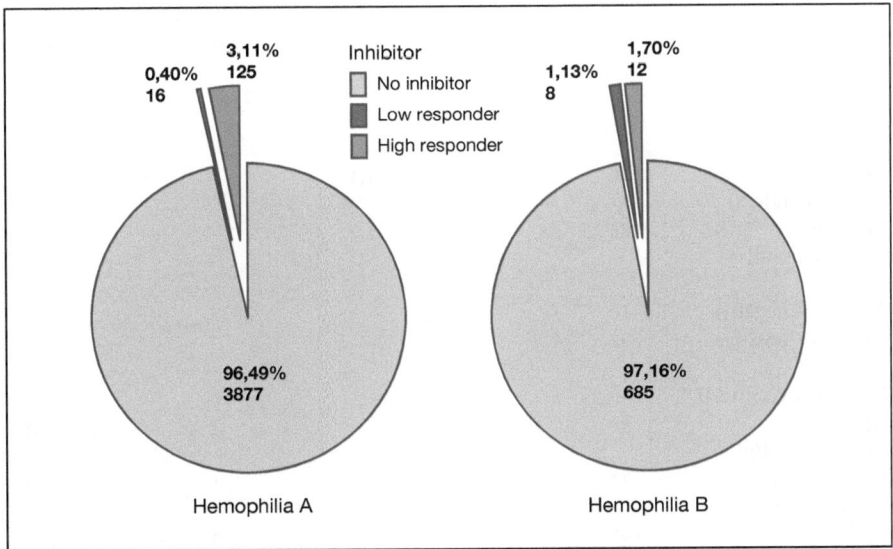

Fig. 4. Distribution of factor VIII/IX activity in patients with hemophilia A and B

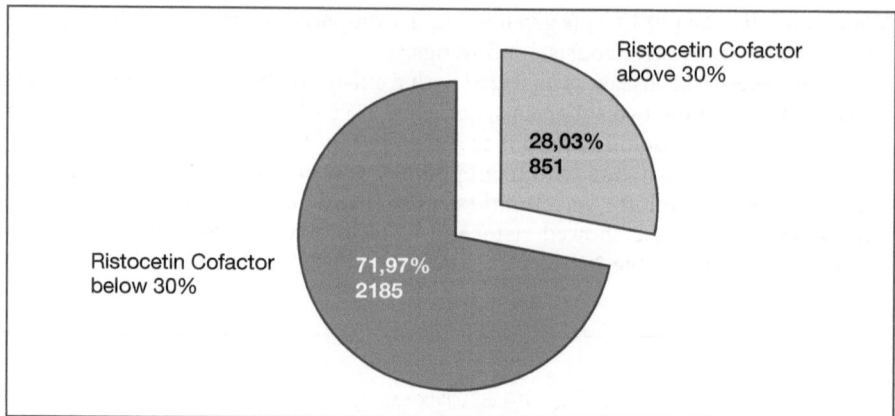

Fig. 5. Distribution of ristocetin Cofactor in patients with von-Willebrand disease

Table 2. Cumulative data from 72 centers as of 2001/2002

	Hemophilia A		Hemophilia B		von-Willebrand disease		Total
	N	%	N	%	N	%	N
Total	3862	47,95	686	8,52	3507	43,57	8055
Factor activity ≤ 2%	2195	54,6	371	52,6	—	—	2566
Factor activity > 2%	1823	45,4	334	47,4	—	—	2157
Ristocetin Cofactor ≤ 30%	—	—	—	—	851	28,0	851
Ristocetin Cofactor > 30%	—	—	—	—	2185	72,0	2185
Inhibitor (low responders)	16	0,4	8	1,1	—	—	24
Inhibitor (high responders)	125	3,1	12	1,7	—	—	137
Total HIV negative	3416	—	618	—	3029	—	7063
Total HIV positive	602	—	87	—	7	—	696
HIV positive, no AIDS	296	—	49	—	0	—	345
HIV positive, CD4<200 cell/μl	82	—	17	—	2	—	101
HIV positive, full blown AIDS	32	—	12	—	1	—	45
HIV positive, no comment	192	—	9	—	4	—	205

HIV Status

Of all reported patients a total of 696 were infected with HIV, equivalent to nearly 9%. Analyzed for HIV distribution in subgroups nearly 15% of all patients with hemophilia A, 12,3% of all patients with hemophilia B, and 0,2% of all patients with von-Willebrand disease were HIV-infected (Fig. 6). A total of 45 patients (6,5% of all HIV positive patients) has reached the stage of full-blown AIDS, compared to 345 patients (49,6% of all HIV positive patients) that have up to now not shown severe symptoms of the immune disease (Table. 3). Unfortunately, 205 HIV positive patients with no further details concerning stadium were reported. As this bates data quality considerable further investigation is needed to fill in the missing information.

Table 3. HIV status

HIV status	Hemophilia A	Hemophilia B	von-Willebrand disease	Total
HIV negative	3416	618	3029	7063
HIV positive, no AIDS	296	49	0	345
HIV positive, CD4+ < 200 cell/µ	82	17	2	101
HIV positive, full-blown AIDS	32	12	1	45
HIV positive, no comment	192	9	4	205
Total HIV positive	602	87	7	696

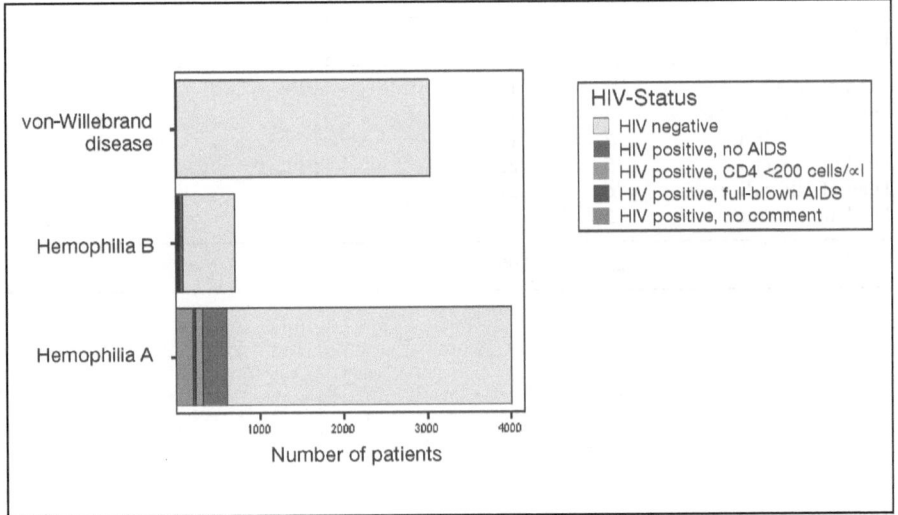

Fig. 6. Distribution of HIV-infected patients

Causes of Death

In the 2001/2002 period a total of 22 patients were reported dead with the distribution of causes of death given in Table 4. Since the beginning of the survey in 1982 a total of 712 patients have been reported dead. The development of mortality and causes of death since 82/83 are depicted in Fig. 9 to Fig. 11. AIDS, liver disease and cancer have been the main causes of death in this year's survey. While AIDS and cancer as causes of death remained relative constant, liver disease declined to a level comparable to that of the preceding years. Up to 1995 the number of AIDS-related deaths increased continuously with decline taking place since. The main reason for this development can probably be attributed to improved antiretroviral therapies. It is striking that cancer launched to become a very important cause of death in our patients (see Table. 4 and Fig. 7e). Arranging data for greater periods, one can see this effect obviously. Clustering data for the years 1982 to 1993 and 1993 to 2002 gives us a statistical significant difference between these periods ($p < 0{,}001$), implicating a gradually rise in cancer deaths (see Fig. 7f). The impact of liver disease on death causes remains uncertain any longer. However clustered data for the years 1982 to 1993 and 1993 to 2002 show a difference close to statistical significance ($p < 0{,}059$, see Fig. 7d), suggesting a future increase. The obvious reason for this may be the increasing number of liver cirrhosis due to Hepatitis C. The same numerical picture shows the HIV/liver disease/cancer deaths expressed as percentage of all deaths per year (see Fig. 8 a–c). Mentionable is the this year's low portion of reported deaths with no comment (see Fig. 10 and Fig. 11), improving data quality clearly. No indications for Creutzfeld-Jakob disease in our patient collective has been reported since 1978.

Table 4. Distribution of death causes

Patients	N	%
Died of AIDS	3	14
Died of liver disease	3	14
Died of bleeding	2	10
Died of cancer	5	23
Died of other diseases	6	27
Died, no comment	3	14
Total	22	100

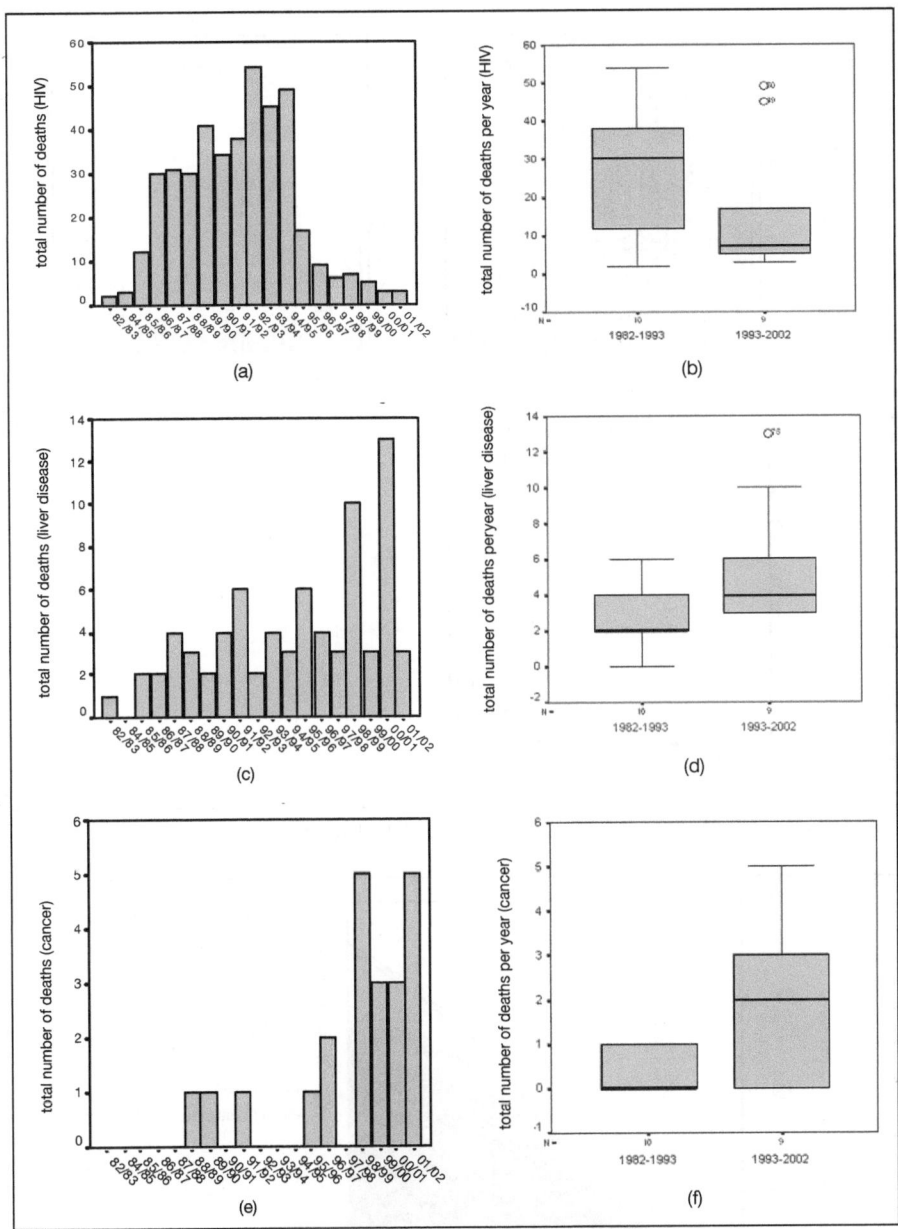

Fig. 7a–f. Comparison total number of deaths of HIV, liver disease and cancer (a–f)

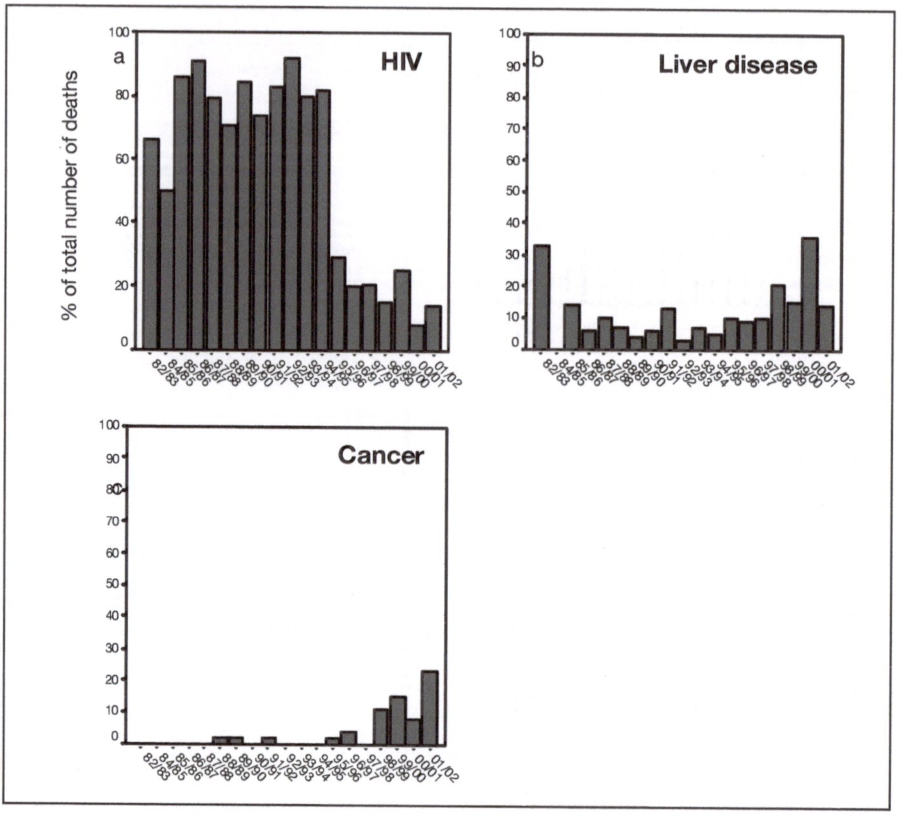

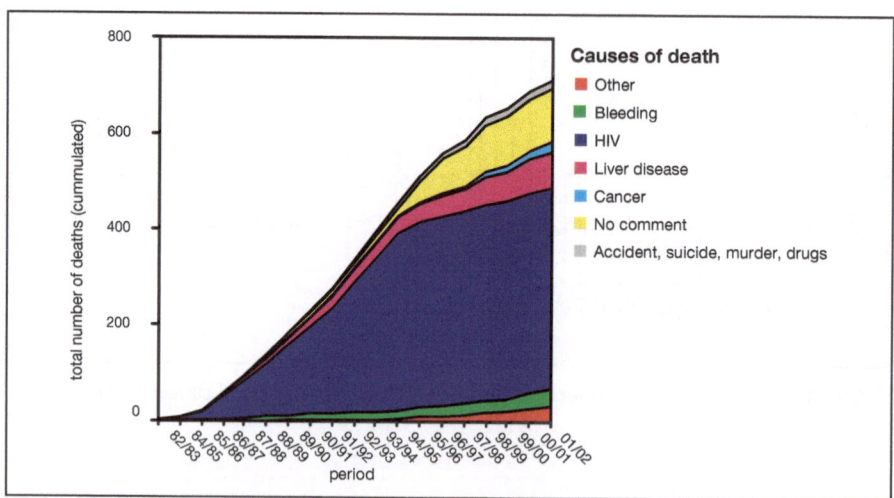

Fig. 8. Comparison % of total number of deaths of HIV, liver disease and cancer (a–c)

Fig. 9. Cumulative chart of deceased patients, separated for causes of death

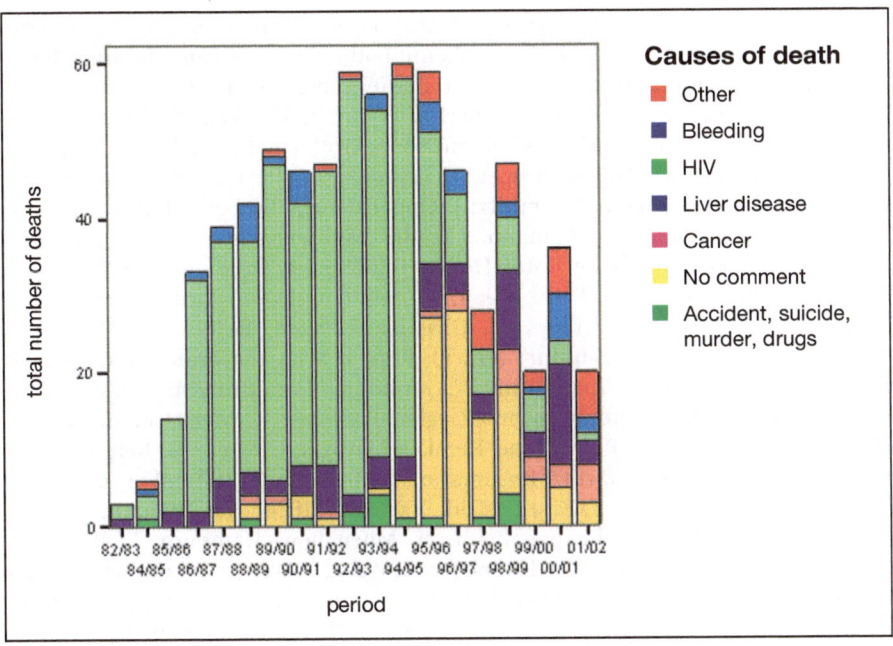

Fig 10. Causes of death since the beginning of the survey

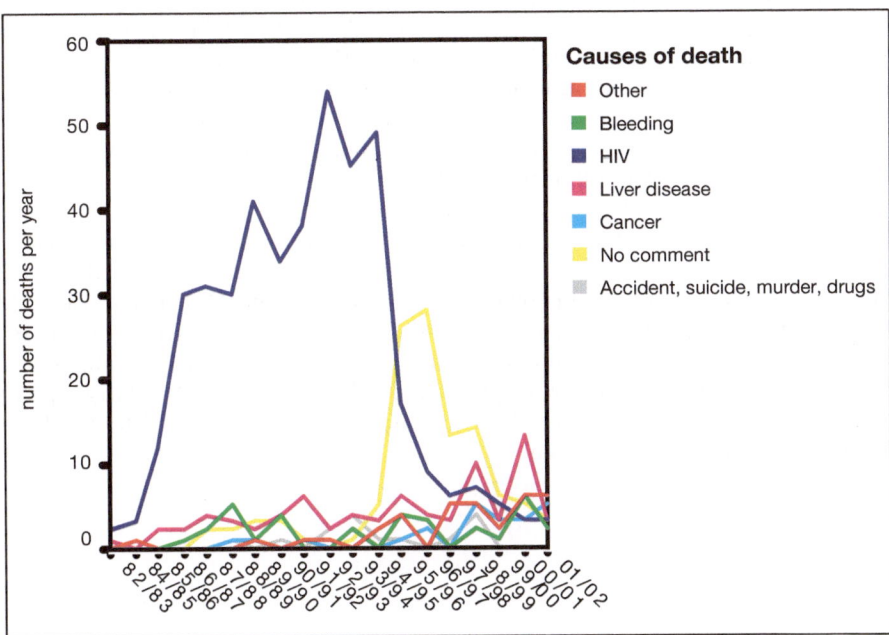

Fig. 11. Chart of deceased patients per year, separated for causes of death

Acknowledgment. Peter Heidemann, Astrid Heidemann, Augsburg; Schlimok, Linné, Augsburg; K. Rager, Bad Mergentheim; Lothar Hempelmann, Berlin; Günter Henze, Frau U. Schulte Overberg-Schmidt, Berlin; Christiane Beck, Dorothea Kroll, Berlin; Ch. Heinrichs, Frau Stumpe, Berlin; H. Koop, M. Klare, Berlin; H. Kiesewetter, Koscielny, Berlin; H.H. Brackmann, Bonn; Wolfgang Eberl, Braunschweig; G. Auerswald, Bremen; Holzhüter, Bremen; H. Leithäuser, Celle; F. Fiedler, Kerstin Wolf, Chemnitz; Klaus Hofmann, Chemnitz; J. Oppermann, Elisabeth Holfeld, Dagmar Möbius, Cottbus; Johann Böhmann, Claudia Niekrens, Delmenhorst; Joachim Mößeler, Dillingen; Wolfgang Kotte, Heiner Güldenring, Dresden; Jörg Wendisch, Dresden; Heiner Trobisch, Duisburg; U. Göbel, Lex, Düsseldorf; G. Vogel, Frau Winterstein, Erfurt; Jens Klinge, M. Girisch, Erlangen; R. Eckstein, Erlangen; Christian Klinkenstein, Frankfurt (Oder); Frau I. Scharrer, Frankfurt/Main; W. Kreuz, Klarmann, Frankfurt/Main; W. Mondorf, Frankfurt/M; Antje Nimtz, Frankfurt/Oder; A.H. Sutor, Barbara Ziegler, Freiburg; R. Mertelsmann, Karola Hasler, Freiburg; Pralle, PD Bettina Kemkes-Matthes, Giessen; G. Berger, Wilke (I Med), Doris Joachim, Görlitz; Rosemarie Schobeß, Halle -Wittenberg/S; Anatol Kurme, Bernhard Pauka, D.K. Hossfeld, Barbara Eifrig, Hamburg; Rolf Kuse, Wittkowsky, Hamburg; Schneppenheim, N. Muenchow, Hamburg; L. Balleisen, Hamm; A. Ganser, M. von Depka, Hannover; K. Welte, C. Wermes, Hannover; Rainer Zimmermann, Heidelberg; E. Wenzel, Pindur, Homburg/Saar; F.C. Sitzmann, Gerd Dockter, Annegret Seider, Homburg/Saar; F. Zintl, Karim Kentouche, Jena; K. Höffken, K. Wollina, Fricke, Jena; Hirschmann, Frau B. Eggeling, Kassel; U.R. Fölsch, H.D. Bruhn, Kiel; Eckhard Lechler, Köln (Lindenthal); Mario Koksch, Leipzig; Harald Lenk, Leipzig; H. J. Siemens, Lübeck; Peter Hellstern, Ludwigshafen; R. Herbert, Lüneburg; D. Franke, Magdeburg; Uwe Mittler, von Aumann, Magdeburg; Volker Kretschmer, Monika Weippert, Marburg; K.U. Freiberger, K. Morgenschweis, Mechernich; Karin Kurnik, München; W. Schramm, München; H. Pollmann, Sr. Heike, Münster; C. G. Lipinski, J. Weisser, Neckargemünd; R. Arndt, Neubrandenburg; B. Berthold, Neubrandenburg; Jürgen Drescher, Oldenburg; Th. Wüst, Pforzheim; M. Karl, Maria Anstadt, Plauen; R. Pasold, Potsdam; Beate Schmeltzer, Potsdam-Drewitz; Prof Andreesen, Karl Huber, Regensburg; H. Konrad, Rostock; I. Richter; Ulrike Kyank, Rostock; M. Freund, O. Anders, Rostock; Bernhard Maak, Saalfeld; P.C. Clemens, R. Schumacher, Schwerin; Rita Subert, Schwerin; F.J. Göbel, Siegen; Osswald, Singen (Hohentwiel); Günter Syrbe, Schw. M.Stephan, Schw. H. Hädrich, Stadtroda; H. Edelmann, Heidrun Schwarz, Suhl; D. Niethammer, H. Scheel-Walter, Tübingen; L. Kanz, Jaschonek, M. Mohren, Tübingen; Debatin, W. Behnisch, Ulm; Dieter Böttcher, Wuppertal; F. Keller, U. Geisen, Würzburg; Speer, Petra Zeitler, Würzburg; Richter, Zella Mehlis; G. Schott, Ute Kreibich, Zwickau; Nentwich, Helga Gräbner, Zwickau

Hemophilia Registry of the Medical Committee of the Swiss Hemophilia Association – Annual Survey 2002

S. HARTMANN

History

The Swiss Hemophilia Registry was founded in 1996 by collecting personal data of hemophilic patients from all the specialists in hemophilia treatment units (so-called centres) in Switzerland. The main goal was the coordination of the centres to achieve optimal medical treatment in emergencies for hemophiliacs throughout the country.

As the selection of data on paper proved to be most difficult, the medical committee (MC) decided to develop a specific software for registration. It was realized by the computer specialist, Mrs. Katja Locher, Weingarten, under the responsibility and medical management of Dr. Serena Hartmann, Chur. The main characteristic is a double interrelated registration:

1. SAFE-domain, complete personal patient data confidential to the hemophilia specialists (selected members of MC), who are responsible for the treatment of the individual patient.
2. REGISTER-domain, automatically correlated with a coding of the name (BGA code) to provide anonymous data, with secondary additional parameters defining the type of hemophilia.

All members have access to the Register-domain. The system is fully compatible with the Swiss law of data protection.

Registration

The inclusion criteria were fixed as follows:
1. Hemophilia A or B with factor VIII/IX level <30%
2. Clinically relevant von-Willebrand disease, with Ristocetin-Cofactor < 10%
3. All other forms of severe plasmatic coagulopathies (single or combined factor deficiencies)

Each year data are collected (by mail or diskette) for an update, the results being analyzed and statistically evaluated by the responsibles of the registry. We present the latest records of October 2002.

I. Scharrer/W. Schramm (Ed.)
33rd Hemophilia Symposium Hamburg 2002
© Springer-Verlag Berlin Heidelberg 2004

Patients

A total number of 729 patients have been reported, including 55 genuine double registrations (i.e. patients having medical control in two centres). There remain 674 patients for evaluation, distributed in 19 participating centres in universities, hospitals and private offices. Only 2 centres take care of >100 patients (109–172), 5 are medium size (41–76), most are small (5–30). Age distribution is following the classification of WFH. Hemophilia A and B: children (0–14) 77, youth (15–24) 77, lower medium age (25–44) 177, upper medium (45–64) 123, older age (65+) 53 patients. Mean age for hemophilia type A was 36.4, for type B 33.4, for von-Willebrand 39 years. The median age does not differ much, 34, 34 and 37 years respectively.

Classification of Hemophilia

The distribution of **hemophilia types** is given in Figure 1: hemophilia A 434 (63%), hemophilia B 98 (15%), von Willebrand disease 86 (13%), other coagulopathies 52 (8%), most relevant deficiencies for Factor VII 16, F XIII 11 and afibrinogenemia 10. For 4 (1%) patients the type remains unknown.

The **severity of disease** is classified strictly following ISTH standards (recommendation of International Society on Thrombosis and Hemostasis: Thromb Haemost 2001, 85: 560). The grading is defined as severe (<1%), moderate (1-5%) and mild (>5%). The corresponding results are for hemophilia A: severe152 (35%), moderate 77 (18%), mild 198 (46%), for hemophilia B: severe 28 (28%), moderate 37 (38%) and mild 30 (31%). A total of 10 (2%) patients have missing results. In our registry, three parameters concerning severity of disease are reported, i.e. the clinical course, the minimum and the maximum percent factor VIII/IX activity. This leads to controversial results for the grading of the disease. The ISTH standard relies only on the minimal level of factor activity. Due to this selecting criteria our results will differ relevantly from the data of the German Hemophilia Registry (see Fig. 2)

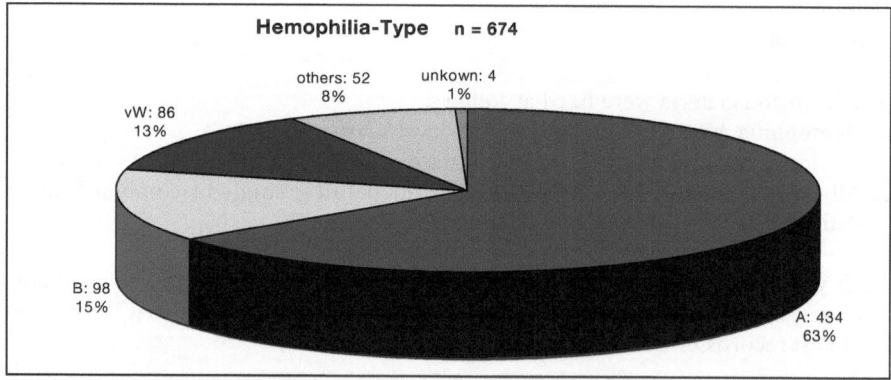

Fig. 1. Distribution of hemophilia type and other coagulopathies

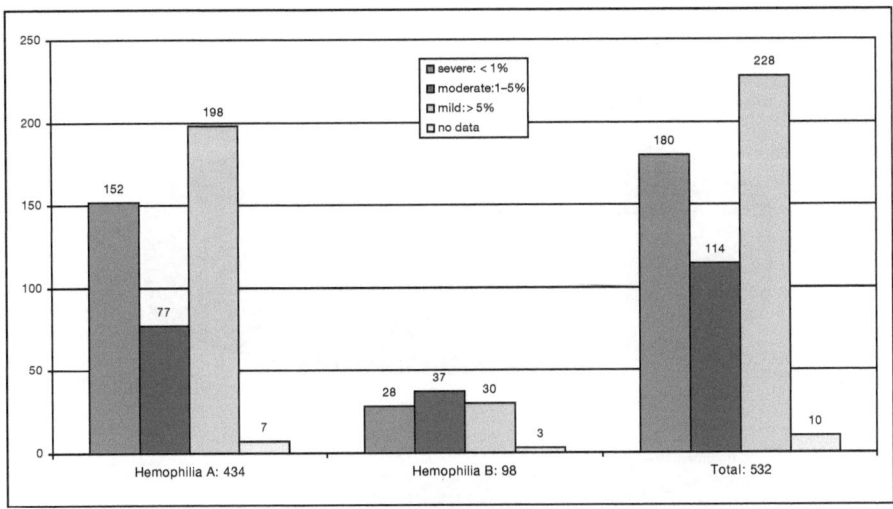

Fig. 2. Severity grading of hemophilia A and B following ISTH standards (Recommendation of International Society on Thrombosis and Hemostasis: Thromb Haemost 2001, 85: 560)

Additionally we register the **mode of substitution,** which is either on demand or prophylaxis (Fig. 3). We still have ³/₄ patients substituting on demand, type A 319, type B 77. Ninety (17%) patients use prophylactic treatment, mostly children. In 46 (9%) there are still no data available. Moreover we can register different **factor substitutes** (Fig. 4). Nearly half of the patients with hemophilia A have adopted treatment with recombinant factor VIII (212/49%), which has increased in comparison to last year (180/42%). Consequently plasma-derived factor VIII sub-

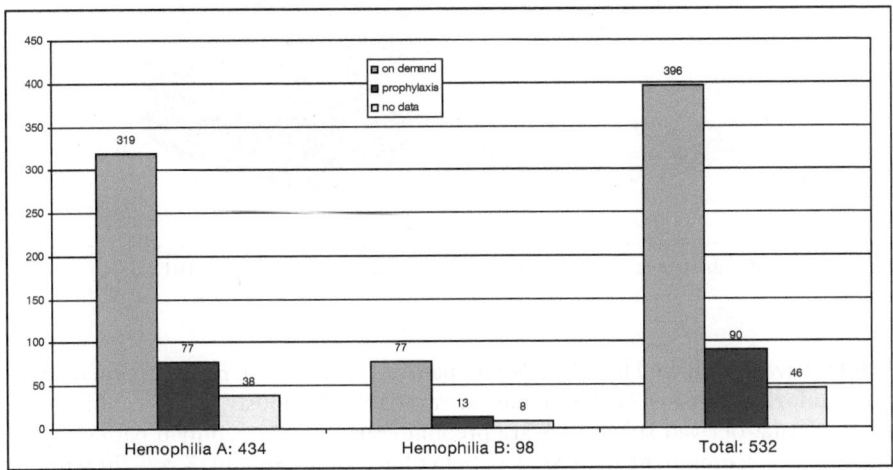

Fig. 3. Mode of substitution on demand versus prophylaxis in hemophilia

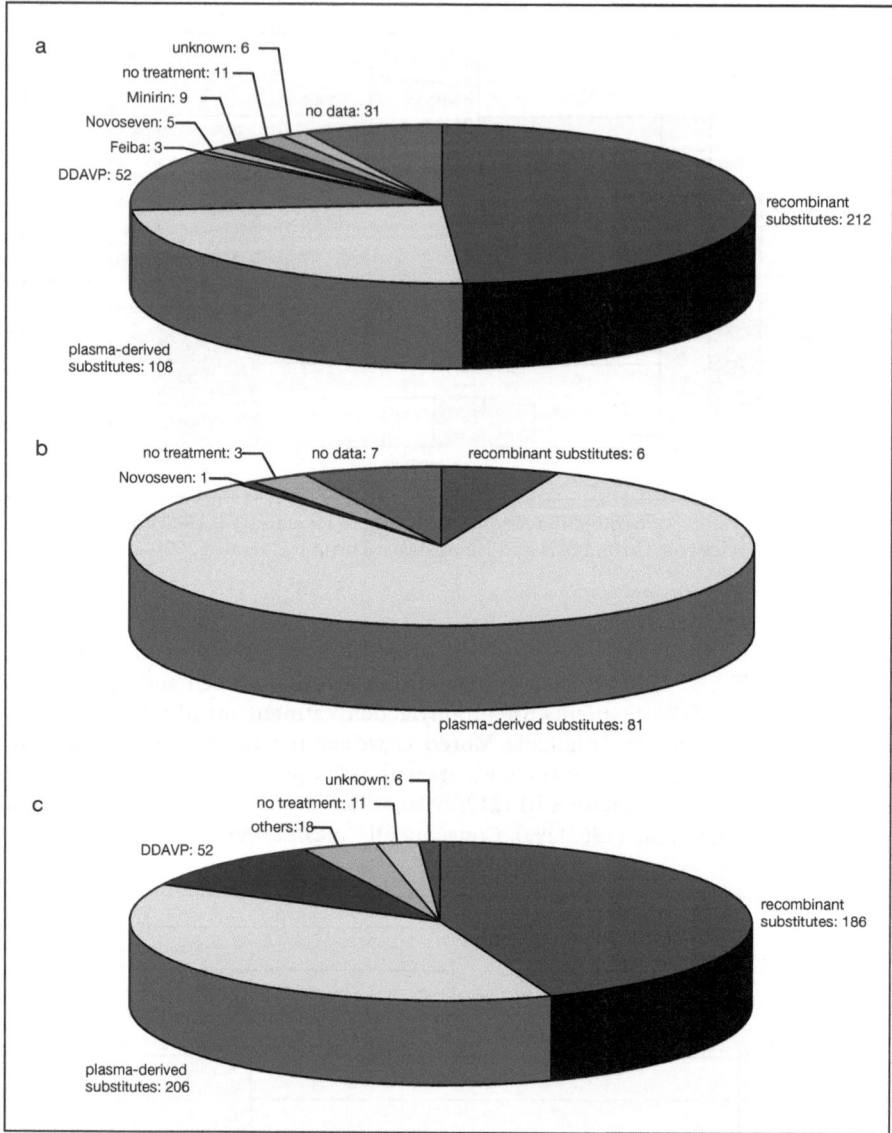

Fig. 4. Range of Substitutes, recombinant versus plasma-derived factor VIII/IX.

stitutes have diminished to 108 (25%). 11 patients remain with no treatment on purpose; unfortunately in 37 cases no data are available. Obviously, for hemophilia type B the plasma-derived substitutes are preponderant (81/83%), only 6 patients have changed to recombinant Benefix. 3 patients have no treatment, 7 remain without data. We are planning to add a module to the software in order to register type and dosage of factor substitutes for the follow up of the total amount of units consumed per year.

The **inhibitor status** is registered as positive or negative: in hemophilia A we find only 20 (5%) inhibitor positive and 1 (1%) in hemophilia B. The results are not representative for the prevalence of inhibitor in our hemophilia population, as there are still 116 (27%) patients without these data. We can differentiate 56 cases former positive that are reported actually negative, on the other hand of the 20 positive cases 16 have already been positive in previous evaluation. We realize that the register does not allow to select patients adhering to immune tolerance treatment.

Table 1. Number of death of hemophilic patients reported in the period 1996–2002

N = 24		mean age
		60 y.
Hemophilia A	19	
Hemophilia B	4	
Von-Willebrand type 3 *	1	
HIV +	7	42 y.
HIV –	16	68 y.
Severe	15 (+1*)	
Moderate	4	
Mild	3	
Inhibitor positive	3	

Table 2. Causes of death of hemophilic patients 1996–2002

		HIV pos.	HIV neg.
AIDS:	opportunistic infection	3	
	Wasting Syndrome	1	
	HIV-assoc. malignancy	1	
Bleeding:	cerebral	1	2
	inner organs		1
	other localization	1	1
Malignant neoplasia			3
Livercell carcinoma			2
Cardiovascular disease			3
Lung disease			1
Infectious disease		1	1
Accident			1
Other causes			1
Unknown			
total N = 24		8	16

Mortality Statistics

In the Swiss Hemophilia Registry number and causes of death are recorded in a separate file. The causes are pre-defined in an official list of diagnosis. We evaluate separately HIV positive and HIV negative patients. Since the beginning of the survey in 1996, a total number of 24 patients have been reported dead (compared to 21 last year), see Table 1: 16 HIV negative (14), 8 HIV positive (7). The mean age at death was 60 years, separately for HIV positive 42, for HIV negative 68 years. Last year we had 1 death of severe von-Willebrand disease. The causes of death are shown in Table 2: In HIV negative patients death was related mainly to bleeding (4, including 1 esophagus bleeding), then malignant and cardiovascular disease (both 3), 2 patients died of liver cancer. Certainly, chronic liver disease is of increasing significance, but our kind of death registration does not allow to define the role of liver disease for mortality.

In general, we believe that the data collected in the Swiss Hemophilia Registry are representative for the actual distribution of hemophiliacs in Switzerland. There is good evidence that only a small number of patients is missing in the registry. We are planning to improve the reporting system in an update of the software by adding new modules and at the same time trying to adopt an online version of internet communication.

»New Viruses« and the Safety of Factor Concentrates and Stable Blood Products: TT Virus and West Nile Virus as Current Examples

T.R. Kreil

Introduction

Although no clinically relevant virus transmissions have been reported for some years [1], reflecting the enormous improvements in the safety margins of plasma derivatives, the potential for virus transmission continues to concern patients. The discovery or emergence of new viruses heightens these concerns and requires extra vigilance to re-establish assurance on the safety of these products. Two new viruses serve as current examples.

TT Virus (TTV) and first Generation Recombinant Factor VIII (rFVIII) Products

When TTV was discovered in 1997 [2] and suggested to be associated with post-transfusion hepatitis, naturally patients, regulatory bodies and the plasma products industry were anxious. Further investigations found the virus to be of no clinical relevance, but revealed a high prevalence of TTV: low viral loads were found in up to 82% of plasma donations, and consequently in many plasma pools [3]. More refined products, e.g. albumin, were, however, consistently TTV negative [4; Baxter-compublished].

The recent suggestion by Azzi et al. [5] that TTV could occur in first-generation rFVIII products, with the stabilizer, human serum albumin (HSA), as its source thus came as a surprise. Upon reinvestigation of recombinant FVIII (Recombinate) and human serum albumin (HSA) using either nested [6] or single-stage PCR assays [7], as earlier described, all the samples tested were negative with each primer set evaluated. The same samples, when tested again after spiking with material from a TTV positive plasma donation, were positive as expected, which controlled against inhibition of the PCR reaction. Altogether, the investigation confirmed earlier results obtained by regulatory bodies and Baxter internally that HSA and thus also first generation recombinant FVIII is not contaminated by TTV [8].

West Nile Virus (WNV) and the Safety of Plasma-Derivatives

The WNV, initially described in 1937, became widely publicized after its first appearance on the East coast of the USA in 1999 [9]. The 2002 epidemic in the USA resulted in approximately 3800 clinical cases and more than 200 case fatalities by the end of the year [10]. Reported transmissions through transplantation of solid organs and transfusion of labile blood components [11] raised concerns over the

I. Scharrer/W. Schramm (Ed.)
33rd Hemophilia Symposium Hamburg 2002
© Springer-Verlag Berlin Heidelberg 2004

safety of plasma derivatives. The effectiveness of virus inactivation processes used during the manufacture of these products was investigated to verify the safety margins, which were initially shown using model viruses very similar to WNV. A newly established infectivity assay with a 1999 New York WNV isolate of the virus was used. The WNV behaved exactly as predicted based on the available data for similar model viruses, i.e. it was readily inactivated by all of the commonly used virus inactivation technologies, such as pasteurization, solvent-detergent (SD) treatment, and vapor heating [12].

Summary

Notwithstanding the advances in the safety of plasma derivatives, the potential for virus contamination continues to concern the patients who use these products. Accordingly, new issues are promptly addressed and investigated. To date these investigations have consistently confirmed the uncompromising safety margins of plasma derivatives, despite challenges by reports that have materialized as questionable rather than based on scientifically sound concerns. The plasma products industry remains committed to providing reassurance for product safety through competent research whenever issues arise, or are perceived as arising.

References

1. CDC: Blood Safety Monitoring Among Persons with Bleeding Disorders – United States, May 1998–June 2002. MMWR January 3, 2003
2. Nishizawa T, Okamoto H, Konishi K, et al. A novel DNA virus (TTV) associated with elevated transaminase levels in posttransfusion hepatitis of unknown etiology. Biochem Biophys Res Commun. 1997; 241: 92–97
3. Pisani G, Cristiano K, Wirz G, et al. Prevalence of TT virus in plasma pools and blood products. Br J Haematol. 1999; 106: 431–435
4. Yu M-Y (CBER, USA), at the »WHO International Working Group on the Standardization of Genomic Amplification Techniques for the Virological Safety Testing of Blood and Blood Products« meeting, Nov. 15, 1998, at the NIBSC
5. Azzi A, De Santis R, Morfini M, et al. TT virus contaminates first-generation recombinant factor VIII concentrates. Blood. 2001; 98: 2571–2573
6. Okamoto H, Takahashi M, Nishizawa T, et al. Marked genomic heterogeneity and frequent mixed infection of TT virus demonstrated by PCR with primers from coding and noncoding regions. Virology. 1999; 259: 428–436
7. Simmonds P, Prescott LE, Logue C, et al. TT virus-part of the normal human flora ? J Infect Dis. 1999; 180: 1748–1749
8. Kreil TR, Zimmermann K, Pable S et al., TT virus does not contaminate first generation recombinant Factor VIII (rFVIII) concentrate. Blood 2002; 100: 2271–2272
9. Petersen LR and Roehrig JT, Emerg Infect Dis [2001] 7(4): 611
10. MMWR [2002] 51/47: 1072
11. MMWR [2002] 51/43: 973
12. Kreil TR, Berting A, Kistner O, Kindermann J, West Nile virus and the safety of plasma derivatives: Verification of high safety margins, and the validity of predictions based on model virus data. Transfusion [2003] 43: 1023

II. New Findings and Possibilities in Therapy of Antibodies

Chairmen:

W. SCHRAMM (Munich)
H.-H. BRACKMANN (Bonn)

A Retrospective Study on the Development of Inhibitors after Continuous Infusion of Factor VIII

CH. V. AUER, J. OLDENBURG, M. V. DEPKA PRODZINSKI,
C. ESCURIOLA-ETTINGSHAUSEN, W. KREUZ, K. KURNIK, H. LENK,
M. VARVENNE, TH. VIGH, and I. SCHARRER

Introduction

The **continuous infusion (CI)** of coagulation factor-VIII (FVIII) concentrates has been used since the early 1990s. Compared to the traditional way of factor application by episodic bolus infusions (BI) the CI had several advantages:

Steady level of missing coagulation factor, avoiding of unnecessary high peaks of FVIII, saving of 30% FVIII concentrate and reduction in treatment costs [1]. Reports of the occurrence of an inhibitor after treatment with CI have raised concerns about this method of factor application.

A **retrospective study** was conducted to investigate inhibitor development after CI of FVIII. 13 hemophilia centres of the Scientific Council of the German Hemophilia Society received the following **questionnaire:**

Age
Severity of hemophilia
Exposure days
Thrombophlebitis
Family history
Genotype
Month/Year of CI
Indication
Infused amount of FVIII
Infusion sets

Inhibitor:
  High responding (HR)
  or low responding (LR)
  Permanent / transient
  Type I / Type II
Immune Tolerance Therapy (ITT):
  Duration of ITT
  Success
Prophylaxis/on demand

Results

In 10 centres CIs were used for treatment of hemophilia A patients. In 5 of these hemophilia centres **10 patients** with inhibitor development after CI were registered and data were collected.

Age of the patients: between 7 months and 57 years (7 Mo., 3.5 y., 5.5 y., 8 y., 11 y., 19 y., 35 y., 45 y., 45 y., 57 y.).

Severity of hemophilia: 5 patients with severe hemophilia (n=5)
1 patient with moderate hemophilia (n=1)
4 patients with mild hemophilia (n=4)

I. Scharrer/W. Schramm (Ed.)
33rd Hemophilia Symposion Hamburg 2002
© Springer-Verlag Berlin Heidelberg 2004

Exposure days:	between 1 and >100 days (1, 5, 10, 13, 16, 28, 30, 3 x >100 days).
Thrombophlebitis:	found in 2 patients
Family history:	one patient's cousin also developed an inhibitor.
Genotype:	missense-mutations (4), intron-22-inversions (2), small deletion (1), 3 were unknown
Indication for CI:	treatment of serious bleeding and surgical procedures
Infused amount before inhibitor development:	between 4300 and > 100000 IE FVIII
Infusion sets:	varied from mini pumps (2) to common infusion sets (7), one unknown
Inhibitors:	alloantibodies, low responding (3) and high responding (7)
ITT:	done in 7 patients, 4 with successful outcome after 26 days, 6 weeks and 3 month of treatment. One ITT-duration is unknown.
Factor concentrates:	plasma derived (6) and recombinant (4) concentrates

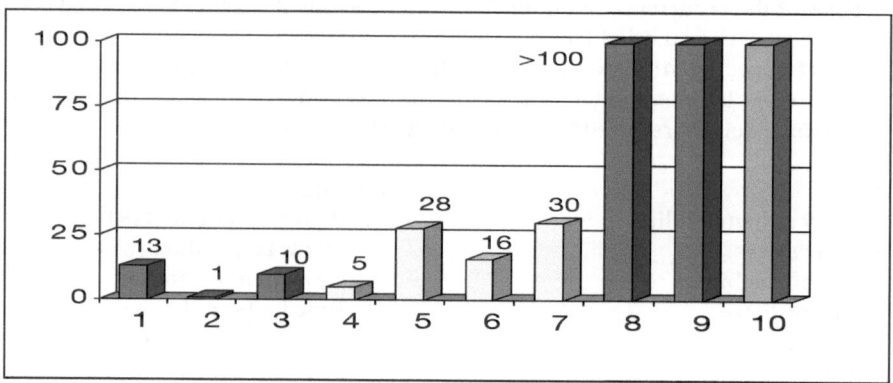

Fig. 1. Exposure days of the 10 patients until the inhibitor development

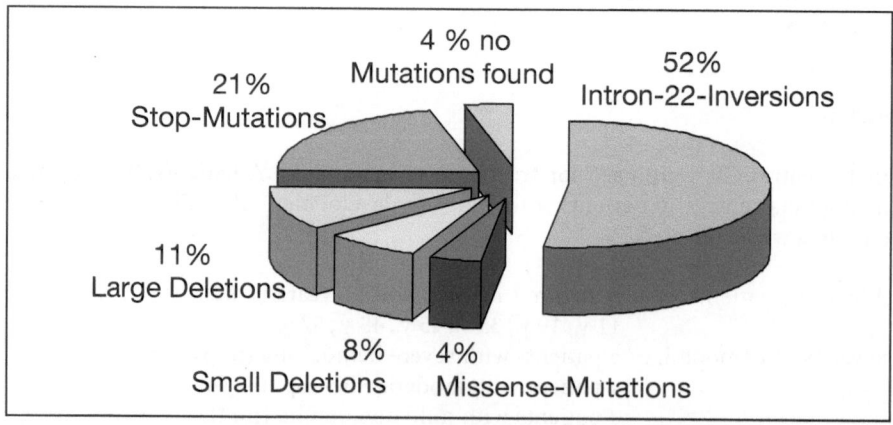

Fig. 2. Distribution of mutations in a common inhibitor patient collective

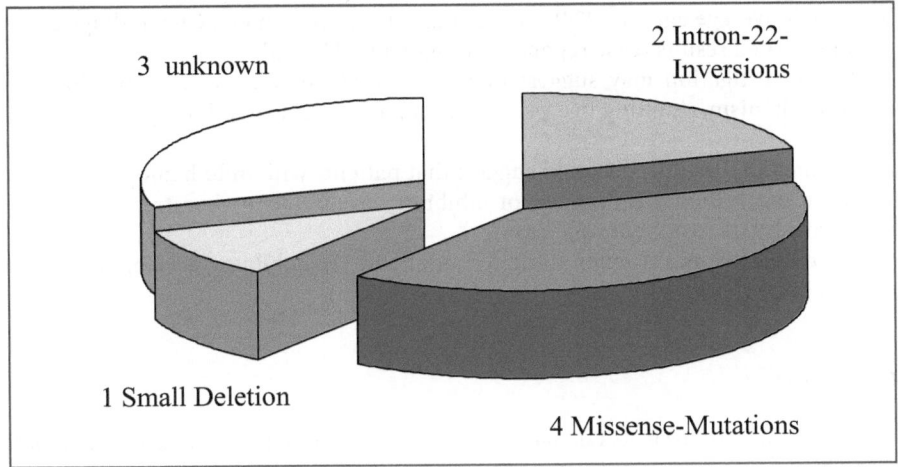

Fig. 3. Distribution of mutations found in our 10 inhibitor patients

Table 1. Survey of our results

Age	Hem. A	Anamn.	HR/LR	p./t.	Exp.-days	Genotype
7 m	severe	PUP	high	perm.	13	Small Deletion
3,5 y	severe	PTP	high	trans.	1	Intron-22-Inversion
5,5 y	severe	PTP	low	trans.	10	Intron-22-Inversion
8 y	mild	PTP	high	perm.	5	Missense Mutation
11 y	mild	PTP	low	perm.	28	Missense Mutation
19 y	mild	PTP	high	trans.	16	Missense Mutation
35 y	mild	PTP	high	perm.	30	unknown
45 y	severe	PTP	high	perm.	> 100	no Intron-22-Inversion
45 y	severe	PTP	low	perm.	> 100	Missense Mutation
57 y	moderate	PTP	high	perm.	> 100	unknown

Discussion

The most common inhibitor development in hemophiliacs is seen in patients with severe hemophilia (often caused by large deletions) that are previously untreated with FVIII-concentrates, at an average age under 5 years and before the 15th exposure day. These patients exhibit an inhibitor prevalence of >**30%** [2]. In our study we found only two patients with the so-called null-mutations (Intron-22-Inversion) where no FVIII protein can be detected. Therefore only the first three patients in our table belong to that group of patients where most commonly an inhibitor development is seen.

In our study strikingly the inhibitors developed very often in patients with **mild hemophilia** and genotypes that exhibit an inhibitor prevalence of < **10 %** [2]. Most of them were previously treated patients and had already more than 15 exposure days, their average age was 22,9 years at inhibitor development. Our findings agree with published results (case reports of 19 patients) [1, 3–5].

Our investigation may suggest that there might be an uncommon inhibitor-pathomechanism, resulting in a peculiar group of patients developing the inhibitor after CI.

On the other hand, one could suggest that patients with mild hemophilia might exhibit a much higher prevalence of inhibitor development when treated with an »intensive FVIII treatment« such as CI.

A prospective multicenter study to investigate the inhibitor development after CI should be conducted.

References

1. Batorova A, Martinowitz U. Continuous infusion of coagulation factors. *Haemophilia* 2002; 8: 170–177
2. Oldenburg J, El-Maarri O, Schwaab R. Inhibitor development in correlation to FVIII geno-types. *Haemophilia*, 2002; 8 (Suppl.2): 23–29
3. Hermans C, Thyn Yee T, Perry D, Lee C. Development of inhibitor in hemophilia patients treated with continuous infusion. *Haemophilia* 2002; 8: 541
4. Koestenberger M, Raith W, Muntean W. High titre inhibitor after continuous factor VIII administration for surgery in a young infant. *Haemophilia* 2000; 6: 120
5. White B, Cotter M, Byrne M, O`Shea E, Smith OP. High responding factor VIII inhibitors in mild hemophilia – is there a link with recent changes in clinical practice? *Haemophilia*, 2000; 6: 113–115

Characterisation of Factor VIII-Inhibitory Antibodies Using Phage Display

C. Mühle, S. Schulz-Drost, A. Khrenov, E.L. Saenko, J. Klinge, and H. Schneider

Abstract

The formation of FVIII-inhibitory antibodies remains a major problem in the treatment of hemophilia. An important step towards understanding the inactivation mechanism and a precondition for the modification of recombinant coagulation factors to reduce their immunogenicity would be the exact localization of immuno-dominant epitopes. To investigate whether such epitopes could be identified using a random peptide phage display library, FVIII antibodies were isolated from plasma samples of three patients by affinity chromatography, followed by several rounds of phage selection. A monoclonal FVIII antibody served as control. The resulting peptides were characterized by alignment with the FVIII sequence and by ELISA binding studies.

Stepwise increasing phage concentrations indicated a selective enrichment of antibody-binding phages in all samples analyzed. The phages isolated after three panning rounds showed high affinity binding to the corresponding antibody preparations and significant homology with the human FVIII sequence, suggesting an epitope of 5 amino acids in the A1 domain for the first patient's sample and overlapping short epitopes in the A2 domain for the second and third patient's samples. In the 3D structural model of human FVIII all three sites are likely to be accessible to antibodies. Immunoprecipitation of the first plasma with radioactively labelled FVIII fragments confirmed antibody binding to the A1 domain, but also revealed two additional reactive domains.

These results provide the proof of principle that random phage display libraries can be used for the mapping of epitopes in a polyclonal antibody preparation. The sensitivity of this method is currently evaluated on patient's antibodies purified by an optimized strategy.

Introduction

Antibodies which inactivate the supplemented exogenous coagulation factor (»inhibitors«) occur in approximately 30% of the patients with severe hemophilia A and represent a serious complication [1–4]. Although certain variables such as the purity of the FVIII product administered and the type of mutation in the FVIII gene are known to play crucial roles in the development of FVIII-inhibitory antibodies [5], the pathogenesis of inhibitors is still not fully understood.

I. Scharrer/W. Schramm (Ed.)
33rd Hemophilia Symposion Hamburg 2002
© Springer-Verlag Berlin Heidelberg 2004

The FVIII molecule is a glycoprotein consisting of a series of repeated, homologous domains A1-A2-B-A3-C1-C2 [6]. The heavily glycosylated B domain with no known function [7] is least immunogenic [8]. In contrast, a large number of inhibitory antibodies have been found to bind to the FVIII domains A2 and C2 [9–11], but until now only a few epitopes have been clearly defined and characterized [12]. Our current study, therefore, aims at the exact localization of inhibitor epitopes in hemophilia A patients by identifying the minimal binding sequence to promote further understanding of the mechanisms of inhibitor development and action. In addition, we hope to identify the critical amino acids of immunodominant epitopes, the modification of which may provide the possibility to reduce the immunogenicity of recombinant FVIII.

Epitope mapping has been performed by different methods including Western blotting or immunoprecipitation of candidate domains [9, 13], site-directed mutagenesis [14], deletion analysis of recombinant FVIII fragments [15], homologue scanning mutagenesis using recombinant hybrid human/porcine FVIII [11] or screening of libraries of overlapping target sequence-specific peptides [16]. However, the use of random peptide phage display libraries may offer advantages over all these approaches, because the precise localization of the antibody binding site could be achieved very rapidly by screening a large number of short random peptides (more than 10^9 different sequences) allowing even for identification of discontinuous epitopes [17]. The phage display method (Fig. 1) is an *in vitro* selection technique which employs peptides genetically fused to a coat protein of a bacterio-

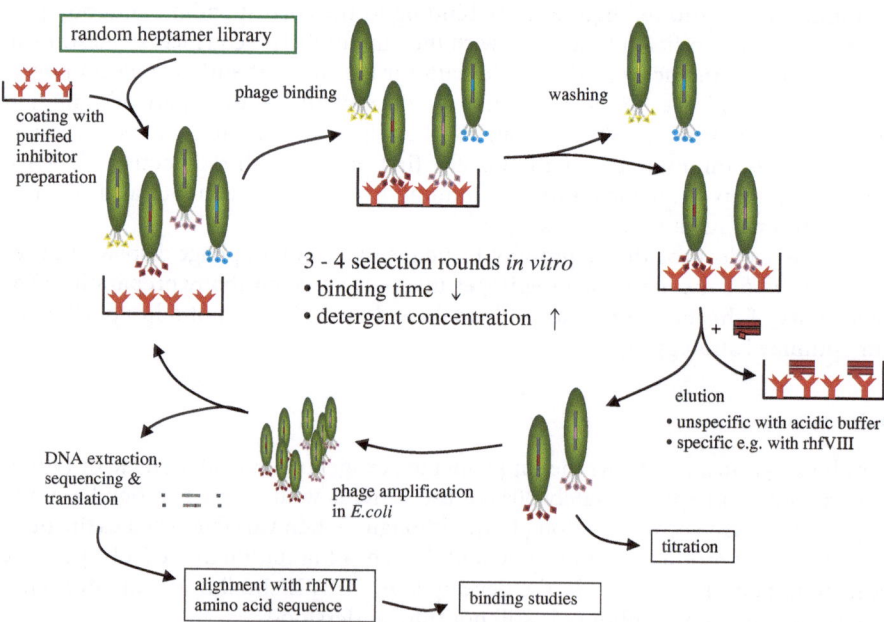

Fig. 1. Scheme of the phage display technology applied

phage resulting in their display on the surface of the virion. The *in vitro* selection (biopanning) is carried out by incubating the pool of phage-displayed peptides with the target molecule immobilized on a plate or beads, washing away unbound phages and eluting bound phages either specifically with the target itself, its ligand or by nonspecific disruption of binding interactions, e.g. with an acidic buffer. Selection and amplification of the phage eluate are repeated several times to iteratively enrich the pool in favor of the best binding partners.

In this study we investigate whether a random peptide phage display library can be used for epitope mapping in polyclonal antibody samples of hemophilia A patients with inhibitors.

Material and Methods

Plasma Samples

Three plasma samples from hemophilia A patients aged 21 months, 3 years and 11 years who had developed inhibitors in response to treatment with purified human or recombinant FVIII were investigated. The inhibitory activity of each plasma sample as quantified by the Nijmegen modification of the Bethesda assay was between 22 and 66 BU/ml.

Antibody Purification

The antibodies were isolated from the patient's plasma samples by affinity chromatography in two steps. After buffer exchange, first the total immunoglobulin content was obtained by chromatography on a protein G column (Amersham) or collected from the flow-through of a DEAE Affi-Gel Blue Gel column (BioRad). In the second step, FVIII-specific antibodies were isolated from the total IgG pool by chromatography on a FVIII column produced by coupling 1000–4000 IU of recombinant human FVIII to the matrix material using either the UltraLink kit (PIERCE) or CNBr-activated sepharose (Amersham). The eluate was dialyzed and concentrated, and the total amount and purity of FVIII-specific antibodies were determined by ELISA using human IgG and a monoclonal FVIII antibody as standards.

Random Peptide Selection by Phage Display

In this study the Ph.D.-7 Phage Display Peptide Library kit (New England Biolabs), a combinatorial library of random heptamers, was used according to the manufacturer's instructions. Biopanning was performed on microtiter plates coated with the purified antibody preparation overnight in a humidified box. For each round of selection, 2×10^{11} phages were applied to a freshly coated plate. Unbound phages were then removed by careful washing, bound phages were specifically eluted with recombinant FVIII (ReFacto; Wyeth).

The eluted phage pool was amplified in *E. coli*, purified and used for three additional binding and amplification cycles (Fig. 1), in which the stringency of the selection was increased by adding the detergent Tween-20 (up to 0.5% final concentration) and reducing the phage binding time from 60 to 10 minutes. Finally, 24 to 48 individual clones were isolated and characterized by DNA sequencing. The corresponding peptides were aligned with the human FVIII amino acid sequence to identify regions of homology.

The human FVIII antibodies B02C11 and F14A12 (a gift of Prof. Saint-Remy, University of Leuven, Belgium, and Sylvie Villard, University of Montpellier, France) served as positive controls.

Phage Binding Assays

The binding of the isolated phages to the purified patient's antibodies was investigated by ELISA on microtiter plates coated with the antibody preparation overnight in a humidified box. After blocking the plates with bovine serum albumin, serial dilutions of the phages were applied to the wells. Unbound phages were removed by careful washing, and the bound phages were detected using an anti-M13 antibody conjugated with horseradish peroxidase (Pharmacia). The color reaction with *o*-phenylendiamine substrate in phosphate-citrate buffer containing 0.03% sodium perborate was quantified by measuring the absorbance at 490 nm.

Radio-Immunoprecipitation

Serial dilutions of the plasma samples were incubated with ^{125}I-labelled recombinant FVIII at a concentration of 0.75 nM which equals the normal concentration in human plasma. Immune complexes consisting of ^{125}I-labelled FVIII and the patient's FVIII antibodies were precipitated using protein G-sepharose, and the bound radioactivity was quantified with a γ-counter. To identify FVIII fragments containing inhibitory epitopes, the FVIII-domains A1, A2, A3, C2 and the light chain were labelled with ^{125}I and used in the same manner for immunoprecipitation.

Results and Discussion

FVIII antibodies to be investigated by biopanning of a combinatorial phage display library of random heptamers were isolated from plasma samples of three hemophilia A patients by affinity chromatography.

To establish and optimize the phage display method, biopanning was first carried out on plates coated with the monoclonal human FVIII antibody F14A12 containing the known epitope DVVRF in the A1 domain. The phage concentrations in the eluates increased from the first to the third round by almost 5 orders of magnitude despite constant input of 2×10^{11} phages, indicating a selective enrichment of antibody-binding phages. After three rounds of panning more than 75% of the isolated phages showed the known or an equivalent motif and high affinity to human FVIII in ELISA binding studies.

In the panning rounds with purified patient's antibodies stepwise increasing phage concentrations also indicated a selective enrichment of antibody-binding phages in all samples analyzed. However, among 32 phages isolated after panning on the first inhibitor preparation (P1) only few consensus motifs were found, and phage W896 containing the peptide with the highest similarity to the human FVIII amino acid sequence (Fig. 2a) was the only one which bound strongly to the corresponding antibody preparation (Fig. 2b). These results suggest an epitope of 5 amino acids in the A1 domain of FVIII. The antibodies of the same patient were characterized additionally by immunoprecipitation with radioactively labeled FVIII fragments. This method revealed antibody binding not only to A1 but also to the A2 domain and the complete light chain (Fig. 2c), whereas no signal was detectable for the domains A3, B and C2. Although there was no C1 domain available for direct testing, the binding to the light chain consisting of A3, C1 and C2, together with the lack of binding to the individual domains A3 and C2 strongly indicates an epitope in the C1 domain. Thus, the immunoprecipitation data support the presence of an

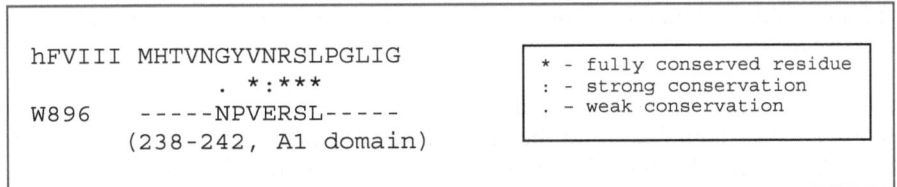

Fig. 2a. Alignment of the peptide W896 with the hFVIII amino acid sequence

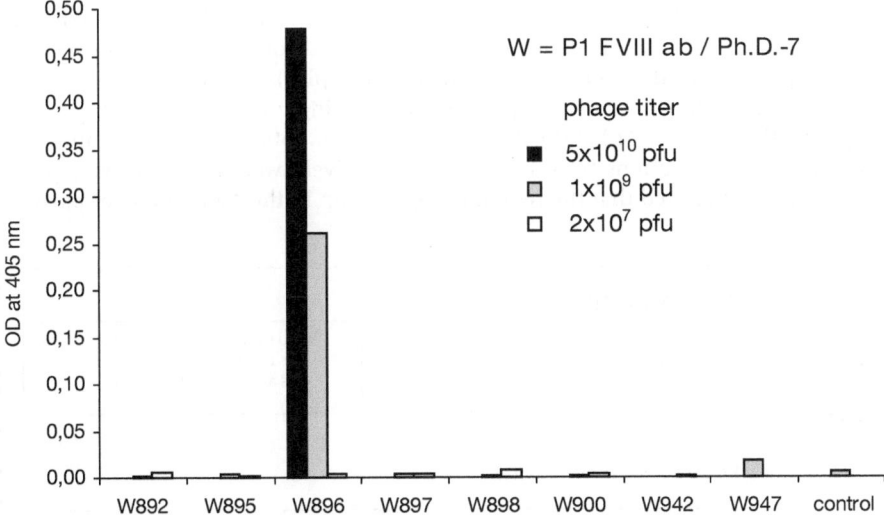

Fig. 2b. ELISA binding analysis of the phages obtained by biopanning with the antibody preparation from plasma P1 (OD values corrected for plastic binding)

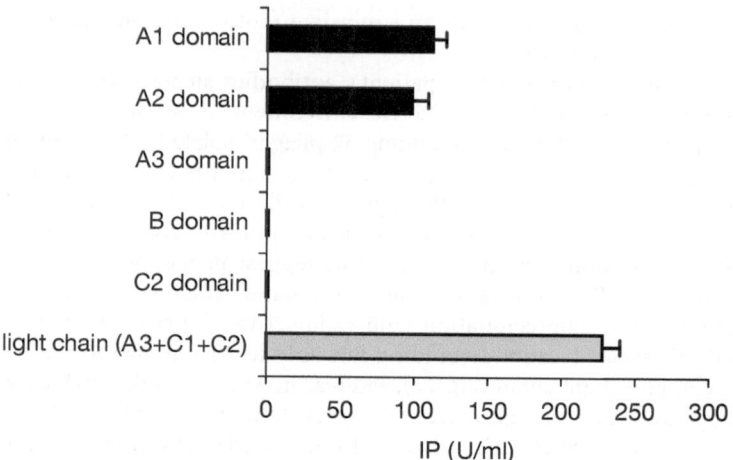

Fig. 2c. Immunoprecipitation of plasma P1 with radioactively labeled FVIII fragments

epitope in the A1 domain as found by phage display, but also suggest two additional reactive domains.

Among the phages obtained by biopanning with the antibody preparation from the second patient (P2), only one of 17 different peptides from a total of 37 phages showed a clear homology with the amino acid sequence of human FVIII (Fig. 3). This phage K412 also bound best to the corresponding immobilized antibodies in the ELISA.

The phages isolated in the panning experiments with antibodies from the third patient (P3) contained four enriched peptide sequences, each present three to five times among the 30 phages analyzed. Although three of them showed some homology with the amino acid sequence of human FVIII, only one phage, L484, which was also the phage with the highest enrichment (five copies), bound with high affinity to the corresponding antibody preparation. Interestingly, the putative epitopes displayed by the phages K412 and L484, which had been obtained by biopanning with the antibody preparations from P2 and P3 respectively, were partially overlapping (Fig. 3). This suggested that the region of the overlap in the A2 domain, in particu-

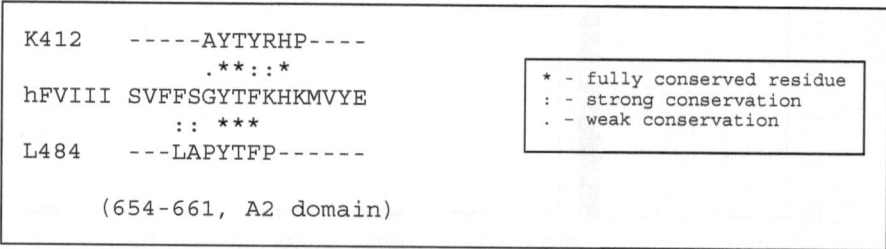

Fig. 3. Alignment of the peptides K412 and L484, obtained by biopanning with the antibody preparations from P2 and P3 respectively, with hFVIII

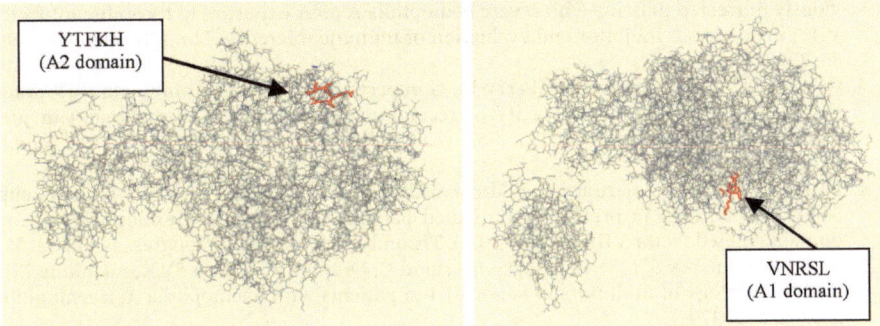

Fig. 4. Localization of the putative epitopes in the three-dimensional structural model of human FVIII

lar the amino acid sequence tyrosine-threonine-phenylalanine, may be part of an immunodominant epitope that could have been responsible for the development of FVIII antibodies in both patients.

Competition assays with recombinant human FVIII to confirm the FVIII specific binding of the phages W896, K412 and L484 to the purified antibody samples, as well as functional tests of the antibody neutralizing activity of the peptides identified are underway.

In the three-dimensional structural model of human FVIII [18] the putative epitopes tyrosine-threonine-phenylalanine-lysine-histidine (YTFKH) and valine-asparagine-arginine-serine-leucine (VNRSL) are located at the surface of the molecule and thus likely to be accessible to antibodies (Fig. 4).

These results provide the proof of principle that random phage display libraries can be used for the mapping of epitopes in polyclonal antibody samples such as inhibitors from the plasma of haemophilia patients. The sensitivity of this method is currently evaluated on patient's antibodies purified by an optimized procedure, in which the second chromatography step was modified. Furthermore, alterations in the phage display protocol such as subtractive panning strategies may be considered.

Acknowledgements. We thank Dr. Auerswald (Bremen) and Prof. Budde (Hamburg) for providing plasma samples and T. Albert (Bonn) for helpful discussions. This work was supported by Wyeth Pharma GmbH, Germany.

References

1. Ehrenforth S, Kreuz W, Scharrer I, Linde R, Funk M, Gungor T, Krackhardt B,Kornhuber B. Incidence of development of factor VIII and factor IX inhibitors in hemophiliacs. Lancet 1992; 339: 594–598
2. Rothschild C, Laurian Y, Satre EP, Borel Derlon A, Chambost H, Moreau P, Goudemand J, Parquet A, Peynet J, Vicariot M, Beurrier P, Claeyssens S, Durin A, Faradji A, Fressinaud E, Gaillard S, Guerin V, Guerois C, Pernod G, Pouzol P, Schved JF,Gazengel C. French pre-

viously untreated patients with severe hemophilia A after exposure to recombinant factor VIII : incidence of inhibitor and evaluation of immune tolerance. Thromb Haemost 1998; 80: 779–783

3. Gruppo R, Bray GL, Schroth P, Perry M, Gomperts ED, for the Recombinate PUP Study Group. Safety and immunogenicity of recombinant factor VIII (Recombinate) in previously untreated patients (PUPs): a 6.5 year update. Thromb Haemost 1997; 162 Suppl.: PD-663

4. Lusher JM, Shapiro A, Gruppo R, Bedrosian CL, Nguyen K, the ReFacto PUP Study Group. Safety and efficacy in previously untreated patients (PUPs) treated exclusively with B-domain deleted factor VIII (BDD rFVIII). Thromb Haemost 2001; Congress Suppl.: 2558

5. Lacroix-Desmazes S, Misra N, Bayry J, Artaud C, Drayton B, Kaveri SV,Kazatchkine MD. Pathophysiology of inhibitors to factor VIII in patients with haemophilia A. Haemophilia 2002; 8: 273–279

6. Saenko EL, Ananyeva NM, Tuddenham EG,Kemball-Cook G. Factor VIII - novel insights into form and function. Br J Haematol 2002; 119: 323–331

7. Pittman DD, Alderman EM, Tomkinson KN, Wang JH, Giles AR, Kaufman RJ. Biochemical, immunological, and in vivo functional characterization of B-domain-deleted factor VIII. Blood 1993; 81: 2925–2935

8. Scandella DH, Nakai H, Felch M, Mondorf W, Scharrer I, Hoyer LW, Saenko EL. In hemophilia A and autoantibody inhibitor patients: the factor VIII A2 domain and light chain are most immunogenic. Thromb Res 2001; 101: 377–385

9. Scandella D, Gilbert GE, Shima M, Nakai H, Eagleson C, Felch M, Prescott R, Rajalakshmi KJ, Hoyer LW, Saenko E. Some factor VIII inhibitor antibodies recognize a common epitope corresponding to C2 domain amino acids 2248 through 2312, which overlap a phospholipid-binding site. Blood 1995; 86: 1811–1819

10. Scandella D. Human anti-factor VIII antibodies: epitope localization and inhibitory function. Vox Sang 1996; 70 Suppl 1: 9–14

11. Healey JF, Lubin IM, Nakai H, Saenko EL, Hoyer LW, Scandella D, Lollar P. Residues 484–508 contain a major determinant of the inhibitory epitope in the A2 domain of human factor VIII. J Biol Chem 1995; 270: 14505–14509

12. Saenko EL, Ananyeva NM, Kouiavskaia DV, Khrenov AV, Anderson JA, Shima M, Qian J,Scott D. Haemophilia A: effects of inhibitory antibodies on factor VIII functional interactions and approaches to prevent their action. Haemophilia 2002; 8: 1-11

13. Fulcher CA, de Graaf Mahoney S, Roberts JR, Kasper CK, Zimmerman TS. Localization of human factor FVIII inhibitor epitopes to two polypeptide fragments. Proc Natl Acad Sci U S A 1985; 82: 7728–7732

14. Ware J, MacDonald MJ, Lo M, de Graaf S, Fulcher CA. Epitope mapping of human factor VIII inhibitor antibodies by site-directed mutagenesis of a factor VIII polypeptide. Blood Coagul Fibrinolysis 1992; 3: 703–716

15. Scandella D, DeGraaf Mahoney S, Mattingly M, Roeder D, Timmons L, Fulcher CA. Epitope mapping of human factor VIII inhibitor antibodies by deletion analysis of factor VIII fragments expressed in Escherichia coli. Proc Natl Acad Sci U S A 1988; 85: 6152–6156

16. Palmer DS, Dudani AK, Drouin J, Ganz PR. Identification of novel factor VIII inhibitor epitopes using synthetic peptide arrays. Vox Sang 1997; 72: 148–161

17. Azzazy HM, Highsmith WE, Jr. Phage display technology: clinical applications and recent innovations. Clin Biochem 2002; 35: 425–445

18. Stoilova-McPhie S, Villoutreix BO, Mertens K, Kemball-Cook G, Holzenburg A. 3-dimensional structure of membrane-bound coagulation factor VIII: modeling of the factor VIII heterodimer within a 3-dimensional density map derived by electron crystallography. Blood 2002; 99: 1215–1223

Rituximab – A new Treatment of Acquired Hemophilia A?

M. Krause, C. Betz, I. Stier-Brück, E. Weidmann, and I. Scharrer

Introduction

The development of inhibitors to factor VIII may cause life-threatening bleedings, and presents a serious clinical management problem. Acquired hemophilia is a rare event, with an incidence of 0.2–1 per million per year and a mortality between 6% and 22%. In the majority of patients no cause can be identified. Up to 50% of the patients with autoantibodies against factor VIII are associated with autoimmune diseases, malignancies, drugs, pregnancies, or the postpartum period. The aims of management in acquired hemophilia are to eradicate the FVIII autoantibodies and to treat the acute bleeding episodes.

Rituximab is a specific anti B-cell chimaeric monoclonal antibody indicated for treatment of CD20-positive non-Hodgkin's lymphoma. CD20 is a B-cell lineage antigenic expressed from pre-B-cells to mature and activated B-cells. Rituximab kills CD20-positive cells via several different mechanisms, which include induction of complement-mediated cytotoxicity (CDC) and antibody-dependent cell-mediated cytotoxicity (ADCC).

Clinical Course in a Patient with Acquired Hemophilia against Factor VIII

A 75-year-old female developed spontaneous giant ecchymoses. The factor VIII level was 1% with a factor VIII inhibitor titre of 21.6 BU. The protocol of our therapy regimens consists of immunoadsorption by Ig-apheresis, intravenous immunoglobulin (IVIG, 0.4 g/kg body weight), steroids (100 mg/day), mycophenolatmofetil (1 g/day), and recombinant activated factor VII (rFVIIa) for acute hemorrhages. After 24 days of the therapy regimes the factor VIII level was 33% with a factor VIII inhibitor titre of 0 BU (Fig. 1). 15 days later we documented relapse of the acquired hemophilia and bleeding episodes. The factor VIII level was 4% and factor VIII inhibitor max. 16.9 BU. The patient received four weekly doses of Rituximab therapy at 375 mg/m² per week. Temporary immunosuppression was achieved with steroids (100 mg/day) and, recurrent soft tissue bleedings were treated with recombinant activated factor VII.

6 days after completion of the therapy, the factor VIII level was 73% and factor VIII inhibitor titre 0 BU. Four months after the fourth infusion, the patient is still in complete remission. The inhibitor titre is 0 BU constantly (Fig. 2).

I. Scharrer/W. Schramm (Ed.)
33rd Hemophilia Symposion Hamburg 2002
© Springer-Verlag Berlin Heidelberg 2004

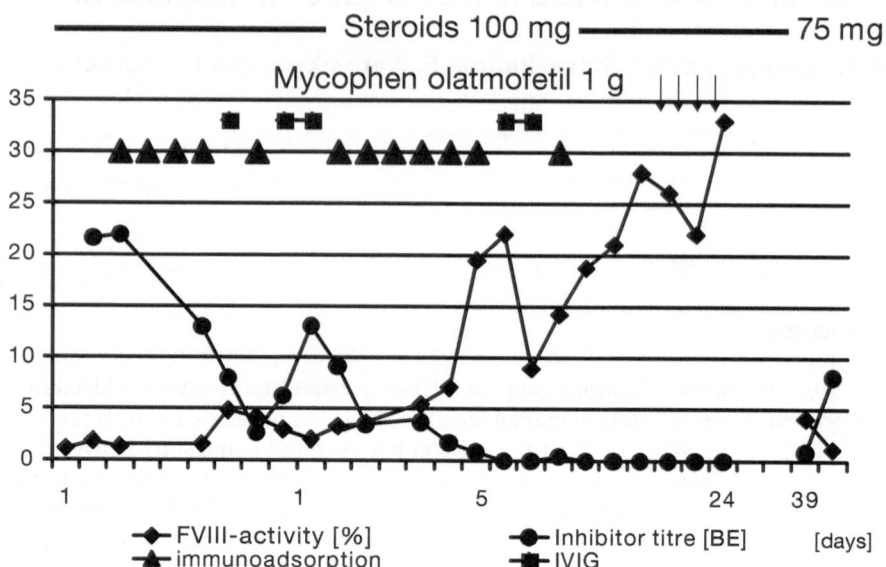

Fig. 1. FVIII levels and FVIII inhibitor – first course –

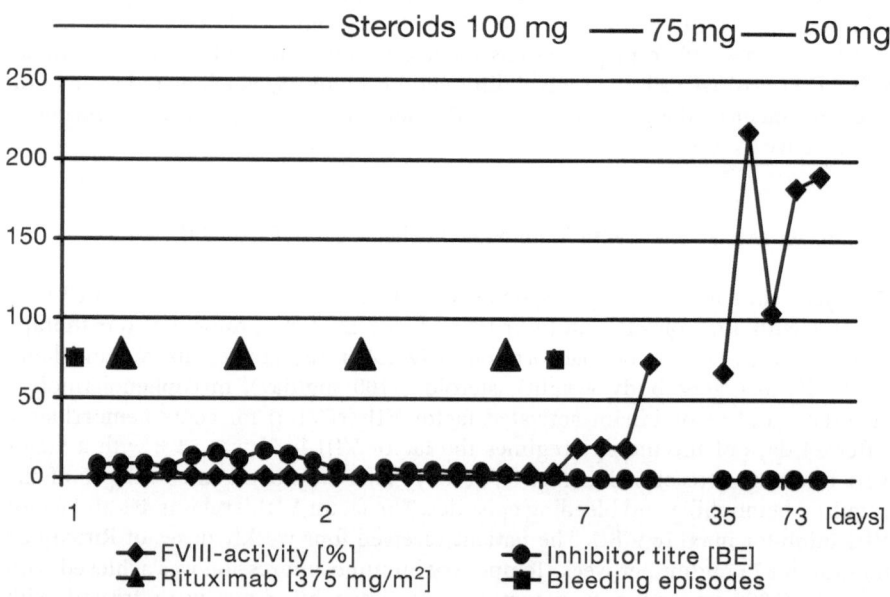

Fig. 2. FVIII levels and FVIII inhibitor – relapse –

The occurrence of the inhibitor against factor VIII seems to be associated with the diagnosis of breast cancer in our patient.

Conclusion

Rituximab appears to be a new and promising drug in the treatment in patients with inhibitors against factor VIII and has an excellent safety profile.

Rituximab seems to be effective in the elimination of inhibitors against factor VIII in patients with acquired inhibitors. The mechanism of response to autoantibodies against FVIII is still unclear.

The combination of Rituximab with steroids may be required for maximal benefit in the relapse of acquired hemophilia in our patient. Further studies are needed to confirm whether Rituximab has an important role in the first line therapy of patients with acquired hemophilia or only in cases unresponsive to other therapy regimens.

References

1. Cohen AJ, Kessler CM. Acquired inhibitors. In: Lee CA, ed. Haemophilia. Bailliere's Clinical Haematology 1996; 9: 331–354
2. Green D, Lechner K. A survey of 215 non-hemophilic patients with inhibitors to factor VIII. Thromb Haemost 1981; 45: 200–203
3. Karwal MW, Schlueter AJ, Zenk DW, Davis RT. Treatment of acquired factor VIII deficiency with rituximab. [Abstract] Blood 2001; 98: 533a
4. Kessler CM, Nemes L. Acquired inhibitors to factor VIII. In: Rodriguez-Merchan EC and Lee CA Inhibitors in patients with haemophilia. Blackwell Science 2002; 98–112
5. Shapiro SS, Hultin M. Acquired inhibitors to the blood coagulation factors. Sem Thromb Haemostas 1975; 1: 336–385
6. Wiestner A, Cho HJ, Asch AS; Michelis AM, Zeller JA, Peerschke EI, Weksler BB, and Schechter GP. Rituximab in the treatment of acquired factor VIII inhibitors. Blood 2002; 100: 3426–3428

Thrombin Generation and Thrombogram: Assays for Monitoring Factor VIII Bypassing Therapies

K. Váradi, H.P. Schwarz, and P.L. Turecek

Inhibitor Bypassing Therapy

Hemophilic patients with inhibitors cannot be treated by conventional substitution therapy, but are usually treated with preparations containing activated coagulation factors that are intended to achieve hemostasis by bypassing FVIII and independently of FVIII [1, 2]. Activated prothrombin complex concentrates such as FEIBA contain vitamin-K-dependent coagulation factor zymogens and a small amount of their activated forms (Table 1).

Activated prothrombin complex preparations have multiple modes of action by initiating the formation of the prothrombinase complex and subsequent thrombin generation, and enhancing the thrombin and FXa-mediated feedback reactions [3]. Recombinant FVIIa, which consists of only a single protein, has also at least two active principles: a tissue factor (TF)-dependent FX activation, and at high doses, a TF-independent reaction in which FVIIa activates FX bound on endogenous phospholipid surfaces [4, 5]. Both therapeutic agents are able to bypass FVIII by inducing thrombin formation in a FVIII-independent manner.

Table 1. Procoagulant protein composition of FEIBA

	Protein	Activity (Units/Unit FEIBA)	Biological half life ($t_{1/2}$)
Zymogens	Prothrombin	1.3	72 h
	Factor VII	0.9	4–6 h
	Factor IX	1.4	20 h
	Factor X	1.1	48 h
Enzymes	Factor VIIa	1.5*	1–2 h
	Factor IXa	0.0004	min**
	Factor Xa	0.006	min**
	Thrombin	0.001	min**

Units are given as the amount of the clotting factors found in 1 ml of normal pooled plasma, determined with appropriate clotting or chromogenic assays. The concentrations of the activated (a) clotting factors are compared with their zymogen forms except for FVIIa (*), which is given in arbitrary units, compared with a recombinant FVIIa as reference [14]. The FEIBA unit is defined as the amount of FEIBA that can shorten the clotting time of a high-titer FVIII inhibitor plasma by 50%. **The half-lives of FIXa, FXa and thrombin cannot be exactly determined, because they are rapidly inactivated by their circulating inhibitors.

I. Scharrer/W. Schramm (Ed.)
33rd Hemophilia Symposion Hamburg 2002
© Springer-Verlag Berlin Heidelberg 2004

Direct monitoring of the effect of the bypassing agents is not possible, not only because some bypassing agents have multiple active components with a broad range of half lives (Table 1), but also because the active ingredients interact immediately with proteins of the hemostatic system to induce activation of the clotting cascade and lead to the thrombin generation required for an appropriate clot formation.

Currently there is no routine test that quantitatively assesses the thrombin forming capacity of a plasma sample. General hemostatic assays, like clotting times (prothrombin time, activated partial thromboplastin time) or thrombelastographic methods, do not reflect the overall thrombin generation and are insensitive to hyper- and in some cases also to hypocoagulation states. Measuring surrogate markers of thrombin, such as prothrombin fragment 1+2, thrombin-antithrombin complex or thrombus-precursor protein, only indicates that thrombin has been formed and interacted with its substrates or inhibitors. Such measurements thus have only a limited value for the assessment of the efficacy of the bypassing agents.

Hemker et al. (1986) were the first to describe the detailed kinetic analysis of prothrombin activation in plasma and introduced the thrombin generation test [6].

Later Hemker et al. introduced the term »endogenous thrombin potential« (ETP) defined as the overall capacity of plasma to form thrombin after induction of coagulation and proposed the use of this parameter as a sensitive indicator of every form of anticoagulation [7]. Using this assay, a linear correlation between the concentrations of recombinant FVIIa and the amount of thrombin generated and between the correction of the ETP and the clinical outcome of the patients was found [8]. In a recent publication Al Dieri et al. [9] showed that all patients with severe bleeding symptoms have a less than normal ETP.

The development and use of an assay system suitable for detecting treatment-dependent changes in the kinetic of thrombin generation and monitoring the pharmacokinetics of inhibitor-bypassing agents during treatment are discussed below.

Kinetics of Thrombin Generation During Clotting

Figure 1 illustrates the changes in plasma thrombin concentrations as a function of the time course of the physiological events of coagulation. Upon exposure of damaged tissue, blood coagulation is triggered by a TF/FVII complex. After FX and FIX activation, enzyme-cofactor complexes assemble on the activated platelet surface, and small amounts of thrombin are generated prompting fibrin formation. The various feedback effects of thrombin's activation of FV, FVIII and FXI, produce a burst of thrombin generation (Fig. 1: Panel A). A short-lived equilibrium of thrombin activation and inactivation follows. After maximum thrombin generation is reached the physiological inhibitor systems [TF pathway inhibitor (TFPI), antithrombin (AT), and the activated protein C-protein S system (APC-PS)] slow down thrombin activation by inactivating the active enzymes and/or degrading their cofactors. Circulating inhibitors, such as α_2-macroglobulin inactivate thrombin directly. The thrombin concentration gradually decreases (Fig. 1: Panel B). The rate of thrombin activation and the amount of peak thrombin depends on the relative rate of thrombin

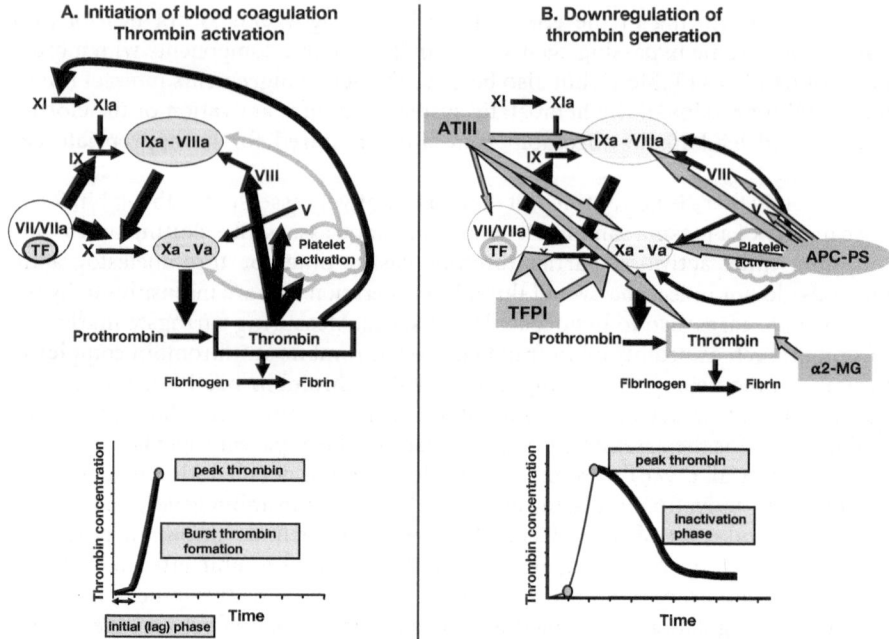

Fig. 1. Kinetic mechanisms of thrombin activation and inactivation during blood coagulation. Principles of thrombin generation assay

activation and inactivation mechanisms. Therefore the »real time« measurement of the thrombin concentration that can be generated in plasma gives valuable information about the homeostasis of the coagulation system.

Measurement Possibilities of Thrombin Generation

To measure the kinetics of the thrombin generation in an ex vivo plasma sample hemostasis has to be triggered and the subsequent time-dependent changes in the thrombin concentration have to be detected. For practical reasons, quantification of thrombin is achieved by measuring the amount of a product generated by thrombin during coagulation from an artificial peptide substrate. The peptide substrate is covalently labeled when it is liberated by thrombin either with a chromophor (para-nitroanilide; pNA) giving a color or with a fluorophor (aminomethyl-coumarin; AMC) group giving a fluorescence signal (Fig. 2).

Thrombin formation can be measured by two basic methods. One is a sub-sampling method using a chromogenic substrate. Coagulation is started in plasma by adding TF, phospholipids and calcium. Subsamples are withdrawn at time intervals, the thrombin activation reaction is stopped and a chromogenic substrate is added to measure the thrombin concentration at the time of subsampling. For this method, plasma samples have to be defibrillated or the fibrin polymerization has to

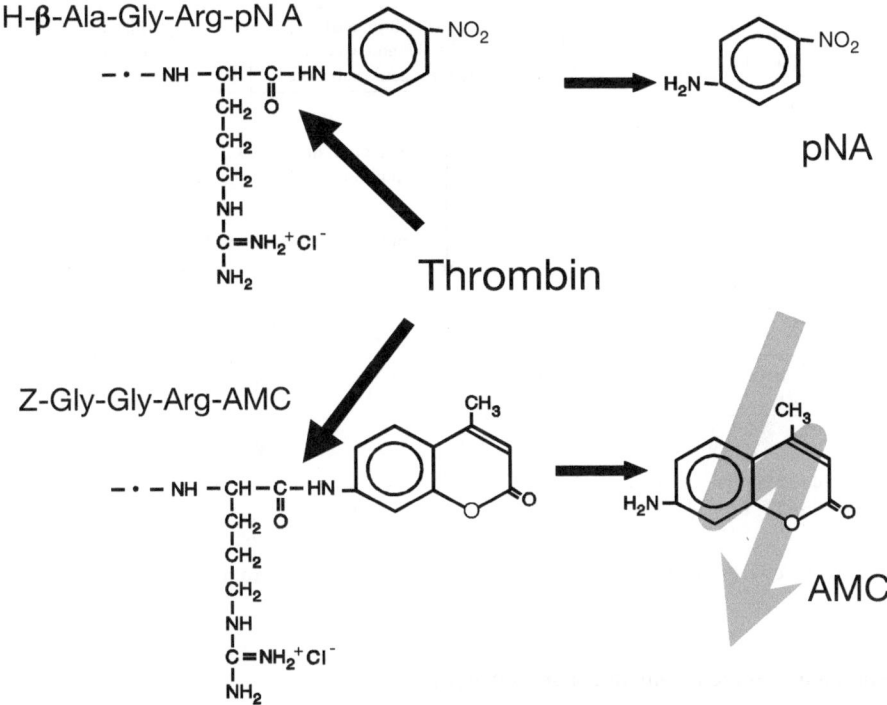

Fig. 2. Thrombin-mediated liberation of the chromophor (pNA) and fluorophor (AMC) groups in the used substrates

be inhibited, since the clotting blocks the subsampling. The second method continuously detects thrombin generation. Coagulation is started in plasma by adding TF, phospholipids and calcium together with a chromogenic or fluorogenic substrate. The low affinity of the substrate results in a slow reaction by the formed thrombin. Chromogenic substrates give changes in the optical density, and to detect this signal an optically clear medium is required. Therefore, the plasma needs to be defibrinated or the fibrin polymerization has to be inhibited. The flow chart in Figure 3 summarizes the assays.

The subsampling method is a complicated, time consuming »three-phase« reaction, which is not suitable for routine use. The continuous method is a simple, one-stage assay. Using a chromogenic substrate has the drawback that fibrin polymerization has to be inhibited either by an inhibitor or by defibrination. Both methods of inhibition result in a manipulated plasma sample, which might give unfeasible results, as fibrin formation has an important regulatory role in thrombin generation [10]. Therefore the recommended method is the continuous method using a fluorogenic substrate. The experimental details of the assay we used are given in the appendix.

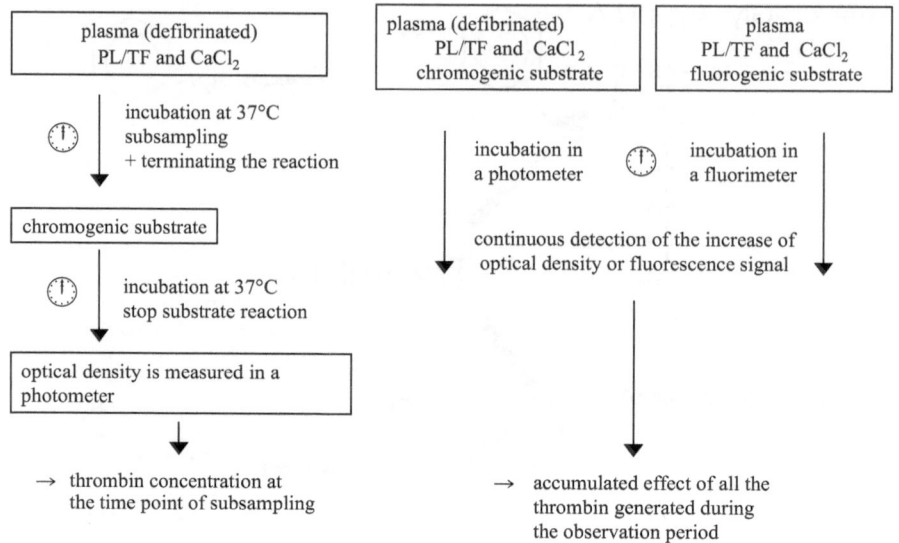

Fig. 3. Procedures of chromogenic and fluorogenic thrombin generation assays

Parameters of the Thrombin Generation Assay

The thrombin generation curve can be characterized by various parameters (Fig. 5 and Table 2). The thrombin potential (expressed in FU) is the amount of thrombin that is formed altogether within a certain period, e.g. 60 min (area under the thrombin generation curve). The peak thrombin is the highest thrombin concentration reached during the time course of thrombin formation and inhibition. The lag phase shows how fast thrombin starts to generate, i.e. when the fluorescent signal starts to increase, and the peak time is the time when the maximum thrombin activity is observed (Fig. 4).

This thrombin generation assay was designed to attain normal thrombin generation in plasma from healthy donors and almost no thrombin generation in FVIII-deficient plasma, which was also well reflected in the characteristic parameters (Table 2).

Table 2. Characteristic parameters of thrombin generation measured in a normal and in a FVIII-inhibitor plasma

	Peak thrombin (nM)	Lag phase (min)	Peak time (min)	Thrombin potential at 60 min (FU)
Normal plasma	214	14.8	20.3	32688
FVIII inhibitor plasma	8.5	39.1	>80	3101

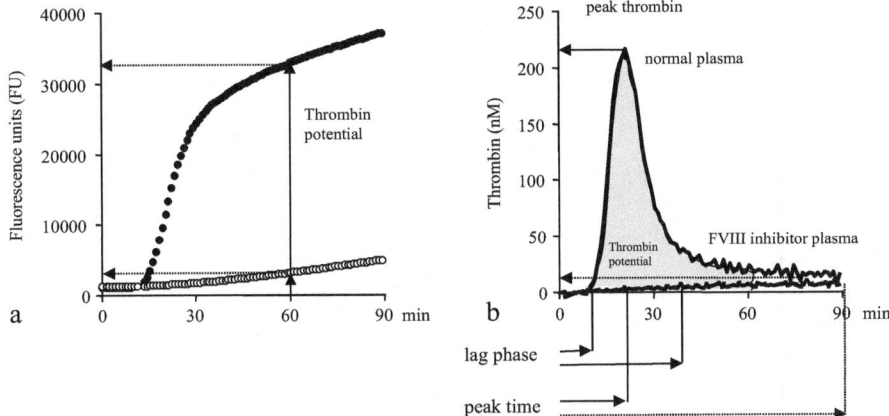

Fig. 4. Continuous determination of thrombin generation in a normal and in FVIII inhibitor plasma. Characteristic parameters of the thrombogram. **a)** Time-dependent accumulation of thrombin, expressed in fluorescence signal as detected in normal plasma (●) and in a high-titer FVIII inhibitor plasma (O) **b)** Thrombin generation curves obtained by calculating the first derivative of the curves seen in Panel a and converted to thrombin equivalent concentrations, as described in the Appendix.

Effect of FEIBA on the Thrombin Generation of FVIII Inhibitor Plasma in vitro

A high-titer FVIII inhibitor plasma was spiked with increasing concentrations of FEIBA, and thrombin generation was measured immediately. The thrombin accumulation and generation curves show the dose-dependent restoration of the thrombin-generating capacity of the FVIII inhibitor plasma resulting in a gradual increase in peak thrombin concentrations and thrombin potentials, and a dose-dependent decrease in lag phases and peak times (Fig. 5).

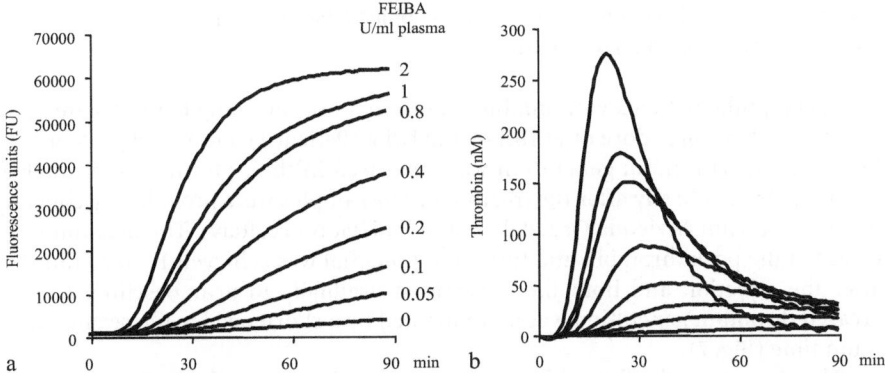

Fig. 5. Continuous determination of thrombin generation in FVIII inhibitor plasma reconstituted in vitro with FEIBA. **a)** Accumulation of the fluorescence signal. **b)** First derivative of the curves from Panel a. Concentrations of FEIBA in plasma increase from the bottom to the top, as marked in Panel a.

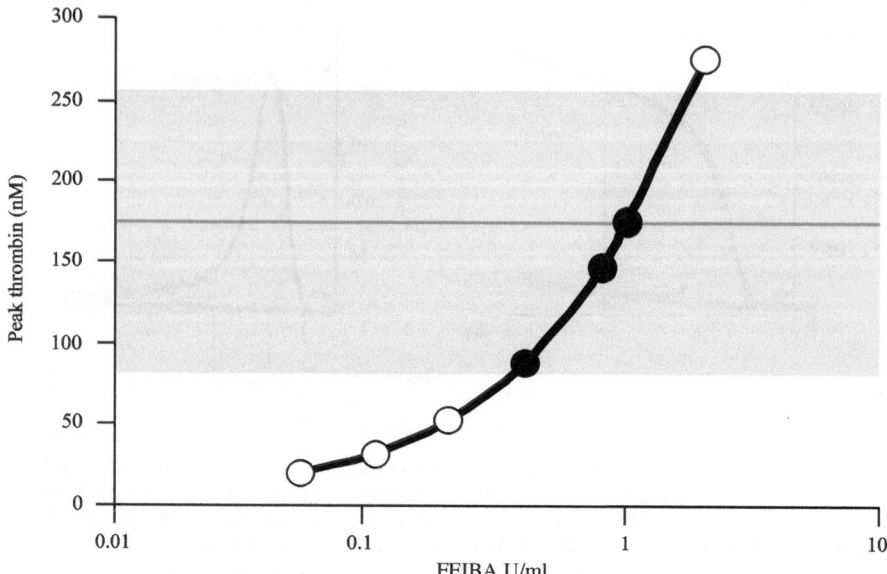

Fig. 6. Dose-dependent increase of maximum thrombin in FVIII inhibitor plasma spiked in vitro with FEIBA. Gray area: Normal range with the mean value of the thrombin peak indicated by a dark gray line. Closed symbols represent the concentrations corresponding to therapeutic doses.

The normal range was reached by plasma concentrations of 0.5–2 FEIBA U/ml (Fig. 6). These concentrations correspond to those that can be achieved with the usual therapeutic doses of 50–100 FEIBA U/kg, calculated on the assumption of a 50 to 100% recovery.

Pharmacokinetics of FEIBA in two Severe Hemophilia A Patients with Inhibitor as Measured by the Thrombin Generation

Two hemophilic patients with inhibitor, both in a non-bleeding clinical state, were injected with a single dose of FEIBA of 100 U/kg (Patient 1) and 80 U/kg (Patient 2) body weight. Thrombin generation was measured in their plasma samples taken before and periodically after the treatment. The samples were provided by courtesy of Dr. M. Morfini (Azienda Ospedaliera Careggi, Florence, Italy). The maximum increase in the peak thrombin and thrombin potential was achieved 15 to 30 minutes after the injection and both then decreased gradually to near baseline. The increased thrombin generation was accompanied by a shortened lag phase and maximum time (Fig. 7).

The changes in the thrombin maximum were time-dependent (Fig. 8a) in both patients but the maximum effect was different.

The half-lives of the thrombin-generation restoration effect, calculated from the declining part of the curves (Fig. 8b), were 4 and 5 hours.

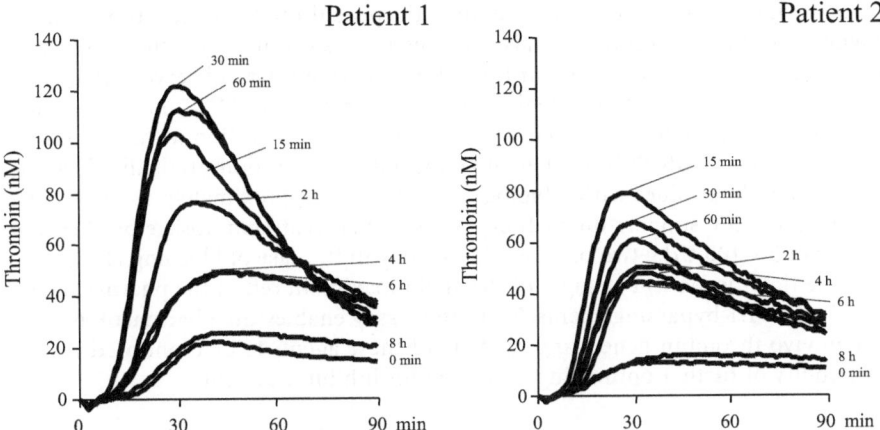

Fig. 7. Thrombin generation curves obtained from the plasma samples of two patients with FVIII inhibitor before and periodically after a single dose FEIBA injection. Thrombin generation measured before FEIBA addition (0 min), 15 min, 30 min, 60 min, 2 h, 4 h, 6 h and 8 h after FEIBA treatment.

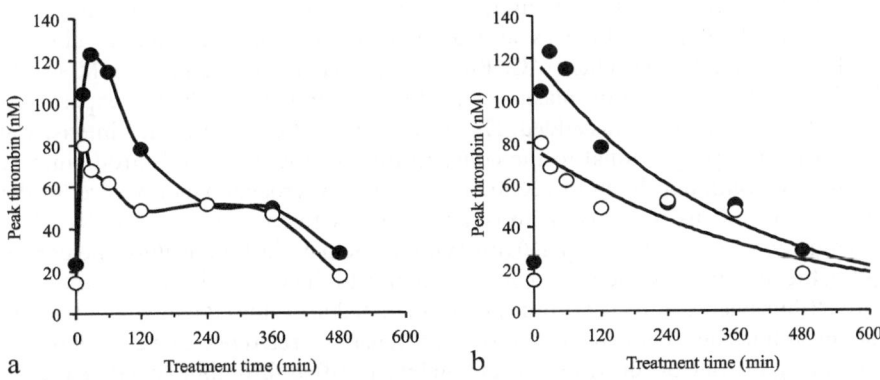

Fig. 8. Pharmacokinetics of thrombin generating capacity of the plasma samples of two FVIII inhibitor patients after a single injection of FEIBA. **a)** Changes in the in peak thrombin. **b)** Fitted curves for calculation of the half-lives Patient 1 (– ● –), Patient 2 (– ○ –)

Conclusions

We present an in vitro assay by which thrombin generation can be continuously followed in plasma after coagulation is triggered with $CaCl_2$ and a low concentration of TF/PL complex. A fluorogenic peptide substrate is used for thrombin generation. The assay conditions mimic in vivo situations with TF release, where sufficient thrombin generation can be achieved by intact hemostasis, but not in severe FVIII deficiency. The assay is easy to use, and can be applied in any laboratory in which coagulation assays or multiplate reader ELISAs are routinely used.

As a characteristic parameter, we chose the peak thrombin concentration, i.e. the highest thrombin concentration raised during the assay time. Using the assay a dose-dependent increase in maximum thrombin generation was observed when FVIII inhibitor plasma was reconstituted in vitro with FEIBA. Two FVIII inhibitor patients were found to have reversed their defective thrombin generation within 30 minutes after treatment with FEIBA. Thereafter thrombin generation gradually decreased back to baseline values with a biological half-life of approximately 4–5 hours. Our results therefore support the viability of the usual treatment dosage of FEIBA, i.e. a dose of 50–100 U/kg two or three times a day in the case of bleeding [11, 12].

The time-dependent changes of thrombin maximum reflect the pharmacological effect of FVIII-bypassing agents. Thus, this assay enables the pharmacokinetics of the in vivo thrombin-generating capacity of these agents to be monitored with the possibility of further optimizing treatment for inhibitor patients.

Appendix

Experimental details of the continuous thrombin generation assay

Thrombin generation was triggered by a relipidated TF preparation, prepared as described elsewhere [13], containing 17.5 pM TF and 3.2 μM phospholipid (PL). A solution of 10 μl TF/PL was added to 50 μl of 1 mM thrombin substrate Z-Gly-Gly-Arg-AMC (Bachem AG, Bubendorf, Switzerland) and 15 mM $CaCl_2$. Adding 40 μl FVIII inhibitor plasma started the reaction. In the control experiment 40 μl of normal plasma was added. The development of the fluorogenic intensity at 37°C, which is proportional to the concentration of the generated thrombin, was monitored continuously up to 120 minutes using a Microplate Fluorescence Reader FL600 (Bio-TEK Instruments, Winooski, VT, USA) with an excitation wavelength of 360 nm and an emission one of 460 nm. With the help of the kinetic fluorimeter program, the maximum velocity, which corresponds to the peak value of the first derivative (fluorogenic units (FU)/min), was calculated and subsequently converted to the thrombin-equivalent concentrations (nM), using a reference curve prepared by measuring the rate of substrate conversion by a purified thrombin added instead of the plasma sample.

Plasma Samples and Reagents

The activated prothrombin complex concentrate preparation, FEIBA, was the product of Baxter, Vienna, Austria. Human thrombin was obtained from Enzyme Research Laboratories (Lafayette, IN, USA), normal plasma from George King Bio-Medical (Overland Parks, KS, USA) and tissue factor (TF) from American Diagnostica (Greenwich, CT, USA). High-titer human FVIII inhibitor plasma was the product of Technoclone (Vienna, Austria). The PL composed of 80% of 1,2-Dioleoyl-sn-glycero-3-phosphocholine (PC) and 20% 1-Palmitoyl-2-oleoyl-sn-glycero-3-phosphoserine (PS), both were purchased from Avanti Polar Lipids (Alabaster, AL, USA). All other reagents and buffer components were made of commercially available reagents of highest purity.

Patients' plasma samples: Blood samples (9 parts added to 1 part of 3.4% Na$_3$-citrate) were taken before and at specified time points after the FEIBA injection. Platelet poor plasma was prepared by centrifuging the blood samples (3000 g for 20 min). The plasma samples were frozen in aliquots at -20°C and thawed at 37°C just before the assay.

Both patients gave informed consent before treatment.

References

1. Lusher JM. Use of prothrombin complex concentrates in management of bleeding in hemophiliacs with inhibitors: benefits and limitations. Semin Hematol 1994; 31 (2 Suppl 4): 49–52
2. Roberts HR. The use of agents that by-pass factor VIII inhibitors in patients with Haemophilia. Vox Sang 1999; 77 (Suppl 1): 38–41
3. Turecek PL, Varadi K, Gritsch H, Auer W, Pichler L, Eder G, Schwarz HP. Factor Xa and Prothrombin: Mechanism of action of FEIBA. Vox Sang 1999; 77 (Suppl 1): 72–79
4. ten Cate H, Bauer KA, Levi M, Edgington TS, Sublett RD, Barzegar S, Kass BL, Rosenberg RD. The activation of factor X and prothrombin by recombinant factor VIIa in vivo is mediated by tissue factor. J Clin Invest 1993; 92: 1207–12
5. Monroe DM, Hoffman M, Oliver JA, Roberts HR. A possible mechanism of activated factor VIIa independent of tissue factor. Blood Coagul Fibrinolysis 1998; 9 (Suppl 1): S15–S20
6. Hemker HC, Willems GM, Beguin S. A computer assisted method to obtain the prothrombin activation velocity in whole plasma independent of thrombin decay processes. Thromb Haemost 1986; 56: 9–17
7. Hemker HC, Beguin S. Thrombin generation in plasma: its assessment via the endogenous thrombin potential. Thromb Haemost 1995; 74: 134–38
8. Madlener K, Gissel B, Brackmann H, Pötzsch B. The endogenous thrombin generation potential (ETP) is an accurate and rapid monitoring method for recombinant factor VIIa. Ann Hematol 2000; 79 (Suppl I): A46
9. Al Dieri R, Peyvandi F, Santagostino E, Giansily M, Mannucci PM, Schved JF, Beguin S, Coenraad Hemker H. The thrombogram in rare inherited coagulation disorders: its relation to clinical bleeding. Thromb Haemost 2002; 88: 576–82
10. Kumar R, Beguin S, Hemker HC: The Influence of fibrinogen and fibrin on thrombin generation – Evidence for feedback activation of the clotting system by clot bound thrombin. Thromb Haemost 1994; 72: 712–21
11. Negrier C, Goudemand J, Sultan Y, Bertrand M, Rothschild C, Lauroua P. Multicenter retrospective study on the utilization of FEIBA in France in patients with factor VIII and factor IX inhibitors. French FEIBA Study Group. Factor Eight Bypassing Activity. Thromb Haemost 1997; 771: 113–19
12. Hilgartner M, Aledort L, Andes A, Gill J, and the members of the FEIBA Study Group. Efficacy and safety of vapor-heated anti-inhibitor coagulant complex in hemophilia patients. Transfusion 1990; 30: 626–30
13. Váradi K, Siekmann J, Turecek PL, Schwarz HP, Marder VJ: Phospholipid-bound tissue factor modulates both thrombin generation and APC-mediated factor Va inactivation. Thromb Haemost 1999; 82: 1673–79
14. Morrissey JH, Macik BG, Neuenschwander PF, Comp PC: Quantitation of activated factor VII levels in plasma using a tissue factor mutant selectively deficient in promoting factor VII activation. Blood 1993; 81: 734–44

III. Hemophilia: Therapeutic Exercise and Sport

Chairmen:

R. ZIMMERMANN (Heidelberg)
A. KURTH (Frankfurt/Main)

Rehabilitation – A Topic for Hemophiliacs?

K. Vermöhlen, H.-H. Brackmann, and W. Kalnins

Introduction

I'm very pleased to start this conference on »hemophilia and sport« with my report about the importance of rehabilitation in connection with complete care of hemophiliacs. Rehabilitation measures often have a primary prophylactic function when treating these patients.

If hemophiliacs go in for sports that takes into account both the individual handicaps and the particular abilities, rehabilitation shouldn't mean the end of a failed career in sport but a further method of treatment. The latter serves as a basis for permanent control, regarding the question whether the sport makes sense or not. It might be that a former decision on a special form of sport has to be adjusted in coordination with patient's hemophilia center.

Rehabilitation also has the purpose to lead older hemophiliacs to therapeutic exercise and sport. Thereby the severity of the disease, the patients' concerns as well as their abilities and preferences must be taken into account by the interdisciplinary team of specialists.

In our rehabilitation hospital we treat persons with mild (factor levels > 5 and <50%), moderate (factor levels 1% to 5%) and severe (factor levels < 1%) hemophilia A and hemophilia B. There are also persons with other clotting disorders as von-Willebrand's disease, platelet dysfunctions and thrombocytopathias, hemophiliacs with inhibitors of factor VIII or IX. Naturally, the emphasis of treatment lies on hemophilia A.

Medical, Vocational an Social Rehabilitation

With regard to rehabilitation measures it is necessary to differentiate between the *medical, social and vocational aspects of rehabilitation*. Talking about a rehabilitation hospital most people exclusively think of medical rehabilitation. This is certainly something we put the main emphasis on. Nevertheless we don't ignore occupational and social rehabilitation programs. According to a complete understanding of rehabilitation, they serve as indispensable components of a far reaching understanding of rehabilitation. This opinion finds expression in an interdisciplinary team-based treatment. I will go into that later.

I. Scharrer/W. Schramm (Ed.)
33rd Hemophilia Symposion Hamburg 2002
© Springer-Verlag Berlin Heidelberg 2004

The *medical rehabilitation* program is designed to help resolve complex problems such as the reduction of motion in case of hemophilic arthropathy, muscle dysfunction, reduced staying-power, pain and psychological handicaps.

In matters of *vocational rehabilitation* the following aspects are central: vocational reintegration, development of coping strategies (with regard to the individual handicaps and remained abilities of the patient), getting into contact with employers and company physicians (only with the patient's agreement), initiation of procedures concerning occupational disability and invalidity pension (life or temporary annuity).

Within the context of *social rehabilitation* the clinic provides for a consulting service and support with regard to social law regulations, organizational help in matters of housing conditions.

The necessity of an interdisciplinary team-based therapy in respect of hemophiliacs has found its latest expression in the work of Scharrer, Kurth and Kreuz published in the German Ärzteblatt 44/2002. They emphasize the fact that a reasonable treatment of hemophiliacs suffering orthopedic problems assumes a close collaboration of hematologists, well versed orthopedic surgeons in treating hemophiliacs, physiotherapists, occupational therapists and orthopedic mechanics.

The comprehensive Care Team

In an efficient rehabilitation hospital this collaborated work of specialists exists under one umbrella. This is an advantage for the patients because the arrangement and coordination of appointments become no longer necessary. The interdisciplinary team of occupational groups, which belong to the clinic, involves the work of physiotherapists, sports instructors, masseurs, medical bath attendants, psychosocial professional/social worker, male and female nurses (activating care!), occupational therapists and a dieticians.

Outside assistance is given by orthopedic mechanics, an orthopedic shoemaker as well as pension consultants and collaborators of the employers' liability insurance associations.

The medical specialist in Rehabilitation Medicine with special experience in treating hemophiliacs is coordinating the team. Together the professionals integrate their unique roles and perspectives into an effective strategy for the patient.

One superior rank task of the medical specialist in Rehabilitation Medicine is to get relevant information about the patient's medical report. He has to keep in touch with the treating hematologist before the patient is admitted to the rehabilitation hospital. The question how intensive the substitution of factor VIII or IX should be during the period of therapy has to be clarified beforehand. To know as much as possible of the preceded treatment is also necessary with regard to spontaneous bleeding episodes.

Thus the treating hematologist becomes an extern member of the comprehensive care team, who takes on the developed mobilization strategies after the patient's return from the rehabilitation hospital. This close collaboration is the key to a long-term process, that is initiated during stay in the rehabilitation hospital.

Normally an intensive rehabilitation program is developed for the patient's individual needs during an assessment program in our special hospital. At this point the program for a patient with hemarthropathy of the knee or the ankle joint is presented exemplarily:

physiotherapy
    1–2 individual therapies daily
    1–2 group therapies daily
medical sport-therapy
swimming and aquajogging
physical therapy,
    »classical« massages, modified massages (according to Terrier), medical baths, compresses, therapeutical ultrasound, short wave diathermy etc.

Substitution of Factor VIII and IX

The patient injects factor VIII or IX every morning before the therapeutic exercise begins. We have close access to the coagulation laboratory of the Hemophilia Center of the University of Bonn. The measure of clotting factor levels is carried out regarding predefined intervals or on demand.

Management of Undercurrent Bleedings

In case of emergency the standby service of this center supports our doctors on duty. Further assistance is given by one of the head physicians of internal medicine who is on duty. In case of serious bleedings the patient could be transferred to the special ambulance for hemophiliacs of the University of Bonn within 30 minutes. If the bleedings should be to serious for this transport the patient could be transferred to a renowned nearby hospital within 15 minutes. But also minor bleedings will be monitored closely. Most patients will treat themselves immediately at the first sign of a minor bleeding to avoid a major bleed. Major bleedings leading to abortion of the therapy have not occurred in the last four years, since I am responsible for the hemophiliacs in our rehabilitation hospital.

Management of Co-Infections

The treatment of hemophiliacs in many rehabilitation hospitals seems to be problematic because of the fear about the co-infections (HIV, HBV, HCV). A permanent information exchange between all members of the comprehensive care team is necessary to prevent improper behaviour towards infected patients and to reduce exaggerated fear regarding the co-infections.

It is a matter of course that these patients are situated in single rooms except they are accompanied by their partners during rehabilitation.

Organizing the Stay in the Rehabilitation Hospital

We try to welcome the hemophiliacs in small groups of 2–4 persons. This practice proved to be very worthwhile. Concentrating them in smaller groups contributes to better feeling of the patients and they mustn't get the impression of being exotic.

The management of rehabilitation measures will become easier in future. Due to the fact that SGB IX was passed by the German Bundestag in the last legislative period (1.7.2001), each county has to establish at least one service team and one service point for affected persons. Amongst other things the purpose of this service is to help patients with the application and to manage all correspondence with the appropriate pension insurance company.

Who Bears the Costs?

For all employed persons initially the appropriate pension insurances (BfA, LVA etc.) have to bear the costs for the rehabilitation. These insurance companies accept such rehabilitation programs as a necessary continuative therapy (AHB) or as a measure within the context of health care (AGM). Normally the treating physician (hematologist, orthopedic surgeon) initiates the rehabilitation by filling in a special printed form. In some cases an informal paper is also accepted.

The health insurance company has to pay the costs for all the other patients. Though there is no need for a formal application many health insurance companies have developed available questionnaires.

It is most important that the takeover of costs with regard to the care and the substitution of the necessary clotting factors or HIV-specific medicaments is guaranteed by a written consent of the cost-bearer. Otherwise the patient can't be accepted because it goes far beyond the financial budget of a rehabilitation hospital to bear the costs for this medical treatment. Although the workgroup »Durchführung der Rehabilitation« (AGDR) has already stated in a conference (20./21.09.1999) that pension insurance companies have to bear the costs for all rehabilitation measures including highly expensive pharmaceuticals, this matter is still problematic.

Statistics: Rehabilitation at the Eifelhöhen-Klinik, 2001

Most of the patients stayed less than 3 1/2 weeks. This was achieved by the arrival of the patients at the beginning of the week, in some cases even on Sundays. Integration into the rehabilitation program started on the second day. The scheduling of the therapy units was determined computer-based under consideration of particular handicaps (e.g. later begin of the therapy due to factor VIII or IX substitution by the patient himself).

As removal dates Fridays or Saturdays were preferred, because the employable patient is able to start his job within the beginning of the next week (Fig.1).

The following diagram shows the distribution of the patients to the different cost bearers (Fig. 2):

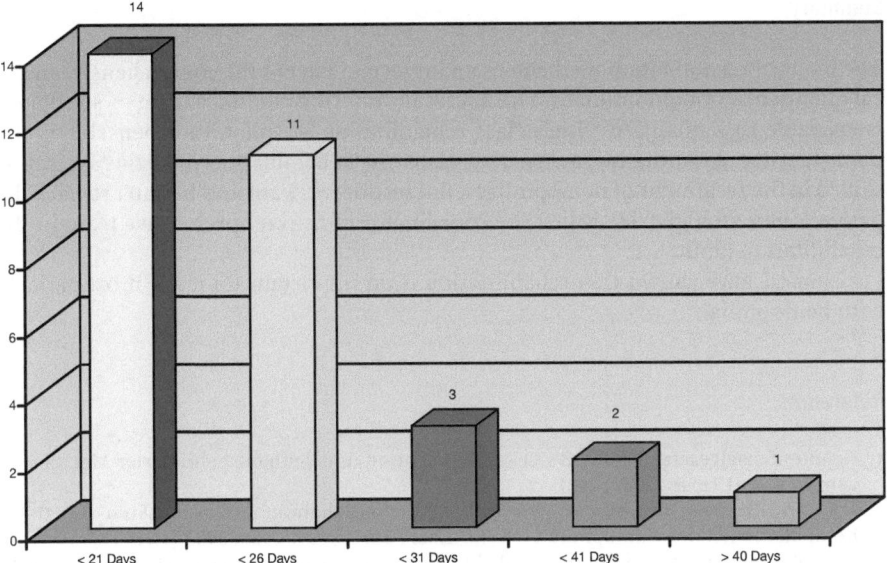

Fig. 1. Duration of stay

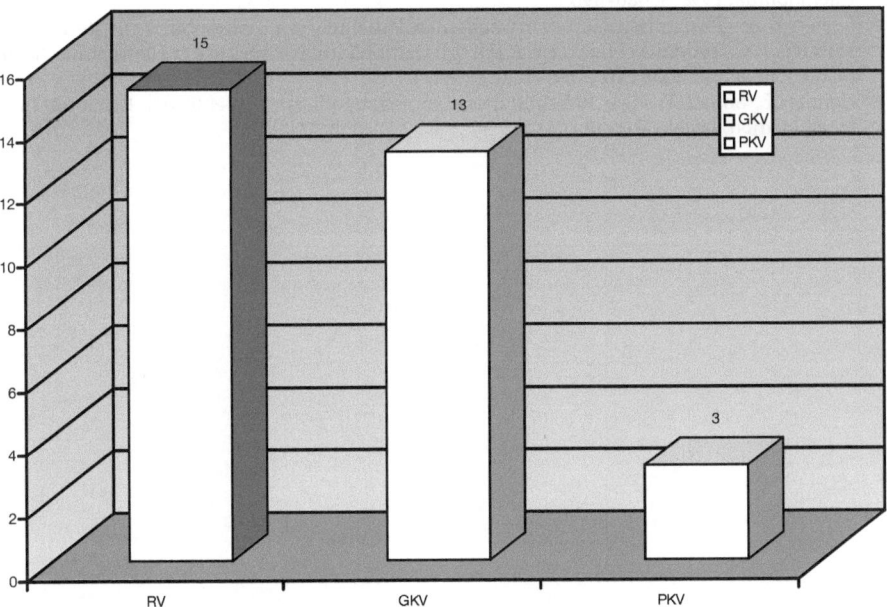

Fig. 2. Cost bearers

Summary

The modern rehabilitation medicine is an important part of the comprehensive medical attendance of hemophiliacs. The necessary multidisciplinary team of specialists is available in a qualitative high-class rehabilitation hospital. Indispensable is the point that the coordinating medical specialist in Rehabilitation Medicine on site is skilled in the treatment of hemophiliacs. But he doesn't want and he can't replace the patient's hematologist. He is just the coordinator of the comprehensive team in the rehabilitation clinic.

I hope I have shown that rehabilitation is an important topic for most patients with hemophilia.

References

1. Neuntes Sozialgesetzbuch (SGB IX) – Rehabilitation und Teilhabe behinderter Menschen – vom 19.6.2001 (BGBl. I, S. 1046)
2. Kurth A, Kreuz W, Scharrer I: »Die orthopädische Behandlung von muskulo-skelettalen Komplikationen der Hämophilie«. Dtsch Arztebl 2002; 99: A 2928–2935 [Heft 44]
3. BAR: Wegweiser – Rehabilitation und Teilhabe behinderter Menschen, 11. Auflage, Frankfurt/Main 2001
4. BAR und Sozialpsychologisches Institut (Köln): Teamentwicklung in der Rehabilitation, Franfurt/Main Juni 2000
5. Buzzard B, Beeton K: »Physiotherapy, Management of Haemophilia«, Blackwell Science, Oxford 2000
6. Rizzo Battistella L: »Rehabilitation in Haemophilia – options in the developing world«, Haemophilia, 1998, 4, 486–490
7. Beeton K S: »Physiotherapie bei erwachsenen Patienten mit Hämophilie«. In Rodriguez-Merchan E C, Goddard N J u. Lee C A (Hrsg): Orthopädische Aspekte der Hämophilie, Stork Medien, Bruchsal 2002 (dt. Übersetzung)
8. Heijnen L, Sohail T: »Die Rehabilitation« in Orthopädische Aspekte der Rehabilitation, Stork Medien, Bruchsal 2002

Functional Analysis as a Basis for Optimizing Physiotherapy in Hemophilic Children

A. Seuser, U. Schulte-Overberg, T. Wallny, G. Schumpe,
H.-H. Brackmann, and B. Dregger

Background

A generation of hemophiliacs with no bleeding-related impairment of the loco-motor system has grown up in Germany over the past two decades. This happy circumstance is the result of preventive treatment of the underlying bleeding dis-order and immediate curative treatment of any bleeding on the basis of ready access to sufficient quantities of coagulation factor concentrates. With no restrictions on their freedom of movement, young hemophiliacs of this generation feel free to exer-cise activities which in the past would have been totally inconceivable.

Before approving these activities, we need to establish whether structural joint integrity correlates with physiological joint function. Initial studies have shown that functional defects were verified by three-dimensional measuring techniques in children with clinically and radiologically normal joints. Functional abnormalities, manifest in some cases as right-left differences in a single individual, may lead to structural defects later on if left untreated. Undetected subclinical bleeds may also eventually cause impairment of joint function.

Patients and Methods

Fifteen children aged 3 to 14 were analyzed consecutively. A wide range of parame-ters was investigated.

Age, factor activity, type of hematological disease, inhibitor, bleedings, previous therapy, orthopedic abnormalities, sporting activities and type of physical therapy were established.

Three-dimensional motion analysis of both knee joints was performed in situa-tions involving differing amounts of strain.

1. Treadmill tests,
2. knee bend tests and
3. overall coordination / proprioception testing using a Posturomed (one-footed testing), a device with a mobile platform which moves in two dimensions.

Relevant biomechanical parameters were analysis of the joint angle, angular velo-city and angular acceleration during locomotion and knee bend, and analysis of the roll and glide profile during a knee bend. Treadmill motion analysis was used to

I. Scharrer/W. Schramm (Ed.)
33rd Hemophilia Symposion Hamburg 2002
© Springer-Verlag Berlin Heidelberg 2004

investigate an everyday activity like walking as an expression of endurance. Treadmill use also involves a minor test of coordination.

Knee bending is a measure of strength which is a suitable basis for documenting the response of the knee joint to major muscle activity.

Curvature Analysis

Sinusoidal curvature is the basis for analysis of curvature in tests of motion. Deviations from sinusoidal curvature indicate functional disorders.

Range of motion of stance and swing phase during locomotion.

We are particularly alert to right-left differences and stance phase parameters. Lateral deviation in abduction and adduction is a criterion for analyzing gait from behind.

Similar criteria apply to knee bend testing. We pay close attention to curve repeatability/variation from knee bend to knee bend and from step to step in lateral and posterior views. Angular velocity and angular acceleration are used to detect the fine points of motion disorders, especially in the form of interim accelerations. The latter are indicative of muscle coordination defects which primarily occur during the transition from extension to flexion and vice versa.

Roll and glide patterns are assessed on the basis of motion repeatability and the steepness of the curve in the diagram from the bottom left to the top right. Roll peaks occur as a result of the continuous increase in roll and glide angle during knee bends.

An unchanging angle indicates an exclusively gliding motion. Decreasing roll and glide curves against the direction of motion are defined as a negative roll. Gliding on its own and negative roll increase the strain on the respective knee joint. Knee flexion and knee extension can be differentiated on the basis of roll and glide analysis in accordance with the respective degree of flexion and extension.

Results

Statistical analysis calls for a large patient population. Due to the fact that we have accrued only 15 test subjects to date, the present paper focuses on individual case reports and reconstruction of therapeutic strategy on the basis of the results of motion analysis.

Case 1

This case concerns a three-year-old boy weighing 12 kg and measuring 94 cm. He has a history of hemophilia A with residual factor activity under 1%. The boy is treated on demand. The most recent bleeding event was a bleed into the left knee joint in October 2000. He is highly active and is encouraged by his parents to keep this up. His main sporting activity is three hours of cycling per week. He had no orthopedic abnormalities and had never had physiotherapy.

An MRI scan was performed which disclosed the remnants of former bleeding events in the synovia of both knee joints, the right more than the left. No cysts or erosions were detected.

Biomechanical Evaluations

Knee a Angle on Treadmill from the Side (Fig. 1)

The figure on the top left is a lateral view of knee angle curvature of the right knee joint while the subject was walking on a treadmill. Analysis of loading/stance phase indicates a very slight loading phase (circle) in occasional gait cycles only. The knee is flexed during heel strike and movement of the knee is only minor in the loading phase. The loading phase can thus be described as variable but is still clearly distinguishable from the swing phase.

The swing phase describes a fairly constant 50° to 60° with no major variability. The knee angle curvature in its entirety can be said to describe a sinusoidal curve.

On the top right we see the knee angle curvature of the left knee joint. There is no detectable loading phase. The knee is flexed during heel strike and proceeds to the swing phase at almost the same angle, indicating that the knee joint is spared. The swing phase is significantly reduced versus the contralateral knee, measuring just 10° to 30°, and its execution is highly variable. Nevertheless, it still describes a sinusoidal curve.

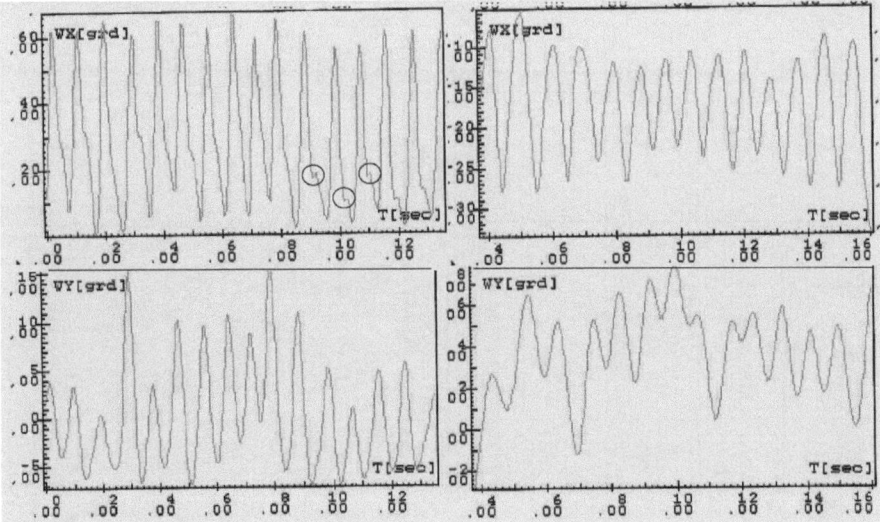

Fig. 1. Treadmill case 1: Knee angle from the side (top) and from behind (bottom), right (left side) and left knee (right side).

Analysis of the knee angle from behind during treadmill testing likewise discloses left-right differences (Fig. 1 bottom right and left).

The right knees (bottom left) lateral deflection in abduction/adduction is highly variable, ranging from 5° to 20°. A posterior view of knee angle curvature for the left knee (bottom right) reveals similar but lower variability, totaling 3° to 6°. This is primarily attributable to an overall reduction in flexibility/motion. Like that of the right knee, the curvature of the left knee is basically sinusoidal.

Analysis of the Knee Bend (Fig. 2)

Knee bends are associated with more strain. This exercise also revealed right-left differences. Analysis of extension-flexion motion (Fig. 2 top) discloses high levels of variation, ranging from 50° to 140° for the right knee (top left). A variable sinusoidal curve was also defined for the left knee (top right), but with significantly lower ranges of motion (30° to 45°).

A look at the acceleration curve during the same knee bend (figure) discloses a variable sinusoidal curve for the right knee (bottom left) with acceleration of +100 to –200°/sec^2 for extension/flexion. The child's third knee bend (140° right knee) displays several changes in the direction of acceleration and significant uncoordination.

The left knee (bottom right) also describes a variable sinusoidal curve and – despite smaller angle sizes – a higher acceleration rate of –150 to +230°/sec^2 in extension and flexion.

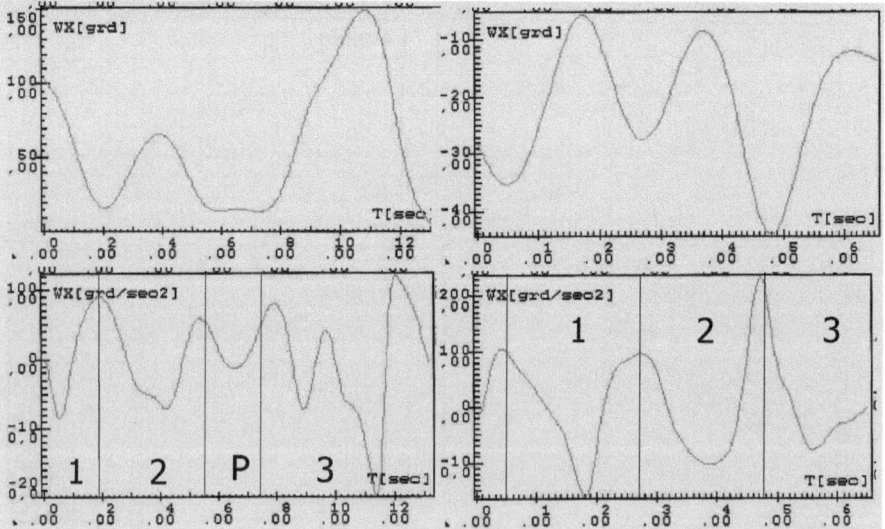

Fig. 2. Knee bend case 1: angle (top) and angular acceleration (bottom), right (left side) and left knee (right side).

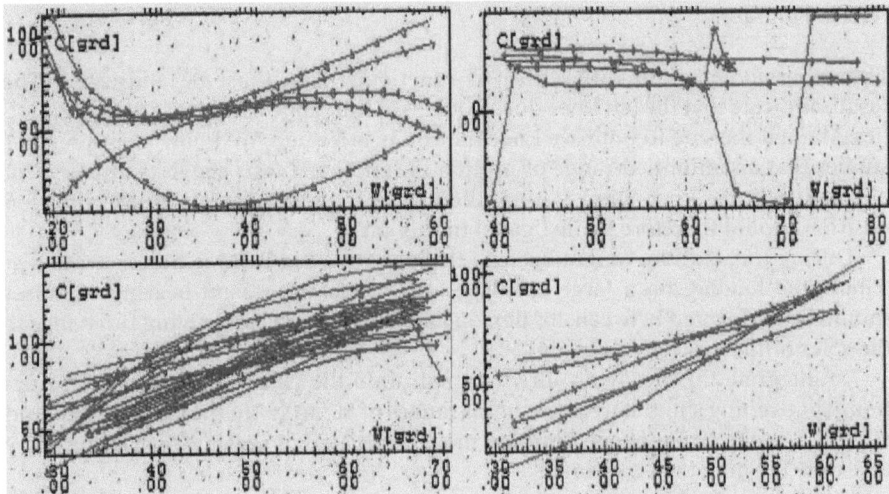

Fig. 3. Roll and glide curve during knee bend. Case 1 (top), case 2 (bottom), right (left side), left (right side).

Comparison of inner joint mechanics on the basis of roll and glide curvature reveals significant left-right differences in terms of the inner kinematics of the knee joints (Fig. 3). Although the right knee (top left) displays variability of curvature from test to test and differences in flexion and extension curves, its motion is more physiological than that of the other knee due to a well developed roll component at angles above 25°.

The left knee (top right) also displays great fluctuation in terms of curvature but without a corresponding roll component. The entire motion is glide-only.

In summary, the left knee is biomechanically inferior to the right knee. This is evident first and foremost in the short angles produced when walking on the treadmill. The left knee joint barely moves in the stance phase. This reduction in joint flexibility/motion is also apparent in knee bend testing and indicates that the left knee joint is being spared. Inner knee joint kinematics, as reflected in the roll and glide pattern, shows that the transfer of physical force between cartilage surfaces is highly variable. As might be expected in young knees, the degree of variability is very high.

A more mature roll component is present in the right knee. The glide component is predominant in the left knee.

An MRI correlate is not apparent in this case. The right knee joint contained more iron deposits than the left knee joint. This did not influence function as tested by kinematics studies. Another disparity is the fact that there is a confirmed history of bleeding into the left knee and none into the right knee.

Further Procedure

The apparent left-right differences in functional tests must be addressed. The results indicate that the left knee does not have a full range of motion in daily activities. Manual therapy to improve knee motion is indicated. We know from previous studies that an unlimited range of motion in functional tests suggests impairment of rotation in the knee joint. Manual therapy to improve rotation in every flexion position should therefore be instigated in this case.

During locomotion, weight bearing throughout a big ROM is necessary to distribute the loading on a large cartilage area, therefore, weight-bearing exercises should be performed between 20° flexion and 5° extension by applying resistance to the soles of the feet (closed chain).

To integrate this newly acquired strength into the gait and improve coordination, gait training should involve motion ranges of 10° to 15° in the stance phase and 40° to 60° in the swing phase. Training may be initiated in slow motion, followed by real-time training on a treadmill.

The child should receive combined strength and coordination training.

Case 2

The second patient is five years old, weighs 17.5 kg and measures 104 cm. He also has severe hemophilia A with residual activity under 1%. He had inhibitor activity (25 BU) when the studies were performed and is on continuous treatment. A number of bleedings in both upper ankle joints were documented in 2002. He is highly active and swims 2 hours a week. He receives average parental encouragement for this activity.

Orthopedic examination disclosed no abnormalities other than physiological bow legs. Physiotherapy had not been performed.

MRI Results

Like Patient 1, patient 2 had residues of old bleedings in the synovia of both knee joints, the right more than the left. No cysts, no erosions, normal cartilage.

Knee angle on treadmill from the side and behind (Fig. 4):

Biomechanical investigation disclosed an equal knee angle profile on both sides in lateral views (top). The knee is flexed during heel strike and no knee movement is detected. The loading phases are static. Sinusoidal curvature is apparent and the swing phase measures 50° to 60° with little variability.

Posterior views of knee angles during locomotion show variable sinus curvature displaying 5% to 15% fluctuation for the right knee (bottom left). Curvature of the left knee also fluctuates, but loss of sinusoidal curvature is more frequent. Variability of 5° to 10° is apparent (bottom right).

Let us look at the results of knee bend testing in extension/flexion (Fig. 5).

The right knee describes a variable sinus curve with flexions ranging from 60° to 80° (top left). The left knee (top right) describes a highly variable sinus curve with flexions ranging from 50° to 80°.

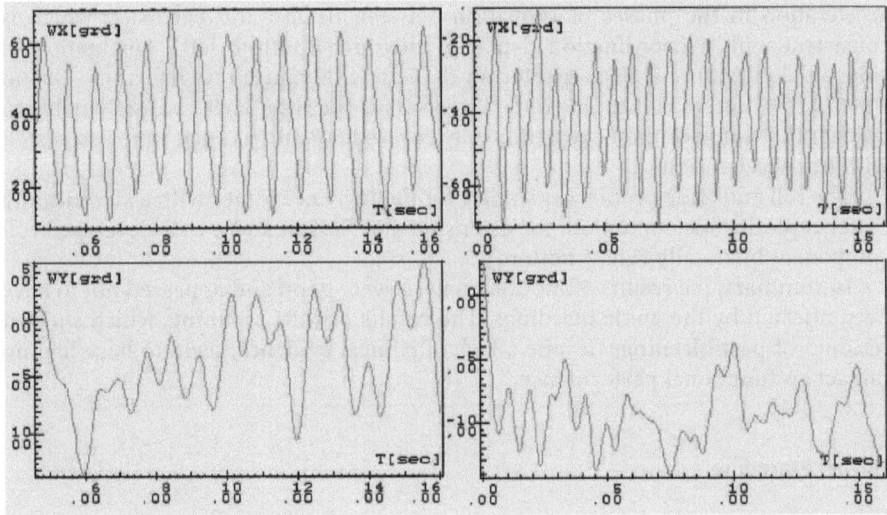

Fig. 4. Treadmill case 2: Knee angle from the side (top) and from behind (bottom), right (left side) and left knee (right side).

Acceleration Patterns During Knee Bends (Fig. 5 bottom)

There are minor right-left differences. On the right we have a variable sinusoidal curve with acceleration rates ranging from +1500 to −1400°/sec^2 and slight interim

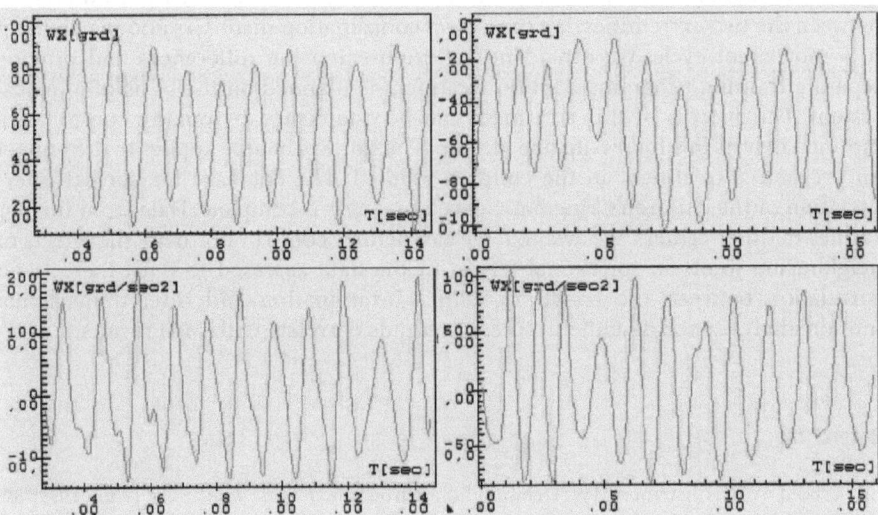

Fig. 5. Knee bend case 2: angle (top) and angular acceleration (bottom), right (left side) and left knee (right side).

acceleration in the phases of transition between flexion and extension which is consistent with a coordination deficit in this area (bottom left). Fluctuation of sinusoidal curvature is even greater on the left, with values ranging from -800 to $+900°/sec^2$ (bottom right). The differences versus the right knee are attributable to the fact that some of the knee bends only covered $50°$ and as such were associated with less acceleration.

The roll and glide profile was similar for the two knee joints, with a significantly better reproducible curve both for extension and flexion and a well-developed roll component bilaterally (Fig. 3 bottom).

In summary, the results of motion analysis were good and appeared not to have been affected by the ankle bleedings. The results of MRI scanning, which showed residues of past bleedings despite a lack of clinical evidence, seem to have had no impact on functional performance.

Further Procedure

Physiotherapy should be performed with an emphasis on coordination training, especially with regard to the turning points between flexion and extension. Slow to fast walking on a deep mat and knee bends on a trampoline would be examples of suitable training in plyometrics. On top there should be a focus and establishing more knee motion in stance phase. This training would be preventive in scope.

Summary and Conclusion

Much remains to be done. What we can do already is detect left-right differences between the two extremities. We can detect coordination disorders and match them to a movement cycle. We can identify flexion-extension differences and provide separate training programs. Motion treatment is planned on the basis of a logical system. The success of this treatment can be established by quality control with motion analysis in a follow-up one year on. The same principle applies to the impact on preventive treatment in the children studied. The database for correct interpretation of the children's kinematic development is incomplete. Data from further studies in other centers are awaited. We can neither confirm nor deny the effects of neighboring joints in functional terms. In the data assessed to date, there is no correlation between the results of clinical examination and three-dimensional motion analysis; nor do either of these methods correlate with MRI results.

References

1. Arnold WD, Hilgartner MW. Hemophilic arthropathy. *J Bone Joint Surg* [Am] 1977; 59: 287–305.
2. Cerny K, Perry J, Walker JM. Effect of an unrestricted knee-ankle-foot orthosis on the stance phase of gait in healthy persons. *Int. Orthopedics* 1990; 13 (10): 1121–1127

3. Cochran GVB. *A Primer of Orthopeadic Biomechanics.* New York, Churchill Livingstone, 1982; 268–293
4. Johnson RP, Babitt DP. Five stages of joint disintegration compared with range of motion in hemophilia. *Clin-Orthop* 1987; 201: 36–106
5. Kadaba MP, Ramakaishnan HK, Wootten Me, Gainey J, Gorton G, Cochran GVB. Repeatability of kinematic, kinetic and electromyographic data in normal adult gait. *J Orthop Res* 1989; 7: 849–860
6. Kapandji IA. *Funktionelle Anatomie der Gelenke: Untere Extremität.* Enke, Stuttgart 1985
7. Pettersson H, Ahlberg A, Nilsson IM. A radiographic classification of hemophilic osteoarthropathy. *Clin Orthop* 1980; 149–153
8. Perry J. *Gait Ananlysis, Normal and Pathological Function.* Thorofare, Slack, USA, 1992; 51–87.
9. Rodriguez-Merchan EC. Effects of hemophilia on articulations of children and adults. *Clin-Orthop* 1996; 328: 7–13
10. Schumpe G: Differenzierung der funktionellen Kniebewegung von hämophilen Patienten mittels Ultraschall-Topometrie. *Dissertation* Bonn, Rheinische Friedrich-Wilhelms-Universität Bonn 1982
11. Schumpe, G. Biomechanische Aspekte am Kniegelenk. *Habilitationsschrift,* Bonn Rheinische Friedrich-Wilhelms-Universität Bonn 1984
12. Seuser, A, Schumpe, G, Eickhoff, HH, Brackmann, H-H, Oldenburg, J. Analyse der Kniekinematik bei Patienten mit Hämarthopathie beim Leg Press Training, In: *24. Hämophilie-Symposium Hamburg.* Springer Verlag, Berlin, 1993; p: 150
13. Seuser A., Schumpe G., v. Deimling U.: Bewegungsanalyse zur Erkennung von Ermüdungserscheinungen und deren Auswirkungen auf die innere Kinematik des Kniegelenkes in: *Regulations- und Repairmechanismen.* 33. Deutscher Sportärztekongreß Paderborn; Hrsg.: Liesen H.et al. Deutscher Ärzte-Verlag Köln, 1993; 429–431
14. Seuser A., Schumpe G., Gäbel H. Quantifizierung von rehabilitativen Therapiemaßnahmen und Qualitätssicherung durch die Verlaufskontrolle mittels Ultraschalltopometrie. *Wien med. Wschr.* 1994;110: 15–18
15. Seuser A, Brackmann HH, Oldenburg J, Effenberger W. Orthopedic outcome of the knee and ankle joints of children and adolescents with severe Hemophilia A: A 12 year follow up. In : *3rd Musculosceletal Congress of the World Federation of Hemophilia,* Herzliya, Israel, 1995; (abstract)
16. Seuser, A, Klein, H, Wallny, T, Schumpe, G, Brackmann, H-H, Kalnins, W. Grundlagen des medizinischen Bewegungstrainings für Hämophile, In: *27. Hämophilie-Symposium Hamburg,* Springer Verlag, Berlin, 1996; p: 266
17. Seuser A, Oldenburg, J, Brackmann, HH . Pathogenese, Diagnose und orthopädische Therapie der hämophilen Gelenkarthropathie. In: *Hämostaseologie: Molekulare und zelluläre Mechanismen, Pathophysiologie und Klinik,* Springer-Verlag, 1999; p: 198
18. Seuser A, Wallny T, Schumpe G, Brackmann HH, Kramer C: Motion analysis in children with hemophilia in: The Haemophilic Joints; New perspectives, Edited by E.C. Rodriguez-Merchan, Blackwell Publishing LTD Oxford 2003, Seite 155–162
19. Spanagel M, Seuser A, Wallny T, Effenberger W, Brackmann HH, Schumpe G: Rotation des hämophilen Kniegelenkes, eine biomechanische Studie. Hämophilie-Symposium Hamburg 1996, Hrsg. I. Scharrer, W. Schramm, Springer-Verlag, Berlin-Heidelberg, Seite 272–279

Sport and Physical Fitness Recommendations for Young Hemophiliacs

A. Seuser, A. Kurme, T. Wallny, E. Trunz-Carlisi, S. Ochs, and H.-H. Brackmann

Introduction

Today's generation of hemophiliac children benefits from adequate substitution and radiologically and clinically healthy joints. With self-confidence on their side, it is natural for these young people to want to take up sports. This natural desire gives rise to a number of questions, such as:

What is the general level of fitness of young hemophiliacs today?

Can suitable sports help prevent musculoskeletal lesions in this patient population?

Further research is necessary before these questions can be answered. An interdisciplinary working group of hematologists, pediatricians, orthopedics and sports scientists was set up in an attempt to explore these issues.

It is difficult to identify suitable sports for individuals with joints that are susceptible to overstrain. In such cases, joint safety has the utmost priority in the search for an appropriate sporting activity.

Where safety is paramount, all the necessary facts need to be collected. Again in an attempt to maximize safety, residual factor VIII activity in excess of 15% was specified as a basic criterion for pursuing sports.

Patients and Methods

Actual joint status is another factor to be considered in the choice of a suitable sporting activity. For each type of sport singled out in advance, the nature of joint involvement qualifying it as suitable or unsuitable needs to be defined.

Example: Rowing

Rowing is conditionally suitable for a child with potential ankle involvement because of the small distance traveled by the joint during rowing and the almost physiological axial strain. However, for a child with knee joint involvement, rowing is unsuitable owing to the enormous strain on the knees (knee flexion in excess of 90°) with each stroke of the oars.

I. Scharrer/W. Schramm (Ed.)
33rd Hemophilia Symposion Hamburg 2002
© Springer-Verlag Berlin Heidelberg 2004

Another criterion for selecting a suitable sporting activity was the motoricity and athletic performance of the individual test subject, made up of factors such as endurance, strength, flexibility/motion and coordination. These elements are scored on a scale from 0 to 5. The personal motor skill profile thus established for an individual subject is checked against the minimum profile defined for each sport.

Each subject's personal motor skill performance profile is established on the basis of a fitness check (see below). Minimum motor skill requirements for each individual sport were defined on the basis of sports science and research data and medical literature.

In addition to the minimum requirements profile, each sport was matched up to a performance/promotion profile (specific aptitude for promoting the relevant motor skills). The minimum requirement profile defines the level of performance a person needs in order to exercise a particular sporting activity and minimize the risks involved. The performance/promotion profile describes the likelihood that the sport will promote or improve a motor skill.

Bleeding Risk

This was the most complex part of the sports medicine search. Various accident statistics of the German Sports Association were used to identify the main injury scenarios and their frequency and to differentiate sports in terms of the risk of bleeding involved. According to these statistics, football is the sport most likely to result in injury, with 0.9 injuries per 1000 hours of play, followed by basketball and handball.

Rollerblading ranks in the bottom third of sporting injury statistics, with 0.24 injuries per 1000 hours of activity. A more detailed breakdown shows that the risk of injury is greatest during the first three months, and that injuries are commonest among adolescents in the 12 to 14 age group. On this basis, it was possible to qualify the risk of injury for each sport, level of activity and age and recommend precautions.

A second criterion was the biomechanical strain associated with any sport. We had access to extensive data from the Institute of Motion Analysis. Sports associated with significant acceleration are associated with a higher risk of bleeding than sports associated with less strain on the joints. Examples are sports involving sudden deceleration, planting, cutting, and jumping, which impose major strain on the joints of the lower extremities. The opposite is true of rollerblading, biking and swimming, which are associated with much lower acceleration and, hence, less of a strain on the joints.

We also attempted to include the »beginner factor« in the assessment of bleeding risk. Some sports are associated with a higher risk for beginners, while other sports are equally low-risk for beginners, more advanced players, and competitive athletes.

We also tested the personal skills profile of the hemophilic children in our study population and, as such, are familiar with their individual resources. The choice of a recommended sporting activity therefore favored sports likely to offset any individual weak points in terms of the demands and strains imposed by the activity.

The bleeding risk for the individual sports was scored 0 to 5. Five indicates a sporting activity with a bleeding risk far in excess of that associated with everyday activities. Scores of up to 3 indicate a bleeding risk slightly above the everyday level. 0–2 indicates a fairly low risk.

Sports with a risk factor above 3 are unsuitable for reasons of safety.

5-Stage Fitness Check

One of the most important principles for recommending suitable sports is to establish the subject's level of personal fitness. This is determined on the basis of a 5-stage fitness test conducted in collaboration with the Institute for Prevention and Aftercare.

Motor skill checks are performed after taking a history including resting heart rate, type of illness, residual factor activity, current factor level, target joints and comorbidities. Assessment is done using a five-point score where 1 represents the poorest value and 5 the best in a reference cohort which is matched for age, gender, bodyweight and body height.

Balance Check (Proprioception)

Balance testing measures balance as a major component of coordination and basic motor skill which is of particular pertinence in hemophiliacs. Testing was performed using a Posturomed, a device which facilitates one-footed testing. The test subject stands with his dominant leg on a mobile platform. The system measures the horizontal oscillations thus generated (leg sway, wobble) for a period of 20 seconds. The data from this new system are differentiated according to age group, with the support of our own database with data from more than 1000 test subjects of all age groups, in agreement with data from the literature from one-footed testing conducted without technological support (Viru, Bös, Rutenfranz, Hollmann/Hettinger and others).

Flex Control (Flexibility/Motion Testing)

Flexibility/motion of the lower and upper extremities is measured in line with the method presented by Janda and Kendall. The flexibility/motion data are compared with literature sources, in particular with Hollmann/Hettinger's papers on mobility in children and adolescents. The data are grouped in accordance with age and gender. An electronic inclinometer which works like a spirit level and is accurate to less than one degree is used for determining flexibility/motion. We opted for measurement of ischiocrural (hamstring) muscles* and chest muscles. The lower

---

* The term »muscles« as used here includes all capsular ligament, muscle and joint structures.

extremity is the major problem area for young hemophiliacs. The upper extremity becomes clinically relevant at a later age following shortening of chest muscles.

Back Check (Trunk Muscle Test)

The back check monitoring device in use for many years in preventive medicine and rehabilitation was used to determine the maximum isometric strength of back and abdominal muscles. The readings were interpreted on the basis of the studies by Ochs and Bathe, in reference to publications by Hollmann/Hettinger. Age, gender and body weight are factored into the analysis as determining variables. In addition to abdominal and back muscle strength in absolute terms, their age-matched and gender-matched ratios are correlated with figures for the healthy basic population.

Fat Check (Analysis of Body Fat)

Fat check analysis is based on frontal infrared measurement on the upper side of the dominant upper arm flexor. This measuring site has been identified as bearing the greatest statistical correlation to hydrostatic weighing as a reference method. Evaluation is based on age-specific and sex-specific percentiles published in the American Journal for Clinical Nutrition.

Aerobic Check (Endurance Test)

IPN endurance testing is a heart rate-based method for determining aerobic performance. The test is based on more general standard endurance data (Rost, Hollmann) which have been broken down to account for age and gender. An indivi-

Table 1. Relative scores for hemophilic youngsters in a 5 stage fitness test versus an age-matched and weight-matched non-hemophilic population

Analysis	> Average	Average	< Average	Mean Score (1–5)
Coordination	19%	43%	38%	2.56
Overall mobility	6%	13%	81%	2.25
Mobility of upper extremities	75%	25%		
Mobility of lower extremities			100%	1.25
Overall trunk strength	6%	69%	25%	1.88
Extension trunk strength	13%	19%	68%	
Flexion trunk strength	19%	6%	75%	
Trunk strength ratio	13%		87%	
Endurance	19%	43%	38%	2.81
Body fat	6%	38%	56%	2.25

dual schedule is calculated on the basis of age, gender, frequency of training and resting heart rate. The schedule comprises two exercise levels each lasting 2 minutes. Comparison of the heart rates thus generated and the subject's exercise performance (watt/kg body weight) are used to draw up an assessment which in turn is used as a basis for individual, heart rate-adapted training recommendations.

Results

The results shown here are for a boy with hemophilia A and a factor VIII concentration in excess of 15% at the time of measuring. His individual test outcome was
• 1 for coordination,
• 2 for mobility,
• 2 for strength,
• 3 for endurance and
• 4 for body fat.

He had no target joints in the upper extremities but did have knee joint involvement in the lower extremity.

The Suitability of Individual Sports was Calculated as Follows:

• Swimming   98%
• Quigong   98%
• Boccia   98%
• Curling   96%
• Bowling   96%
• Skittles   96%
• Cycling   96%
• Sailing   96%
• Scuba diving   96%
• Marksmanship   94%
• Walking   91%

The Following Sports Were Rated »Conditionally Suitable«:

• canoeing,
• table-tennis,
• hill walking,
• golf,
• jogging,
• horseback riding,
• tobogganing and
• cross-country skiing.

The Following Activities Were Rated as Being »Unsuitable Sports«:

- dancing,
- karate,
- taekwon-do,
- wing chung,
- rowing,
- badminton,
- rollerblading,
- ice skating,
- basketball,
- tennis,
- track and field (jump disciplines),
- downhill skiing,
- windsurfing,
- volleyball,
- mountain climbing,
- surfing and
- springboard diving.

The patient said that tennis was the sport he wished to pursue. Tennis is associated with a bleeding risk slightly above everyday levels. In a subject with knee joint involvement, tennis would have qualified as »conditionally suitable« if the patient had met all the other minimum fitness criteria for this sporting discipline.
However, the boy achieved only one point instead of the minimum two points in coordination tests. Tennis was therefore rated »unsuitable« in this subject.

The patient was given tips for improving his coordination and trunk muscle strength. The following scenario was presented:
An increase in coordination by one point in a repeat test to the minimum level of 2 points would requalify tennis as a »conditionally suitable sport«. The range of suitable sports would extend to include
- mountain climbing   92%,
- walking   91%,
- golf   87%,
- horseback riding   77%,
- tobogganing   76%
- cross-country skiing   63%.

Tennis could never be classed as a suitable sport given the particular circumstances and knee joint involvement.

* Minimum criteria for tennis: strength 2, coordination 2, endurance 1, mobility 1

Results of Initial Patient Testing

16 children were studied, 9 with hemophilia A and 7 with hemophilia B. Age range 8 to 18, mean 12.25 years. Weight range 27 kg to 105 kg, mean 55.75 kg. Height range 137 cm to 185 cm, mean height 158 cm.

Analysis shows that young hemophiliacs in most cases perform less well than the healthy population (non-hemophilic adolescents). 56 percent generated below average results and not a single test subject produced above average results.

Analysis of individual tests discloses striking disparities: 19% of hemophilic children scored above average for coordination in their age group but 38% were well below average.

94% had below average scores in trunk strength tests. Only 6% were above average. This outcome mainly reflects an unfavorable extension-flexion ratio, which is supposed to be approx. 100 to 70 for boys and 100 to 60 (back to abdominal muscle) in girls (back check).

Mobility testing showed that 100% did not reach reference values for an age-matched healthy population as regards the lower extremities. 75% of hemophilic youngsters achieved levels above the norm for the upper extremities. Average fitness was poorer than in the reference population in 56% of cases.

Scores were poorest for lower extremity flexibility/motion, followed by trunk strength, body fat, and coordination. Endurance was the best developed criterion.

Conclusion

The desirability of establishing suitable sports and maximizing safety is obvious in day to day practice. The primacy of safety is surely self-evident when it comes to recommending suitable sports for children with a chronic illness. An important insight from the studies to date is that young hemophiliacs have healthy joints but are by no means physically fit.

The most striking deficits are short hamstrings and significant trunk muscle imbalance. Advice on suitable sports should be linked with preventive training. This training should on the one hand lay the groundwork for a suitable sport and on the other hand preserve healthy joints on a long-term basis.

References

1. Beaten K, Corneal J, Alter J. Muscle rehabilitation in hemophilia. Haemophilia 1998;4: 532–7
2. Buzzard BM. Proprioceptive training in hemophilia. Haemophilia 1998; 4: 528–31
3. Corbin Dr Ch B, Lindsey Dr R. Concepts of physical fitness 7th edition. Editor: WCB Wm C Brown Publishers 1990; p. 78–81
4. Falk B, Portal S, Tiktinsky R, Weinstein Y, Constantini N, Martinowitz U. Anaerobic power and muscle strength in young hemophilia patients. Med Sci Sports Exerc 2000; 32: 52–7
5. Greene WB, Strickler EM. A modified isokinetic strengthening program for patients with severe hemophilia. Dev Med Child Neurol 1983; 25: 189–96
6. Roosendaal G, Mauser-Bunschoten EP, De Kleijn P et al. Synovium in hemophilic arthropathy.Haemophilia 1998; 4: 502–5

7. Lagerstrom D, Trunz E, IPN – Ausdauertest. Gesundheitssport und Sporttherapie 13, Nr. 3 (1997): p. 68–71
8. Laskowski ER, Newcomer-Aney K, Smith J. Proprioception. Phys Med Rehabil Clin N Am 2000; 11: 323–40
9. Rodriguez-Merchan EC. The destructive capabilities of the synovium in the haemophilic joint. Haemophilia 1998; 4: 506–10
10. Roosendaal G, TeKoppele JM, Vianen ME, van den Berg HM, Lafeber FP, Bijlsma JW. Blood-Induced joint damage: a canine in vivo study. Arthritis Rheum 1999; 42: 1033–9
11. Ochs S, Froböse I, Trunz E, Lagerstrom D, Wicharz J. Einsatzmöglichkeiten und Perspektiven eines neuen Screeningsystems zur Objektivierung des Funktionszustandes der Rumpfmuskulatur (IPN-Back Check). Gesundheitssport und Sporttherapie 14 (1998): p. 144–150
12. Pietri MM, Frontera WR, Pratts IS, Suarez EL. Skeletal muscle function in patients with hemophilia A and unilateral hemarthrosis of the knee. Arch Phys Med Rehabil 1992; 73: 22–8
13. Seuser A, Hallbauer T, Schumpe G: 3D Gang- und Bewegungsanalyse des Kniegelenkes beim medizinischen Muskelaufbautraining, in Proceedings zum Europäischen Symposium über klinische Ganganalyse 1992 in Zürich, (Laboratorium für Biomechanik der ETH Zürich Hrsg.), Hans Beusch, Schlieren / Schweiz 1992, S. 192–195
14. Seuser, A, Schumpe, G, Eickhoff, HH, Brackmann, H-H, Oldenburg, J. Analyse der Kniekinematik bei Patienten mit Hämarthopathie beim Leg Press Training, In: 24. Hämophilie-Symposium Hamburg. Springer Verlag, Berlin, 1993; p: 150
15. Seuser A., Schumpe G., v. Deimling U.: Bewegungsanalyse zur Erkennung von Ermüdungserscheinungen und deren Auswirkungen auf die innere Kinematik des Kniegelenkes in: Regulations- und Repairmechanismen. 33. Deutscher Sportärztekongreß Paderborn; Hrsg.: Liesen H.e.a.; Deutscher Ärzte-Verlag Köln, 1993; 429–431
16. Seuser A, Brackmann HH, Florijn YCK, Oldenburg J, Sandow U: Bewegungstraining für Hämophilie, (Wissenschaftliches Institut der Ärzte Deutschlands (WIAD e.V.), Hrsg.), 1995, Rheinischer Landwirtschafts-Verlag, Bonn
17. Seuser, A, Klein, H, Wallny, T, Schumpe, G, Brackmann, H-H, Kalnins, W. Grundlagen des medizinischen Bewegungstrainings für Hämophile, In: 27. Hämophilie-Symposium Hamburg, Springer Verlag, Berlin, 1996; p: 266
18. Seuser A: Biomechanik der Wirbelsäule beim Fechter in Zusammenfassung der zweiten fechtspezifischen sportmedizinischen Weiterbildung für Ärzte, Trainer und Physiotherapeuten am 25./26.09.1999 in Dillingen/Saar, Vortrag Seite 33–38
19. Seuser A, Wallny T, Schumpe G, Brackmann HH, Ribbans WJ: Biomechanical Research in Haemophilia in: Musculoskeletal Aspects of Haemophilia, Edited By E. C: Rodriguez-Merchan, N. J. Goddard & C. a. Lee, Blackwell Science 2000, Seite 27–36
20. Seuser A, Wallny T, Schumpe G, Brackmann HH, Kramer C: Motion analysis in children with hemophilia in: The Haemophilic Joints; New perspectives, Edited by E.C. Rodriguez-Merchan, Blackwell Publishing LTD Oxford 2003, Seite 155–162
21. Stroh S. Methoden zur Erfassung der Körperzusammensetzung. Ernährungs-Umschau 42 (1995) Heft 3; p. 88–94

Pain Versus Clinical and Radiological Assessment in Hemophilic Arthropathies

T. WALLNY, L. LAHAYE, H.-H. BRACKMANN, A. SEUSER, and C. N. KRAFT

Introduction

There seems to be a general consensus in the literature that clinical and radiographic findings correctly depict the severity of hemophilic arthropathy [1–3]. Though joint pain is known to be the symptom that encumbers the hemophiliac most [4], this valuable indicator of the patients quality of life [5] usually attains little attention from the physician during routine clinical and radiographic follow-up. Only in recent years have studies focussed more on these important aspects [5–11].

With our study we would like to focus the physicians understanding of and awareness towards the importance of joint pain for the hemophiliac. A particular focus of our work lies in determining whether there is a statistically significant correlation between clinical and radiographic results in hemophilic arthropathy and the patients subjective joint-pain status. We hereby pursue the suggestion brought forward by Miners et al [8] to more closely scrutinize the relationship between hemophilic arthropathy and the patients quality of life by assessing possible correlations between objective parameters and patient self-evaluation.

Materials and Methods

Using a questionnaire [12], we interviewed 112 hemophiliacs in January 2000 concerning their subjective joint pain (visual analogous scale, VAS), social status and quality of life related to the year 1999. All patients had been in the regular hematological and orthopedic care (4 times per year) of the Hemophilia Care Unit at the Institute for Experimental Hematology and Transfusion Medicine, University of Bonn, for a minimum of 10 years, and all had at some stage at least one clinically painful joint. Prior to distribution by post, the non validated questionnaire was read and evaluated by 3 hemophiliacs to judge whether it was understandable and self-explanatory. The questionnaire was self-administered, yet all patients had the possibility of contacting a specialist by telephone. 79 of 112 patients (70.5%) returned the questionnaire and gave written consent as to the use of their data for research.

The age of the 79 hemophiliacs involved ranged from 18 to 63 years with an average of 42.0 years and a median of 43.5 years. 96.2% (76/79) suffered from hemophilia A (74 severe, 2 moderate), the rest were hemophilia B patients. 82.3% suffered from a chronic hepatitis C, and 49.4% from an HIV-infection.

I. Scharrer/W. Schramm (Ed.)
33rd Hemophilia Symposion Hamburg 2002
© Springer-Verlag Berlin Heidelberg 2004

At the time of questioning, 72 of 79 hemophiliacs (91.1%) substituted factor concentrate regularly, and not only in case of bleeding episodes. This was in general at least 3000 IU factor VIII/factor IX per week.

Clinical Score

All available clinical and radiographic data concerning the typically afflicted joints (ankle-, knee-, elbow-, hip- and shoulder joint) of these 79 patients from the year 1999 was collected. Any data, standing in connection with an acute bleeding episode or a trauma was not evaluated. The clinical assessment of the patients was performed by experienced physicians who know and have looked after this group for many years. Joint damage was quantified by a score-system which used the parts »clinical examination« and »pain« of the WFH (World Federation of Hemophilia) [13] score-system, incorporating criteria such as »swelling«, »muscular atrophy«, »frontal plane axial deviation«, »crepitation on movement«, »range of motion«, »flexion-contraction«, »joint instability« (0–12 points) and »pain« (0–3 points). The total sum of these criteria is defined as the *clinical joint-score* (range 0–15 points), whereby a joint with 0 points is clinically healthy and one with 15 points is clinically massively impaired. We then went on to define a *clinical patient-score*, which is the sum of the patients ankle-, knee- and elbow *joint-scores* and has a range from 0–90 points.

Radiographic Measurements

In 75.9% (60/79) of patients we were able to evaluate complete X-rays of the ankle-, knee-, and elbow joint from the year 1997-2000. In the remaining 19 hemophiliacs either X-rays of all clinically damaged joints were not complete (14 cases) or radiographs could no longer be evaluated for our study because of the implantation of artificial joints (5 cases). The severity of hemophilic arthropathy on the X-ray was determined utilizing the Pettersson-score [14]. The Pettersson-score incorporates the following 8 criteria: »osteoporosis«, »enlargement of epiphysis«, »irregularity of subchondral surface«, »narrowing of joint space«, »subchondral cyst formation«, »erosion at joint margins«, »incongruence between joint surfaces« and »deformity (angulation and/or displacement) of articulating bones«. The sum of these 8 criteria leads to the *radiographic joint-score* (range 0–13), whereby 0 points suggest no radiographically evident pathological finding and 13 points shows a massively damaged joint on the X-ray. The *radiographic patient-score* was defined as the sum of the radiographic joint scores of ankle-, knee and elbow joint (range 0–78 points). Clinical and radiological score were assessed by one doctor.

Questionnaire

Using a visual analogous scale (VAS) in the questionnaire (Fig. 1) [12] which ranges from 0–10 (0 being no pain and 10 the most severe pain the patient can imagine),

Please consult the following visual analogue scale (VAS), concerning your pain threshold, and then answer the following questions: (a 10 on the scale is the worst pain you can imagine, and a 0 is no pain at all)

0	1	2	3	4	5	6	7	8	9	10

no
pain

worst imaginable
pain

Localization	Major pain region?	Where else do you suffer from pain?	What is the quality of your pain? (a = stabbing, b= persistent, c= burning, d = sudden-onset, e= dull, f = bright)
Shoulder right			
Shoulder left			
Elbow right			
Elbow left			
Hip right			
Hip left			
Knee right			
Knee left			
Ankle right			
Ankle left			
Other joints			
Spine			

What is the most frequent reason for your joint pain?
O bleeding episodes   O chronic joint pain   O pain after rest
O pain during movement   O „wrong" movement   O climbing stairs   O other

Do you have pain throughout the day?
a) without medication: O yes   O no   O occasionally
b) after injection of factor: O yes   O no   O occasionally
c) after factor and use of other medication: O yes   O no   O occasionally

At what time of day are your pain-symptoms worst?
O   morning   O   midday   O   afternoon   O   evening   O   night

Did your pain symptoms alter your daily activities as well as your requirements over the past year?
O   no   O   occasionally   O   moderately   O   significantly

Were you in low spirits over the past year because of your pain-symptoms?
O no   O occasionally   O frequently   O constantly

Fig. 1a. Pain-questionnaire

Please estimate the pain level you find tolerable in daily life (circle the appropriate number):

0   1   2   3   4   5   6   7   8   9   10
no   worst imaginable
pain   pain

Were you able to alleviate your pain?
O no   O slightly   O markedly   O completely

Are you in constant need of medical treatment because of joint pain (apart from bleeding episodes)?
O yes   O no

Which treatment was performed to alleviate pain in joints?
(please use a 1 for regular and a 2 for occasional treatment)

Localization	Factor-concentrate	Pain killers	Cortisone	Ointments	Stabilizing bandages	Orthopedic shoes
Shoulder right						
Shoulder left						
Elbow right						
Elbow left						
Hip right						
Hip left						
Knee right						
Knee left						
Ankle right						
Ankle left						
Other joints						
Spine						

If you take pain killers, what drug do you use? Please name all medication below:

_____

_____

in which doses
O 1x daily   O 2x daily   O 3 x daily
O more frequently   O only when needed

Do the pain killers sufficiently alleviate your pain?
O yes   O no

Do you perform exercises / physical therapy to train muscles and joints (i.e. cycling, swimming, gymnastics)?
O daily   O 2-3 times per week   O once per week   O less than once per week

Were you ill from work more than two times in 1999 because of joint pain?
O yes   O no

Have you prematurely been retired because of your joint pain?
O yes   O no

Fig. 1b. Pain-questionnaire

patients were asked to evaluate the individual pain level of their ankle-, knee-, hip-, elbow and shoulder joints. We called this point-score (VAS) for each individual joint the *subjective joint-score*. The sum of the subjective joint-scores of the ankle-, knee- and elbow joints then gave us the *subjective patient-score* (range 0–60 points).

A section of the questionnaire, offering answers from which the patient could choose, aimed to determine the main reasons for pain, at what time of the day patients usually suffered the most intense pain, what was usually done to alleviate pain and the efficacy of pain-alleviating measures. Furthermore we were interested in the type of pain-killers taken as well as how the hemophiliacs subjectively judged their usefulness. We questioned patients as to the influence of pain on daily activities and to what degree they felt psychologically impaired because of pain. A further aspect we evaluated was whether the patients social status was subject to change because of the pain-status or skeletal deformities.

Statistics

The clinical review on the one hand and the radiographic evaluation on the other served as our objective parameters concerning assessment of the severity of hemophilic arthropathy. Data collected from the questionnaire delivered all subjective patient-derived factors in connection to pain status and quality of life. Statistical evaluation was performed on a PC using the »Statistical Package of the Social Sciences« (SPSS, Version 9.0). Possible correlations between the clinical score and subjective pain-score as well as between radiographic score and subjective pain-score were assessed by means of the Spearman´s-coefficient. Using the Mann-U-Whitney test we tested for significance between the clinical respectively the radiographic patient-score and different answers of the patients to our questions. The level of significance was set at $p \le 0.05$.

Results

Clinical, radiographic as well as subjective findings showed the ankle joint to be the most afflicted joint in the hemophiliac (= clinical respectively radiographic joint-score >0; VAS >0). The second most frequently damaged joint was the knee, followed by the elbow, hip and then the shoulder (Table 1).

Table 1. Number of affected joints

Joints	Subjectively		Clinically		Radiographically	
	right	left	right	left	right	left
Ankle	67% (53/79)	70% (55/79)	86% (68/79)	82% (65/79)	83% (50/60)	75% (55/79)
Knee	61% (48/79)	66% (52/79)	75% (59/79)	75% (59/79)	65% (39/60)	66% (52/79)
Elbow	44% (35/79)	41% (32/79)	62% (49/79)	61% (48/79)	53% (32/60)	50% (30/60)
Hip	9% (7/79)	8% (6/79)	14% (11/79)	14% (11/79)	12% (7/60)	12% (7/60)
Shoulder	9% (7/79)	11% (9/79)	10% (8/79)	10% (8/79)	5% (3/60)	5% (3/60)

Table 2. Average points of VAS, clinical and radiographic score

Joints	Subjective Score (VAS)		Clinical Score		Radiographic Score	
	right	left	right	left	right	left
Ankle	2.7	2.7	3.9	3.6	5.7	6.1
Knee	2.4	2.4	3.9	4.0	5.0	5.4
Elbow	1.5	1.3	3.2	2.9	3.8	3.7

The average point score of the subjective VAS as well as the clinical and the radio-graphic score is depicted in Table 2. The ankle was the most painful joint for our patients and also showed the most marked radiographic changes. The clinical damage was found to be similar to that of the knee. The largest discrepancy between objective and subjective assessment was found for the shoulder joint. Hip and shoulder joints were most seldomly involved in hemophilic arthropathy. They were also the joints with the least clinical and radiographic impairment and were subjectively associated with the least pain (average values in the clinical and radiographic joint-score as well as in the VAS <1).

Table 3. Spearman-correlation: VAS (subjective) vs. clinical and VAS vs. radiographic assessment

Joints	VAS vs. clinical score		VAS vs. radiographic score	
	right	left	right	left
Ankle	0.512	0.474	0.365	0.479
Knee	0.641	0.663	0.710	0.663
Elbow	0.460	0.411	0.426	0.483

On average our group had 4.4 clinically and 4.0 radiographically damaged joints. Averagely 3.5 joints were claimed to be manifestly painful. This value relates to the ankle-, knee- and elbow joint (min.: 0; max.: 6). The clearest correlation between subjective and objective results was found for the knee, then followed by the ankle. The elbow did not show any useful correlation in this respect. In Table 3 the Spearman's coefficients are shown regarding the target joints: a coefficient lower than 0.5 was considered to be too low to demonstrate a strong correlation.

Fig. 2 and 3 compare the joint-scores of the clinical and radiographic data as well as the score of the subjective pain status (VAS) for the right knee joint. The linear regression demonstrates the correlation: the more clinical impairment (Fig. 2) respective radiographic damage (Fig. 3) was found, the more the patient claimed to suffer from pain. Interestingly the intersection of the linear regression with the y-axis lies above 0 in the positive area. This indicates that patients only suffer from pain with a certain degree of clinical or radiographic damage to the joint (Fig. 2 and 3).

45.6% (36/79) of our patients claimed to have pain throughout the day if they did not take any pain killers. Despite the use of factor concentrate and analgesic

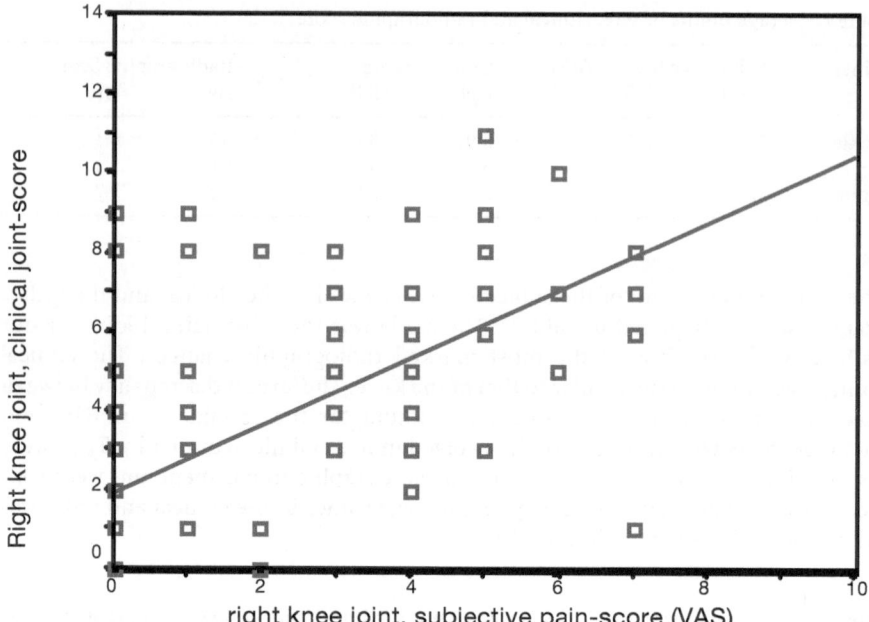

Fig. 2. VAS versus clinical score (WFH)

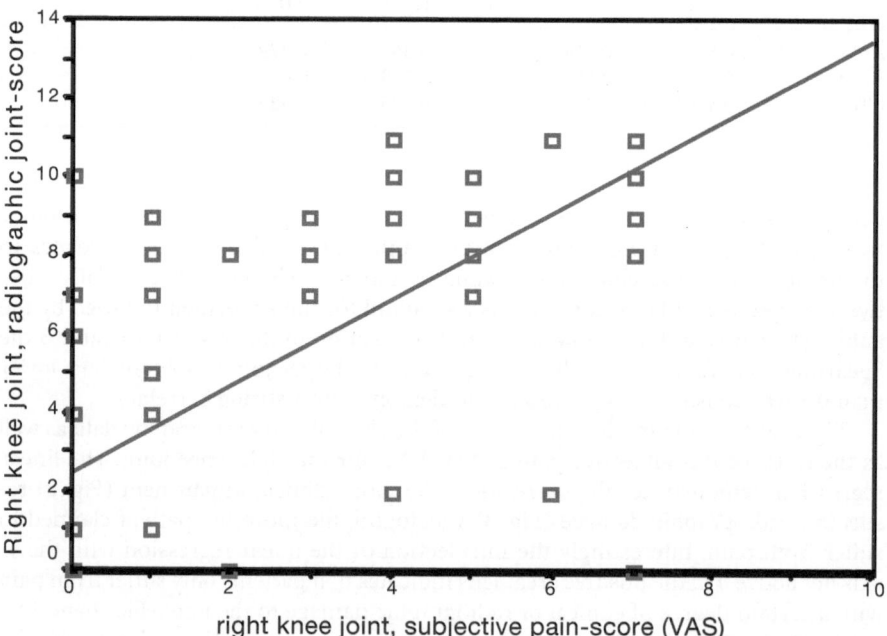

Fig. 3. VAS versus radiographic score (Pettersson)

drugs still 11.4% (9/79) of the hemophiliacs suffered pain throughout the day. The most severe pain was either in the morning (38/132 answers = 28.8%) or in the evening (47/132 answers = 35.6%). In declining frequency factor concentrate, non-steroidal anti-inflammatory drugs (NSAID) and modified orthopedic shoes were used to curb pain (157/227 answers = 69.2%).

Of the 48/79 patients using oral pain killers, 21/48 (43.8%) did this on a regular basis. The most popular analgesic drugs were the NSAID acemetacin and diclofenac.

Almost a third of all hemophiliacs (15/48 = 31.3%) claimed that the analgesic effect of oral pain killers was not sufficient, and 43/79 (54.4%) stated that they were frequently not able to curb pain at all. Concerning the patient-score the following became evident: The more damaged ankle-, knee- and elbow joint were found to be, the more difficult it was to achieve adequate pain-relief. The comparison of the medians of the patient-score and the radiographic score in those patients with poor pain-relief (median 24.0 patient-score and 35.0 radiographic-score) and those with sufficient pain-relief (median 18.0 patient-score and 27.5 radiographic-score) showed a marked divergence of these values. Yet these discrepancies were not found to be significant in the Mann-U-Whitney-test.

Half the patient group (40/79 = 50.6%) acknowledged to be significantly or even massively encumbered in activities of daily life because of constant or recurrent pain and disclosed that their quality of life was moderate due to frequently being in low spirits. A connection between the patients moods and his joint status (sum of the joint-scores of ankle-, knee- and elbow joint) was found. The higher the clinical- and radiographic-scores, the more the patient claimed to suffer from depressive spells and acute changes of mood as well as decrease of daily activities: patients with relatively low objective scores (median clinical-score 18.5 and median radiographic-score 25.0) alleged to predominantly be in good spirits, while those with clinically and radiographically more severely damaged joints (median clinical-score 24.0 and median radiographic-score 36.0) suffered markedly from depressive spells. According to the Mann-U-Whitney test, this discrepancy was found to be significant (p=0.031).

35.4% (28/79) of our hemophiliacs had been on sick-leave from work more than twice in 1999 or were prematurely retired because of their joint-pain. These patients showed a significantly higher clinical (p=0.001) and radiographic (p=0.003) joint-score (median clinical-score 30.5 and median radiographic-score 43.0) than those patients who regularly attended work (median clinical-score 17.0 and median radiographic-score 26.0). Patients who had prematurely retired from work were found to have all 6 joints damaged (clinical and radiographic median of 6.0 damaged joints), hereby on average having 2 more joints severely damaged than those patients who were still able to work (clinical and radiographic median of 4.0 damaged joints).

Discussion

Subjective Versus Objective Measurements

In general it should be mentioned that clinical score and questionnaire are not validated. The Pettersson-score is validated but this does not seem to have an influence on the clinical outcome: only clinical and radiological scores > 2 points are associated with pain. For the knee joint the correlation between subjective pain-score (VAS) and clinical evaluation respectively between subjective pain-score (VAS) and radiographic findings showed a clear association. Though not as pronounced, an association between clinical result and subjective pain-score (VAS) was also found for the right ankle. In these joints the treating physician can therefore deduce that with increased radiographic damage and clinical impairment the patient will in fact suffer increased joint pain. Why this relationship is particularly manifest for the right knee remains speculation.

Our results underline the findings of Erlemann and Wörtler [15] that the hemophiliac experiences his arthrotic joint as particularly painful, far more than he is troubled by a damaged ankle. This may be explained by the larger range of motion of the knee-joint as well as the fact that in the knee motion is primarily controlled by muscles and ligaments.

The ankle has the highest density of receptors of all human joints. Initial motion and load induction occur here. Minor false movements and increased stress are usually completely absorbed by the healthy ankle, with the effect that excess strain is taken from neighboring joints [16].

In parallel to our findings, Aznar et al. [5] as well as Erlemann et al. [17] found the ankle to radiographically be the most damaged joint in the hemophiliac. This is attributed to the increase of daily life and sport activities made possible by the massive progress in factor substitution-therapy [13]. The result is that injury-induced bleeding into the ankle joint occurs more frequently. While a less severe bleeding episode into the knee joint will usually cause significant pain and subsequent immobilization, this is often not the case with minor bleeding into the ankle-joint, where the patient may continue to weight-bear [15]. The ensuing minor inflammatory reactions which may subjectively go unnoticed are considered particularly damaging for the joint and may explain why the ankle is most frequently and most severely arthropathically afflicted [18]. With the ankle joint playing such a key role in estimating the severity of hemophilic arthropathy, it seems all the more important to point out that patients considered modified orthopedic shoe wear to play an important role in reducing pain. The effect of the shoe wear is chiefly on the ankle joint in that the foot and ankle is stabilized and strain and impact absorbed.

Parameter »Daily Activities« in Other Studies

Insofar as one can compare this study to others, Miners et al. [8] also found a high negative correlation between the parameter »physical functioning« and the intensity of »bodily pain« in hemophiliacs. Yet in the aforementioned study the value of this comparison is diminished due to the fact that the two criteria were evaluated solely by means of a patient-questionnaire, therefore representing only the subjectively flawed patient standpoint, therefore seems more feasible. Solovieva [11] mentions the association between the degree of invalidity and the pain-status measured by VAS: the more pronounced the invalidity is, the more intensive the pain is claimed to be. Solovieva asked patients to determine their level of invalidity on a 5-point-scale, with an increase of points suggesting an increased restriction of the hemophiliacs bodily activity. In a sense this level of invalidity reflects the clinical impairment of patients and in analogy to our results correlates positively with their pain-status.

There is a tendency that with increased clinical and radiographic patient-score an augmented restriction of the hemophiliacs quality of life can be found; an aspect that has been highlighted in numerous studies [5, 7–9, 11]. Every second patient questioned could not adequately curb joint-pain despite the use of factor concentrate, non-steroidal anti-inflammatory drugs (NSAID), modified orthopedic shoes, ointments, stabilizing bandages or cortisone, and almost one third of patients regularly taking oral analgesic drugs claimed that pain relief was not sufficient. This calls for more efficient methods to combat the pain of hemophilic arthropathy. Apart from the optimization of drug therapy, a further solution may be cognitive behavioral therapy. Some studies [19–21] have revealed the positive effect of this psychological approach to the management of arthritis pain. Whether this management option is practicable will have to be shown in larger surveys.

Conclusion

Particularly older hemophilic patients are chronic pain patients. Depending on the afflicted joint, the more pronounced the objectively assessed joint damage in patients with hemophilia is, the higher the subjectively claimed joint-pain and loss of quality of life can be expected. This statement is limited insofar as that in this study statistically significant correlations were only found for the knee- and ankle-joint.

Our results underline that the treatment of painful symptoms from arthropathies is frequently insufficient. Scores and questionnaires may help to adequately define the hemophiliacs pain-status, thereby offering a possibility of assessment and long-term observation.

References

1. Brown IS, Toolis F, Prescott RJ. Haemophilic arthropathy: A ten year radiological and clinical study. *Scott Med J* 1982; 27: 279–283
2. Greene WB, Wilson FC. The management of musculoskeletal problems in haemophilia. Part II. Pathophysiologic and roentgenographic changes in hemophilic arthropathy. *Instr Course Lect* 1983; 32: 217–223
3. Wood K, Omar A, Shaw MT. Haemophilic arthropathy. A combined radiological and clinical study. *Br J Radiol* 1969; 42: 498–505

4. Frommer EA, Ingram GIC. Pain in hemophilia. *Lancet* 1973; 1:931-932
5. Aznar JA, Magallon M, Querol F, Gorina E, Tusell JM. The orthopaedic status of severe haemophiliacs in Spain. *Haemophilia* 2000; 6: 170-176
6. Ahlberg A. Haemophilia in Sweden. *Acta Orthop Scand* 1965; Suppl. 77: 20-45
7. Dalyan M, Tuncer S, Kemahli S. Hemophilic arthropathy: evaluation of clinical and radiological characteristics and disability. *Turk J Pediatr* 2000; 42: 205-209
8. Miners AH, Sabin CA, Tolley KH, Jenkinson C, Kind P, Lee CA. Assessing health-related quality-of-life in individuals with haemophilia. *Haemophilia* 1999; 5: 378-385
9. Molho P, Rolland N, Lebrun T, Dirat G, Courpied JP, Croughs T, Duprat I, Sultan Y. Epidemiological survey of the orthopaedic status of severe haemophilia A and B patients in France. *Haemophilia* 2000; 6: 23-32
10. Schoenmakers MAGC, Gulmans VAM, Helders PJM, van den Berg HM. Motor performance and disability in Dutch children with haemophilia: A comparison with their healthy peers. *Haemophilia* 2001; 7: 293-298
11. Solovieva S. Clinical severity of disease, functional disability and health-related quality of life. Three-year follow-up study of 150 Finnish patients with coagulation disorders. *Haemophilia* 2001; 7: 53-63
12. Wallny, T, Hess, L, Seuser, A, Zander, D, Brackmann, HH, Kraft, CN. Pain status of patients with severe haemophilic arthropathy. *Haemophilia* 2001; 7: 453-458
13. Pettersson H, Gilbert MS. Hemophilic Arthropathy. In: Pettersson H, Gilbert MS, (eds.). *Diagnostic Imaging in Hemophilia.* Musculoskeletal and other hemorrhagic complications. Berlin-Heidelberg-New York-Tokyo: Springer, 1985: 23-68
14. Pettersson H, Ahlberg A, Nilsson IM. A radiologic classification of hemophilic arthropathy. *Clin Orthop* 1980; 149: 153-159
15. Erlemann R, Wörtler K. Bildgebende Diagnostik der hämophilen Osteoarthropathie. *Orthopäde* 1999; 28: 329-340
16. Seuser A, Wallny T, Klein H, Ribbans WJ, Schumpe G, Brackmann HH (1997) Gait analysis of the hemophilic ankle with silicon heel cushion. *Clin Orthop* 343; 74-80
17. Erlemann R, Pollmann H, Reiser M, Almeida P, Peters PE. Staging of hemophilic osteoarthropathy using the Pettersson score. A study of 40 children and adolescents. *ROFO Fortschr Geb Rontgenstr Nuklearmed* 1987; 147: 521-526
18. Houghton GR, Duthie RB. Orthopedic problems in hemophilia. *Clin Orthop* 1979; 138: 197-202
19. Bradley LA, Young LD, Anderson KO, McDaniel LK, Turner RA, Agudelo CA. Psychological approaches to the management of arthritis pain. *Soc Sci Med* 1984; 19: 1353-1360
20. Varni JW. Self-regulation techniques in the management of chronic arthritic pain in hemophilia. *Behav Ther* 1981; 12: 185-194
21. Varni JW, Gilbert A. Self-regulation of chronic arthritic pain and long-term analgesic dependence in a haemophiliac. *Rheumatol Rehabil* 1982; 21: 171-174

IV. Laboratory Diagnostics

Chairmen:

M. Spannagl (Munich)
U. Budde (Hamburg)

Endogenous Thrombin Potential in Platelet-Rich Plasma – New Insights Regarding the Different Action of FVIII and FIX

A. Siegemund, T. Siegemund, U. Scholz, S. Petros, and L. Engelmann

Background

The cascade model of coagulation [1] has been used for the last 38 years to describe the coagulation process. In the new cell-based model of blood coagulation [2] activated platelets play an important role, because the surface of activated platelets provides the platform for the assembly of the tenase and prothrombinase complexes catalyzing the generation of activated factor Xa and IIa. In this model patients with hemophilia A or B have a markedly decreased ability to generate F Xa on the platelet surface followed by an insufficient thrombin generation. To describe the process of insufficient thrombin generation we measured the thrombin generation in platelet-rich plasma in patients with severe and moderate forms of hemophilia A and B. The aim of our investigations was to describe especially the role of platelets in the thrombin generation process.

Materials and Methods

ETP was measured as described by Hemkers [3] and Wielders et al. [4] with some modifications in substrate and activator concentrations.

Fresh drawn citrate blood was centrifuged for 10 minutes at 170 g. Platelet count was adjusted at a predefined level by dilution with autologous Platelet Poor Plasma (PPP) that was prepared by double centrifugation of Platelet Rich Plasma (PRP) at 2860 g each time for 20 minutes. Fluorescence intensity was detected using the Fluoroscan Ascent 2.2 (Labsystems Helsinki, Finland) at wavelengths of 340 nm (excitation wave length) and 440 nm (emission wave length). As fluorogenic substrate we used Z-Gly-Gly-Arg-AMC (Bachem, Heidelberg, Germany) at a concentration of 0.24 mM. 100 µl of PRP were mixed with 25 µl of substrate at predefined platelet count. The fluorescence intensity was measured over 120 minutes. ETP was given as arbitrary units of fluorescent activity (FU).

Plasma coagulation factor activities were measured by one-stage clotting assay using Pathromtin SL and the corresponding deficiency plasma at the BCS (all Dade Behring Marburg GmbH, Germany).

I. Scharrer/W. Schramm (Ed.)
33rd Hemophilia Symposium Hamburg 2002
© Springer-Verlag Berlin Heidelberg 2004

Patients

Patients with severe and moderate hemophilia A and B visiting the Hemophilia Center of the University of Leipzig were investigated. The control group are healthy blood donors and patients with history of thrombosis and elevated levels of coagulation factors VIII and IX to describe the overall concentration range for this coagulation factors.

Mathematical Computation

In plasma, free thrombin builds a complex with α_2-macroglobulin (α_2M) that has no known biological activity. The free thrombin curve is obtained by a mathematical processing of the signal (29, 30). In order to subtract the hemostatically inactive α_2M-thrombin complex the following recursive equation was applied:

$$f_n(t) = f_0(t) - k_n \int_0^t f_{n-1}(s)ds$$

where, $f_n(t)$ is ETP (n^{th} recursion step), $f_0(t)$ is the data curve, and k_n is the binding rate of free thrombin to α_2M.

$$k_n = \frac{f_0'(t_{max})}{f_{n-1}(t_{max})}$$

ETP is then $f_n(t_{max})$.

In addition to ETP measurements, the maximal reaction velocity (Vmax), the lag phase and the end of reaction were also analyzed.

Results

The thrombin generation is a function of several parameters. The most important parameters are the number of platelets, the number and functionality of receptors on platelets and the components of the coagulation system. In this work we investigate especially the relation between the number of platelets and the activity of the coagulation factors VIII and IX. The ETP is a function of platelets (Fig. 1) and a function of coagulation factors (Fig. 2).

The interactions between thrombin generation, platelet count, F VIII or F IX is more complex, because both, the platelet count and the activity of F VIII/F IX determine the thrombin generation and the related parameters like time to peak or start/end of the reaction (Fig. 3). With a model calculation we subdivided the ETP in two parts. One part is the ETP as function of platelet count at constant F VIII (F IX) or ETP as function of F VIII (F IX) at constant platelet count (Fig. 4).

Our investigations show that the influence of platelets on ETP is different in patients with hemophilia A and B. Platelets increase the ETP in hemophilia B patients

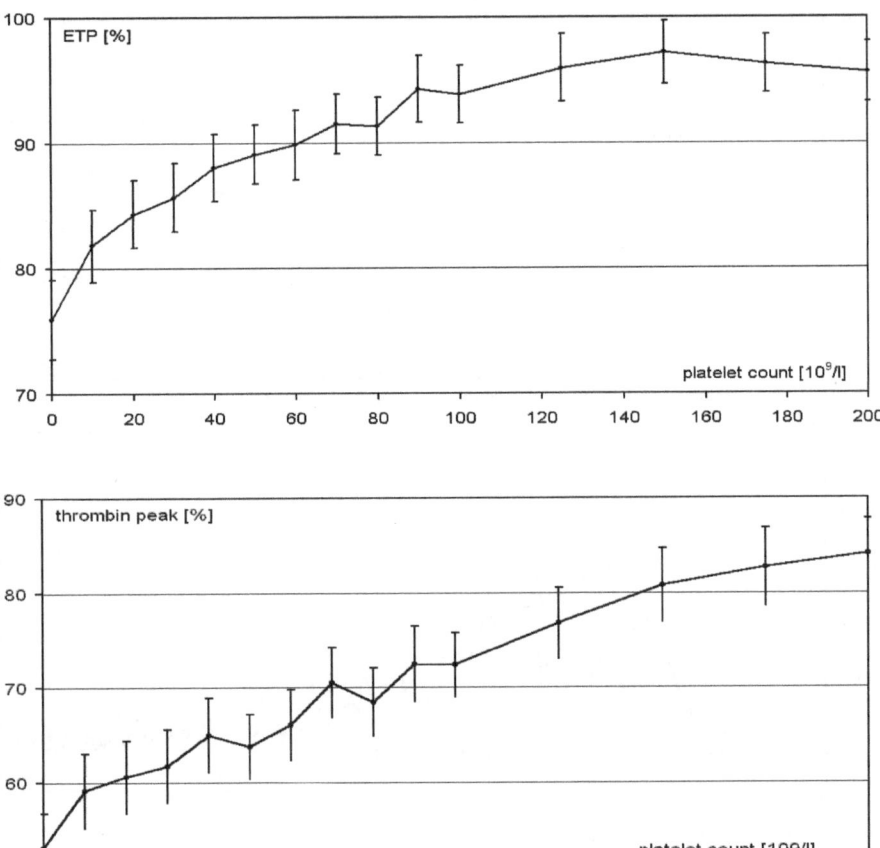

Fig. 1a, b. ETP (1a) and thrombin peak (1b) as function of platelet count

more than in hemophilia A patients. On the other side a theoretical calculation of the relation between ETP, platelets and F VIII/F IX give a higher ETP value at low platelet count in hemophilia A patients. With increasing platelet counts the influence of platelets on the ETP increases stronger in hemophilia B than in hemophilia A (Fig. 4). To describe the overall concentration ranges of F VIII and F IX and platelets and ETP we include patients with thrombophilia in our investigations. In the normal range between 70 and 130% the influence of platelets and coagulation factors (F VIII and F IX) is equal. At high concentrations of coagulation factors the influence of platelets is higher in case of elevated F VIII comparable to elevated F IX (Table 1).

In order to demonstrate the share of platelets to thrombin generation the following experiment was done: PRP from a hemophilia B patient (F IX< 2%) was mixed with platelets from a healthy volunteer at predefined platelet counts. To

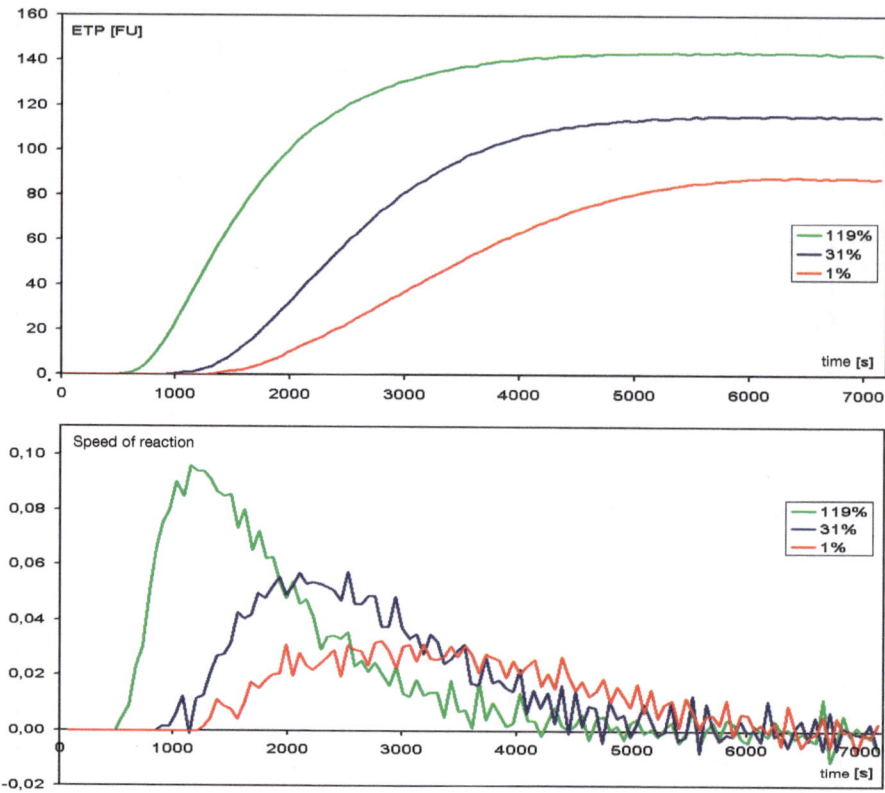

Fig. 2a, b. (ETP (2a) and v_{max} (2b) as function of FIX

Table 1. Influence of coagulation factors and platelets on the ETP – Comparison of FVIII and FIX

	0 – 35%	35 – 60%	60 – 140%	> 140%
Endogenous thrombin potentional	VIII > IX	VIII > IX	VIII = IX	VIII ≥ IX
Dependence on platelets	VIII << IX	VIII < IX	VIII = IX	VIII > IX
Thrombin peak	VIII > IX	VIII ≥ IX	VIII = IX	VIII < IX
Dependence on platelets	VIII < IX	VIII = IX	VIII = IX	VIII > IX

eliminate the influence of FIX, PPP from patient and volunteer was mixed in the same way. The area between both dotted curves reflects the contribution of platelets to thrombin generation. This effect can only be shown in patients with severe hemo-

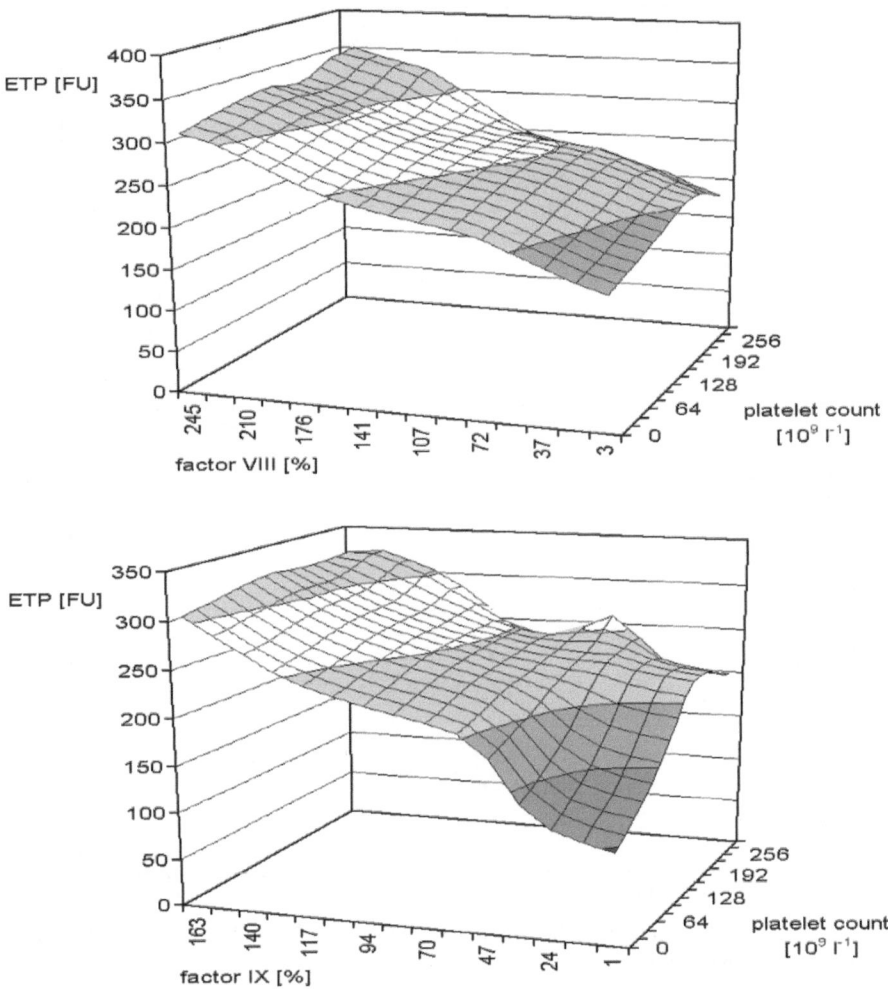

Fig 3a, b. Thrombin generation in dependence of F VIII (3a) and F IX (3b) and platelet count

philia B. After substitution with F IX concentrate the effect of platelets from healthy volunteers on thrombin generation is negliable because of normal thrombin generation followed by the factor substitution (Fig. 5).

Discussion

Measurement of thrombin generation is gaining an increasing importance in the field of hemostaseology. The ETP demonstrates the overall potential of the hemostatic system and represents the interactions between coagulation factors and platelets. The

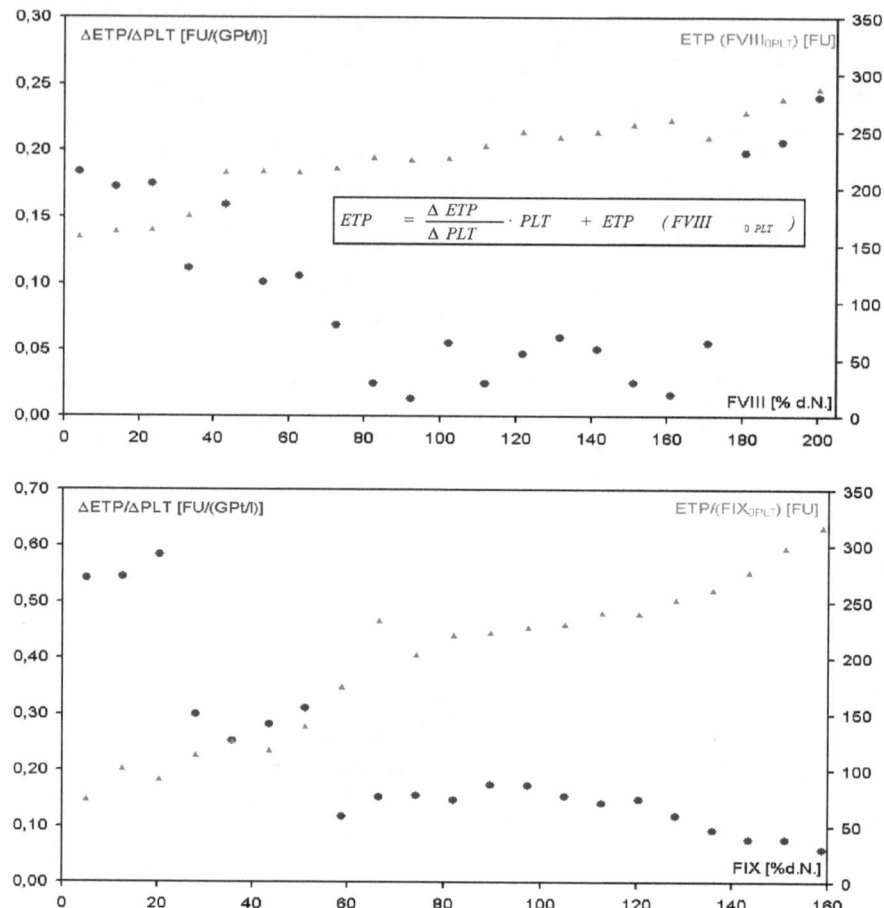

Fig. 4a, b. Thrombin generation in dependence of FVIII (4a) and FIX (4b) and platelet count – model calculation

results confirm that the major defect in hemophilia A and B is the decreased ability to generate enough thrombin. The reduced thrombin generation is more obvious in hemophilia B than A.

Summarizing our data show a high FVIII-related thrombin generation in hemophilia A and a high platelet-related thrombin generation in hemophilia B. On the other side, in case of elevated FVII we obtain a high platelet-related thrombin generation with a moderate FVIII related thrombin generation. In cases of elevated FIX levels platelets play a minor role. In contrast to FVIII the elevation of FIX directly contributes to the thrombin generation.

Our data emphasize the cell based model of thrombin generation. But the effect of platelets on thrombin generation at low concentrations of the enzyme FIX and a normal concentration of the cofactor VIII seems to be stronger than that of low concentration of the cofactor VIII at a normal concentration of the enzyme FIX.

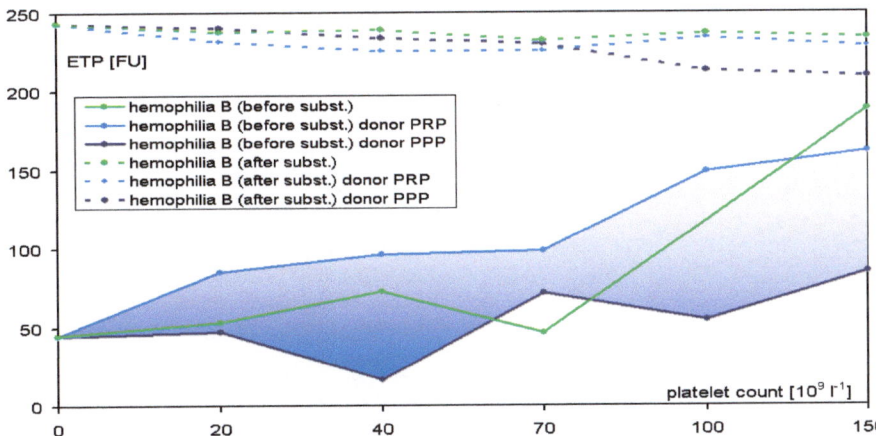

Fig. 5. Influence of F IX-substitution on the platelet-dependent ETP

Measuring thrombin generation in platelet rich plasma is a good method to describe such interaction between coagulation factors and platelets. Platelets are involved in the thrombin generation process and should be enrolled in discussion of bleeding episodes also in patients with hemophilia.

At this time the method is not suitable in routine laboratory practice. Platelet rich plasma is not easy to prepare because of the short stability. But with the flurogenic measurement method we have a very sensitive method to describe the interactions between cellular and humoral components. Further investigations are necessary to recognize the effect of fluorescence quenching by the blood components or drugs.

References

1. Dawie EW, Ratnoff OD. Waterfalkl sequence for intrinsic blood clotting. Science 145: 1310–12, 1964
2. Hoffman M, Monroe DM: A cell based model of hemostasis. Thromb Haemost 85: 958–65, 2001
3. Hemker HC, Béguin S: Thrombin generation in plasma: its assessment via the endogenous thrombin potential. Thromb Haemost 74: 134–38, 1995
4. Wielders S, Mukherjee M, Michiels M, Rijkers DTS, Cambus JP, Knebel RWC, Kakkar V, Hemker HC: The routine determination of the endogenous thrombin potential, first results in different forms of hyper- and hypocoagulability. Thromb Haemost 77: 629–36, 1997

References

V. *Pediatric Hemostaseology*

Chairmen:

A. H. SUTOR (Freiburg)
G. AUERSWALD (Hamburg)

Interactive and Case-Based Training of Diagnostic Skills and Therapeutical Management of Coagulation Disorders with CAMPUS, a Computer-Based Program

K. Selke, H. Gaspar, B. Zieger, A. Sutor, R. Klar, F. J. Leven, U. Budde, L. B. Zimmerhackl, M. Brandis and the consortium of casereport [1]

Introduction

Up to now medical education mainly involves the teaching of theoretical knowledge about diseases. However, new teaching strategies as the problem- and case-based learning are becoming more and more important in the modern curriculum in medical school. The computer program CAMPUS was designed to present the student a more practical training using virtual scenarios. Aim of this new learning approach is to give students a better possibility to apply their knowledge and to correctly diagnose the patient's disease.

New technologies like multimedia, the World Wide Web and computer-based training systems provide advantages and new possibilities for establishing these up-to-date learning strategies. In this context case-based training systems are an important supplement to traditional medical education. Therefore, the MediCase working group [2] in the laboratory for Computer-Based Training in Medicine of the University of Heidelberg/Heilbronn (Prof. F.J. Leven et al.) developed CAMPUS, an interactive, computer- and case-based multimedial learning system.

CAMPUS – an Interactive, Computer- and Case-Based Program

With CAMPUS, authentic medical cases can be used for medical training in an interactive and almost realistic way. All cases have the same structure: First the student has to take the patient's history, then to examine the patient »physically«. After these steps he has to determine differential diagnoses. To confirm the correct diagnosis the student can use one or several diagnostic loops in the program for further investigations. These loops include lab work, ultrasound, x-ray etc. After the student has identified the correct diagnosis he has to initiate the adequate therapy. At the end, the program provides the student an overview of the medical case including information about the prognosis of the patient.

At all these steps the users can get help via expert comments or context-sensitive systematic knowledge which is available in addition to the case data on demand. Questions can be defined by the author to enhance active knowledge processing and

Supported by CASEPORT, a project of the Bundesministerium für Bildung und Forschung (BMBF), Förderkennzeichen 08NM111A

I. Scharrer/W. Schramm (Ed.)
33rd Hemophilia Symposion Hamburg 2002
© Springer-Verlag Berlin Heidelberg 2004

interactivity. By using different multimedia components like text, picture, sound or animation complex medical interactions can be better understood.

Demonstration of a CAMPUS-Case: Presenting a Patient with a Coagulation Disorder

We designed an interactive case report to introduce the student to an efficient diagnostic and therapeutic proceeding in a medical case with a patient who presents with a coagulation disorder. Further aims of this interactive case-report include teaching the student about the pathophysiology of the coagulation system. A variety of laboratory tests in hemostaseology and the differential diagnoses in a case with bleeding symptoms are explained. Furthermore, therapy and complications of hemophilia are described.

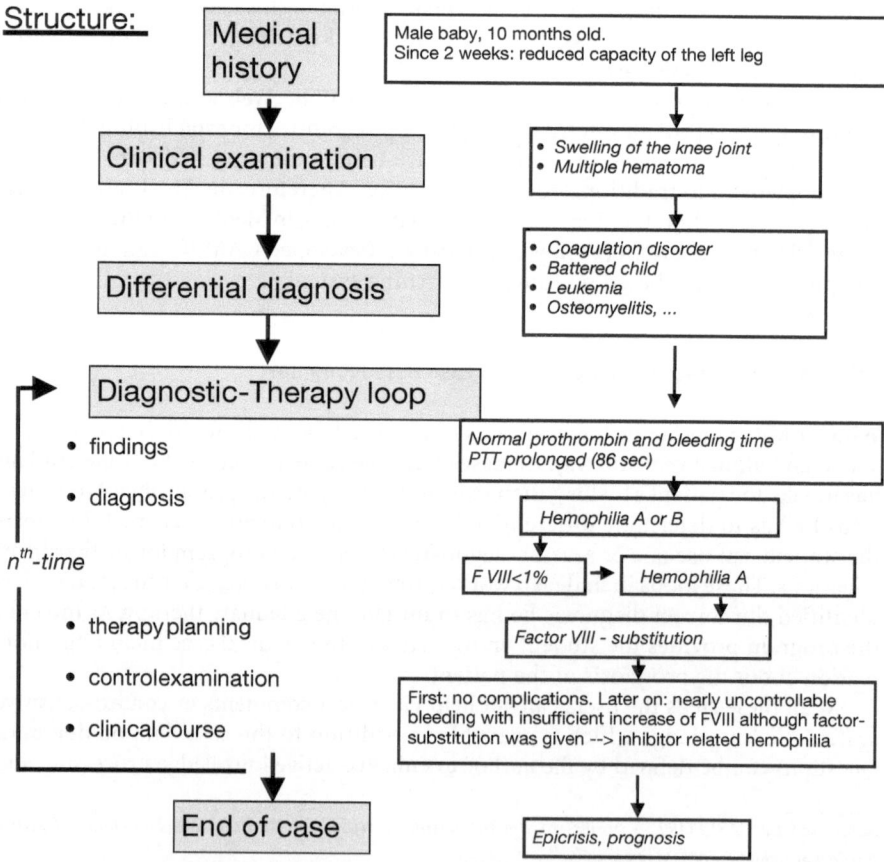

Fig. 1. Schema of the general and specific case handling in CAMPUS

We present a 10-months old male baby who has favored his right leg for the past two weeks. The physical examination shows a significant swelling of the left knee and multiple hematomas on both legs, arms and on the back.

Based on this information, the student has to determine differential diagnoses such as e.g. coagulation disorder, battered child, leukemia or osteomyelitis. These differential diagnoses should be excluded or confirmed step by step by a systematic, diagnostic approach: After a detailed tracking of the medical history, the student should first initiate the routine coagulation test. Then, depending on the appropriate results, the student must initiate the extended and more specific diagnostic coagulation tests. In our case prothrombin time and bleeding time was normal, however the partial thromboplastin time was prolonged (86 sec).

These results are characteristic of a disorder in the intrinsic coagulation system (e.g. factor VIII or factor IX deficiency). The following analysis of the factor VIII-activity showed a factor VIII-activity below 1%. This result confirms the diagnosis of hemophilia A. Now the student has to determine the adequate therapy. In the following the program shows that the patient was successfully treated with a factor VIII-concentrate. However, two months later the boy suddenly develops a mucosal bleeding which does not stop although FVIII-concentrate has been applied first at

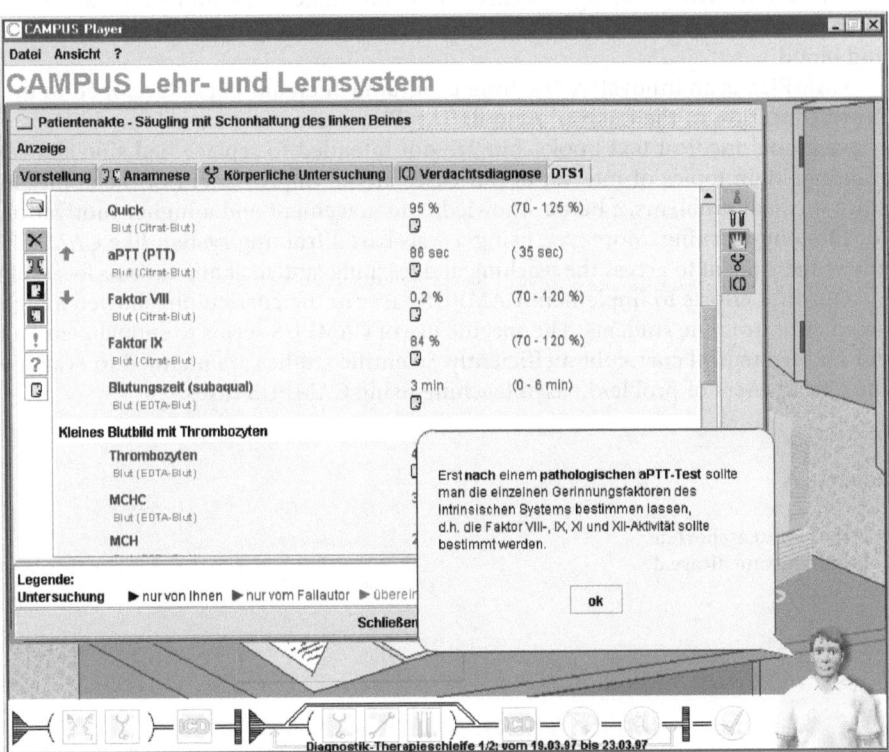

Fig. 2. screenshot of the labor results within the first diagnostic-therapy loop

prophylactic and then at therapeutic levels. The student is asked for an explanation of this phenomenon. The student now has to suggest a screening for a FVIII-inhibitor. The test for a FVIII-inhibitor is positive. These new circumstances require a new therapy strategy (e.g. an immune tolerance therapy with high-dose FVIII-concentrate). The program shows that after several months of immune tolerance therapy no FVIII-inhibitor is measured anymore and the FVIII-recovery is back to normal.

At the end, the program provides the student an overview of the medical case including information about the prognosis of the patient.

Summary and Outlook

This CAMPUS-case involves students in a virtual situation in which they are faced with handling a patient with a coagulation disorder. The interactive design of this CAMPUS-case avoids passive learning, but supports the active learning process. To intensify the student's knowledge links to further related information are implemented in this case report. Questions concerning this medical case additionally enhance the student's knowledge. By using different multimedia components like text, picture, sound or animation, these complex medical interactions should be better understood. After solving this case report the student should be able to handle a coagulation disorder in a logical manner thereby saving unnecessary costs, tests and blood.

CAMPUS is an innovative teaching program which has been developed to improve education in the medical school. CAMPUS cases can be used in addition to conventional medical text books, but are not intended to replace bed side clinical training. Main topics of interest of our cases are an improvement of the ability to solve medical problems, a better knowledge-management and a higher motivation for life-long-learning. Moreover, using a web-based training system like CAMPUS allows the student to access the teaching and learning system at any time or location.

Our first efforts to implement CAMPUS cases in the curriculum showed a high acceptance from the students. The specific use of CAMPUS seems to supplement and enrich the medical curriculum efficiently. Scientific studies are planned to evaluate the effectiveness of problem based teaching using CAMPUS cases.

References

1. http://www.caseport.de
2. http://www.medicase.de

Elevated Fibrinogen is a Risk Factor for Arterial Thrombosis in Children

C. WERMES, K.-W. SYKORA, A. CZWALINNA, K. WELTE, A. GANSER, and M. VON DEPKA PRONDZINSKI

Background

Several authors reported about the role of an elevated fibrinogen level as a risk factor for arterial and venous thromboembolism in adults [1–5]. In children elevated fibrinogen levels also are discussed to be a risk factor for thrombus development, but no special pediatric studies exist, which confirm this hypothesis [6].

Patients and methods

We investigated fibrinogen levels in children with arterial and venous thrombosis and two groups of healthy children which served as controls. Inclusion criteria and exclusion criteria are presented in Table 1.

Table 1. Inclusion and exclusion criteria

Inclusion criteria	
Patients	Controls
• Documented thrombosis ≥8 weeks ago	• No thromboembolism in the own history (and in the family)
• Age ≤18 years	• Age ≤18 years
• No infection at the time of investigation	• No infection at the time of investigation
Exclusion criteria	
Patients	Controls
• Thrombosis < 8 weeks ago	• Defects of hemostasis (von-Willebrand disease, hemophilia, M. Glanzmann, and others)
• Chemotherapy	
• Infections	• Dysfibrinogenemia in the family
• Dysfibrinogenemia	• Infections
	• Other diseases

I. Scharrer/W. Schramm (Ed.)
33rd Hemophilia Symposion Hamburg 2002
© Springer-Verlag Berlin Heidelberg 2004

Patients

Forty-four children with thromboembolism (TE) were included in the study. Twenty of them developed a deep vein thrombosis (DVT), 6 of them were catheter related. Four patients suffered from a thrombosis of the portal vein, three had purpura fulminans and two children developed a thrombus in a cerebral vein. In 10 children a cerebral insult took place. In addition 5 children with peripheral arterial thrombosis could be included.

A total of 29 children suffered from venous and 15 from arterial thrombosis.

In 29 children with **venous** thromboembolism, the median age was 8 years (range 0.3–18 years). 15 of them (51,7%) were female. In 14 children no underlying diseases were found. 6 patients suffered from cancer and 9 patients had other underlying diseases. The investigation of fibrinogen took place 0.95 years after the thrombotic event had occurred (range 2 months – 8.5 years).

Fifteen patients had **arterial** thrombosis. They had a median age of 6.1 years (1.0–14.8 years) at the time of the event. 46.7% (n=7) of them were female. Twelve of them had no diseases, one child suffered from cancer and two others had other underlying diseases. Fibrinogen was measured about 1.3 years (median) after the development of the thrombosis (range 0.2–7.6 years later). All children were older than one year at the time of the investigation.

Controls

Seventy-eight healthy children without thromboembolism in their own history, but with a positive family history of thrombosis were included in the „control group A". The median age of them was 7.9 years (0.3–16.1 years). Forty-four of them (56,4%) were female. The „control group B" consists out of 156 healthy subjects without thrombosis in their own or in their family histories. About the half of them were female (n=81, 51,9%). The median age was 5.6 years (0.2–16.5 years).

These children were investigated during preoperative screening before surgery of the tonsils and adenoids, while being clinically free of acute infections. In addition, in most of the patients C reactive protein was measured and was negative.

Laboratory Methods

Fibrinogen was measured by the method of Clauss (Sigma Diagnostics).

Statistic Analysis

Statistical analysis was performed with SPSS for windows 11.0. T-test in independent samples and chi-square-test were used to compare the fibrinogen levels in the patients and in the control groups.

Results

In Table 2 and Figure 1, the mean values of fibrinogen in the patient and the control groups are shown. The patients were separated in two groups depending on the kind of the thrombosis. In patients with arterial thrombosis, the mean of the fibrinogen level was 3.19 g/l. This level was significantly higher than in the control groups, where the mean fibrinogen level is 2.71 g/l in control group A, or 2.77 g/l in control group B, respectively (p<0.001 control group A; p<0.002 control group B), although the values themselves are not extremely high (range 2.2–4.6 g/l in the patients with arterial thrombosis).

Table 2. Fibrinogen (Clauss) in patients and controls

Fibrinogen (g/l)	Venous TE (n=29)	Arterial TE (n=15)	Control group A (n=78)	Control group B (n=156)
Mean	2.94	3.19 * / **	2.70 *	2.77 **
Range	1.7–5.0	2.2–4.6	1.9–3.9	1.8–4.6
Standard deviation	0.87	0.68	0.46	0.47

* p<0.001; ** p<0.002

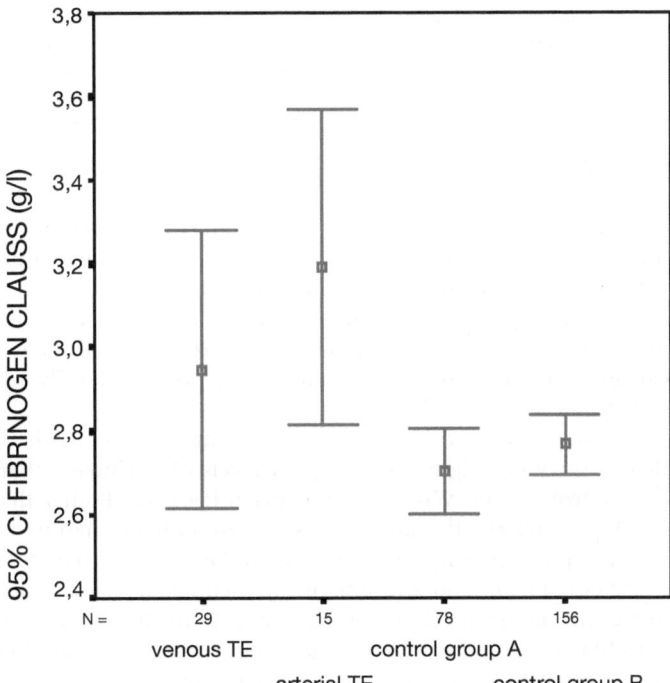

Fig. 1. Fibrinogen (Clauss) in patients and controls (arterial TE versus control group A: p<0.001; arterial TE versus control group B: p<0.002)

Table 3. Fibrinogen (Clauss) in patients and controls older than one year of age

Fibrinogen (g/l)	Venous TE (n=25)	Arterial TE (n=15)	Control group A (n=76)	Control group B (n=153)
Mean	2.92	3.19 * / **	2.71 *	2.77 **
Range	1.7-5.0	2.2-4-6	1.9-3.9	1.8-4.6
Standard deviation	0.88	0.68	0.46	0.47

* $p<0.001$; ** $p<0.002$

The values were calculated a second time after exclusion of the children, which were younger than one year (Table 3). Again the fibrinogen levels in patients with arterial thrombosis were significantly higher than in the control groups ($p<0.001$ control group A; $p<0.002$ control group B).

In addition, the relative risk was calculated to obtain a thrombotic event if the fibrinogen level was higher than 3.5 g/l. The relative risk was 3.0 for the development of venous, and 5.3 for arterial thrombosis (Table 4).

Table 4. Relative risk for the development of venous or arterial thrombosis if fibrinogen is higher than 3.5 g/l. Comparison with healthy controls (group B).

| | Relative risk | 95% CI | |
		Low	high
Venous thrombosis	3.0	1.0	9.6
Arterial thrombosis	5.3	1.4	19.7

Discussion

The aim of the study was to examine the role of the fibrinogen levels as a risk factor for thrombophilia in childhood. Therefore, we investigated pediatric patients with venous and arterial thrombosis in their history.

We chose two control groups of healthy children, one with a positive family history of thromboembolism and one where the families had no thrombophilia to exclude genetic factors. Children with a positive family history of dysfibrinogenemia were also excluded.

In conclusion, we could demonstrate that children with arterial thrombosis in their history had significantly higher levels of fibrinogen than healthy children of the control groups. When the fibrinogen level was higher than 3.5 g/l, the risk to develop an arterial thrombosis was 5.3 times higher than in control group B. There was no significance in comparison with the control group A.

Children with venous thrombosis in their history showed only a tendency towards higher fibrinogen levels in comparison with the healthy controls. But for the group with fibrinogen higher than 3.5 g/l, the relative risk to develop a thrombosis, is 3.0 times higher than in control group B. Once more there is no higher risk in comparison with the control group A. Possibly, patients with a positive family history for TE have already higher fibrinogen levels, as was published by Jastrzebska et al. [1].

It is known that young children in the first year of their life have different fibrinogen values in comparison to older ones. In addition during the first year of life most of the thrombotic events in childhood occur. Therefore, a second calculation after exclusion of all children younger than one year was performed. It could be shown, that the results are similar when the children younger than one year were excluded. Furthermore, in all patients with arterial thrombosis fibrinogen levels were examined later, when the children were older than one year. Therefore, we conclude, that the higher fibrinogen levels are independent of the age.

Because children with infections were excluded from the study, and patients with cancer were examined later, when chemotherapy was terminated and the children were in remission, we propose that the higher fibrinogen levels in the patient group do not depend on acute phase reactions.

This is the first study concerning the clinical relevance of elevated fibrinogen levels as prothrombotic risk factor in childhood. These data have to be confirmed in a larger number of patients in a multicenter study.

References

1. Jastrzebska M, Torbus-Lisiecka B, Honczarenko K, Foltynska A, Chelstowski K, Naruszewicz M. Von Willebrand factor, fibrinogen and other risk factors of thrombosis in patients with a history of cerebrovascular ischemic stroke and their children. Nutr Metab Cardiovasc Dis 2002 Jun; 12 (3): 132–140
2. Ceriello A, Pirisi M, Giacomello R, Stel G, Falleti E, Motz E, Lizzio S, Gonano F, Bartoli E. Fibrinogen plasma levels as a marker of thrombin activation: new insights on the role of fibrinogen as a cardiovascular risk factor. Thromb Haemost 1994; 71: 593–95
3. Ernst E. Fibrinogen: an important risk factor for atherothrombotic disease. Ann Med 1994; 26: 15–22
4. Humphries S. The genetic contribution to the risk of thrombosis and cardiovascular disease. Trends Cardiovasc Med 1994; 4: 8–17
5. Koster T, Rosendaal FR, Reitsma PH, van der Velden PA, Briet E, Vandenbroucke JP. F VII and fibrinogen levels as risk factors for venous thrombosis. Thromb Haemost 1994; 71: 719–22
6. Nowak-Göttl U, Kosch A, Schlegel N, Salem M, Manco-Johnson M. Thromboembolism in children. Curr Opin Hematol 2002 Sep; 9 (5): 448–53

Increased von-Willebrand-Factor-Binding to Platelets in Neonatal Plasma

T. Rehak, G. Cvirn, B. Roschitz, and W. Muntean

Introduction

Platelets of newborns aggregate poorly in-vitro [1, 2]. However, newborns have efficient hemostasis, as illustrated by their short skin bleeding time. It has been demonstrated that elevated von-Willebrand-factor (vWF) concentrations and unusually large vWF multimers, not present in normal adult plasma [3], allow sufficient vWF-collagen binding, probably contributing to the clinically observed effective primary hemostasis of neonates.

Subsequently to the binding to collagen, vWF causes platelet adherence by binding to the glycoprotein Ib receptor (GP Ib) on the platelet membrane. To our knowledge, no data exists about the ability of neonatal vWF to bind to GP Ib as compared to adult vWF.

Therefore, it was the aim of our study to determine the amount of GP Ib on the neonatal platelet membrane compared to that on adult platelets and to quantify vWF-binding to both neonatal and adult platelets. Conformation change of vWF due to the binding to collagen, enabling binding of vWF to platelets, was stimulated in our experiments by incubating platelets with ristocetin [4]. Quantification of vWF binding to platelets was performed by means of FACScan flow cytometry using mouse-anti-human-vWF and FITC-conjugated rabbit-anti-mouse antibody.

Methods

Blood sampling

Blood was taken from umbilical cord of term neonates immediately after vaginal delivery. For normal adult controls blood was collected by cubital venipuncture from healthy volunteers who had not taken aspirin or other drugs for at least 10 days. In both cases blood was collected into 0.1M citrate-containing tubes.

Platelet Isolation

Platelet-rich plasma (PRP) was prepared by centrifugation of citrated blood at 1300 rpm for 10 min, PRP was centrifuged at 2300 rpm for 10 min and plasma was removed. Platelet pellet was resuspended in 2 ml of phosphate buffered saline (PBS) and centrifuged at 2000 rpm for 10 min at room temperature. Washing procedures were repeated three times. Platelet counts were determined on a Sysmex counter and suspensions were adjusted to $50*10^3$ cells/μl.

GP Ib-staining

Platelet suspensions (40 μl) were incubated with a FITC-conjugated anti-CD42b antibody (Immunotech) or with a FITC-conjugated IgG1 control, respectively, for 30 min at room temperature, then diluted with 300 μl PBS.

VWF-staining

Platelet-poor plasma was diluted 1:10 with PBS containing 0.1% Na-azide and incubated with mouse-anti-human-vWF antibody (Dako) for 30 min in the dark and subsequently with a FITC-conjugated rabbit-anti-mouse antibody (Dako) for 30 min in the dark.

Tubes were prepared with 40 μl of platelet suspension, 50 μl of plasma dilution containing antibody-stained vWF and 20 μl Ristocetin (final concentration: 0,3; 0,4; 0,7 mg/ml) or PBS, respectively. After 10 min at room temperature samples were diluted with 300 μl of 2% paraformaldehyde solution.

Flow cytometry

GP Ib- and vWF-samples were analyzed on a FACScan® flow cytometer (Becton-Dickinson), Median was taken for further statistical analysis.

Results

- Neonatal platelets showed similar expression of GP Ib as adult platelets (Fig. 1).
- Fluorescence-intensities of neonatal vWF bound to neonatal platelets were significantly higher than those of adult vWF bound to adult platelets (Fig. 2).
- Fluorescence-intensities of neonatal vWF bound to neonatal or adult platelets were similar (Fig. 2, 3).
- Fluorescence-intensities of adult vWF bound to adult or neonatal platelets were similar (Fig. 2, 3).

Conclusions

Despite similar GP Ib expression on both neonatal and adult platelets, the ability of neonatal vWF to bind to platelets is markedly increased compared to that of adult

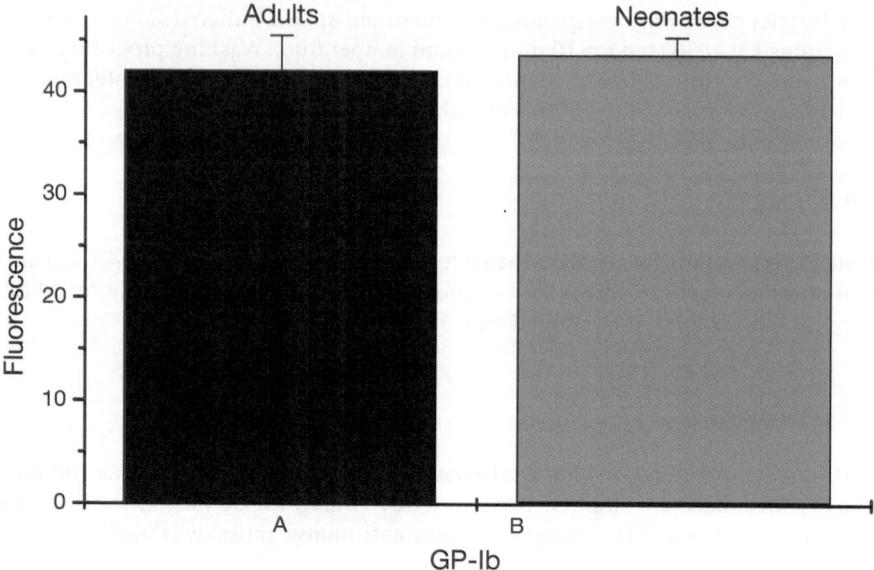

Fig. 1. Expression of GP Ib on neonatal and adult platelets.

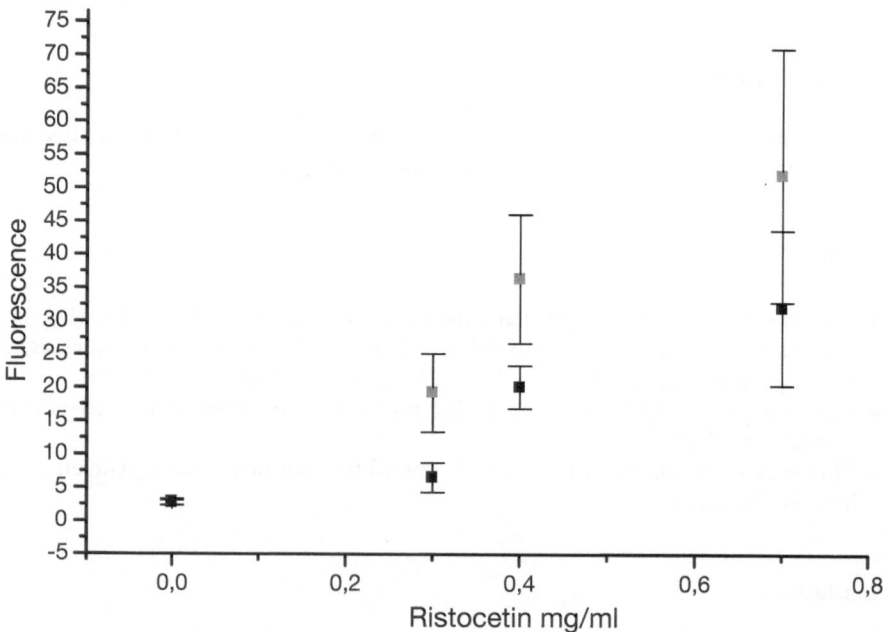

Fig. 2. Medians of neonatal vWF bound to neonatal platelets (grey) and adult vWF bound to adult platelets (black).

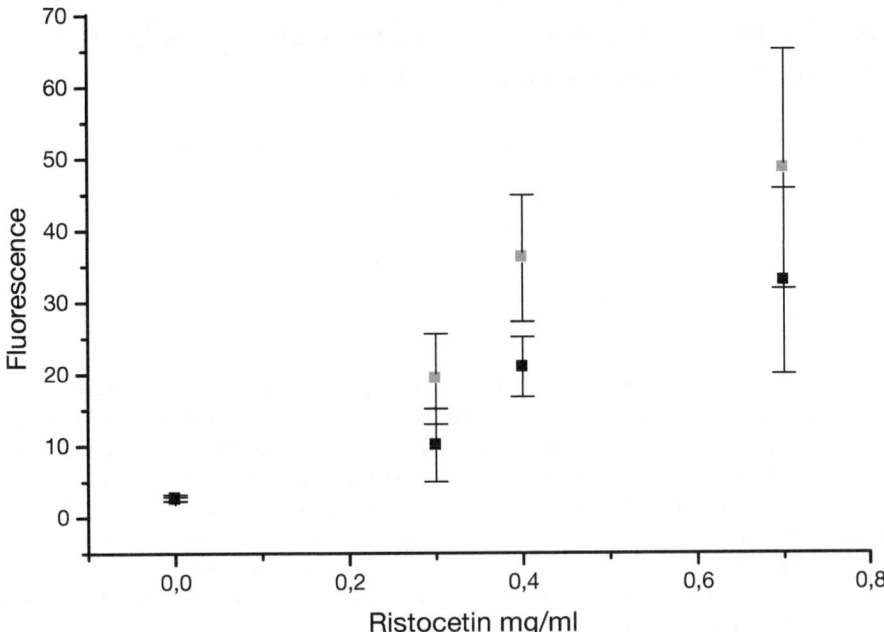

Fig. 3. Medians of neonatal vWF bound to adult platelets (grey) and adult vWF bound to neonatal platelets (black).

vWF. This increased binding is attributable to the large vWF multimers present in neonatal plasma. Both effective neonatal vWF-collagen binding and efficient neonatal vWF-GP Ib binding, as demonstrated in our study, contribute to the excellent hemostasis of neonates despite poor in-vitro aggregation of neonatal platelets and low levels of hemostatic proteins.

References

1. Rajasekhar D, Kestin AS, Bednarek FJ, Ellis PA, Barnard MR, Michelson AD. Neonatal platelets are less reactive than adult platelets to physiological agonists in whole blood. Thromb Haemost 1994 Dec; 72 (6): 957–63
2. Michelson AD. Platelet function in the newborn. Semin Thromb Hemost 1998; 24 (6): 507–12
3. Fischer BE, Kramer G, Mitterer A, Grillberger L, Reiter M, Mundt W, Dorner F, Eibl J. Effect of multimerization of human and recombinant von-Willebrand-factor on platelet aggregation, binding to collagen and binding of coagulation factor VIII. Thromb Res 1996 Oct 1; 84 (1): 55–66
4. Dong JF, Berndt MC, Schade A, McIntire LV, Andrews RK, Lopez JA. Ristocetin-dependent, but not botrocetin-dependent, binding of von-Willebrand-factor to the platelet glycoprotein Ib-IX-V complex correlates with shear-dependent interactions. Blood 2001 Jan 1; 97 (1): 162–8

Neonatal Protein C Deficiency after
massive thromboembolic Event of the right upper Limb –
Treatment with Protein C Concentrate

J. Dinger, R. Knöfler, D. Müller, G. Hahn, P. Goebel, and G. Siegert

Introduction

Neonatal thromboembolic events, both arterial and venous, are rare but increasingly recognized problems in tertiary care neonatology. The pathophysiology of these events in the context of the neonatal hemostatic system and the importance of both inherited and acquired prothrombotic disorders remain poorly defined [2, 7]. Today we have certain knowledge about a number of hereditary factors which change the hemostatic balance of their carriers toward a tendency to develop embolism. Typically the first manifestation occurs frequently without any recognizable cause at a young age and in the majority of cases as thrombotic or embolic occlusion of the deep veins or arterial vessels [1, 2, 10].

Aortic and massive venous thrombosis in the newborn are usually associated with umbilical vessel catheterization, inherited or acquired thrombophilia [5]. It may lead to death or such severe complications as intestinal necrosis, oliguria, renal hypertension, paraplegia and peripheral gangrene, depending on the size and localization of the thrombus. Medical and surgical therapies have been attempted with varying results [3, 4, 5, 7, 10]. Standardized therapeutic guidelines have not yet been established.

Acquired deficiencies of protein C and protein S appear to be relatively common in sick, preterm infants and there are some limited data to suggest an increased risk of thrombosis in these patients [5, 7].

The approval of commercially available protein C concentrate increases the importance of protein C diagnostics for the detection of protein C deficiencies and the monitoring of a therapy now possible.

We report the presentation, treatment and follow up of a newborn with massive renal vein and inferior vena caval thrombosis followed by a thromboembolic arterial event of the right upper limb treated with protein C concentrate (Ceprotin, Baxter, Germany).

Case report

The male infant was born at 40 weeks from a healthy mother by cesarean section for fetal distress (birth weight 3440 g, Apgar 7/7/8, umbilical cord-pH = 7.04, BE = -11 mmol/l). The infant was referred to neonatal care unit because of mild respira-

I. Scharrer/W. Schramm (Ed.)
33rd Hemophilia Symposion Hamburg 2002
© Springer-Verlag Berlin Heidelberg 2004

Table 1. Laboratory data before, during and after treatment with protein C concentrate

day of life	1. (at birth)	6. (before treatment)	7. (day 1 of treatment)	10. (day 3 of treatment)	14. (day 7 of treatment)	21. (day 14 of treatment)	28 (7 days after treatment)	age related reference range
CRP	–	18.4	–	12.3	11.3	4.3	2.2	< 5 mg/l
Platelets	44	74	115	161	260	348	454	150--400 x 10 9 /l
aPTT	32	66	87	67	47	47	37	68 ± 17 s
Fibrinogen	3.0	2.1	1.2	2.2	2.8	2.5	2.7	2.8 ± 0.7 g/l
AT	63	42	73	126	87	86	91	53 ± 22 %
D-dimer	–	1.245	>19.000	1.290	11.931	1.419	201	< 115 ng/ml
Protein C	57	28	87	86	94	84	106	50 ± 15 %
Creatinine	–	55	61	62	52	–	41	< 115 µmol/l

(aPTT = activated partial thromboplastin time; CRP = C reactive protein)

tory distress syndrome. At birth an acute ischemia of the right upper limb was noticed. The limb appeared pale, cold, atonic and areflexic. Thromboembolic occlusions of the right radial and ulnar arteries were confirmed by ultrasonography. At that time the protein C activity was in the age-related normal range (Table 1). Treatment with low dose unfractionated heparin (200 IU/kg/d) was started. Pain was treated with analgesic therapy, and motor impairment required physiotherapy. During the next days peripheral gangrene of the fingers progressed and the child was sent to our tertiary neonatal care unit on day 6 of life for intensification of therapy.

The Doppler ultrasonography which was performed at admission to our hospital showed a massive, partially recanalized renal vein and inferior caval vein thrombosis of prenatal onset which most likely resulted in the thromboembolic events of the right radial and ulnar artery immediately prior birth. Because of the extension and the age of the peripheral gangrene there was no indication for surgical treatment. Compared to the laboratory findings immediately after birth a marked decrease of the protein C activity was noticed (Table 1). Therefore treatment with protein C concentrate and antithrombin (AT) was started to achieve a protein C activity of over 70% and an AT concentration of over 80%. CEPRO-TIN (initial dose of 80 IU/kg, during the next five days 3 doses of 40 IU/kg/d and for the next nine days 2 doses of 60 IU/kg/d were given, cumulative dose = 4375 IU) was intravenously administered for 14 days and AT (initial dose of 85 IU/kg, during the next eight days 2 doses of 35 IU/kg/d were given, cumulative dose = 2550 IU) for 8 days. Additionally the dose of unfractionated heparin was increased up to 500 IU/kg/d resulting in an appropriate prolongation of the activated partial thromboplastin time.

As shown in Table 1, the protein C activity increased and remained over 70% at the time of treatment with protein C concentrate and beyond it. As a marker of enhanced fibrinolysis, the d-dimer concentration increased very rapidly after starting therapy with protein C concentrate. Unfortunately the gangrene and the loss of the fingers could not be prevented. However, skin defects of hand and arm markedly

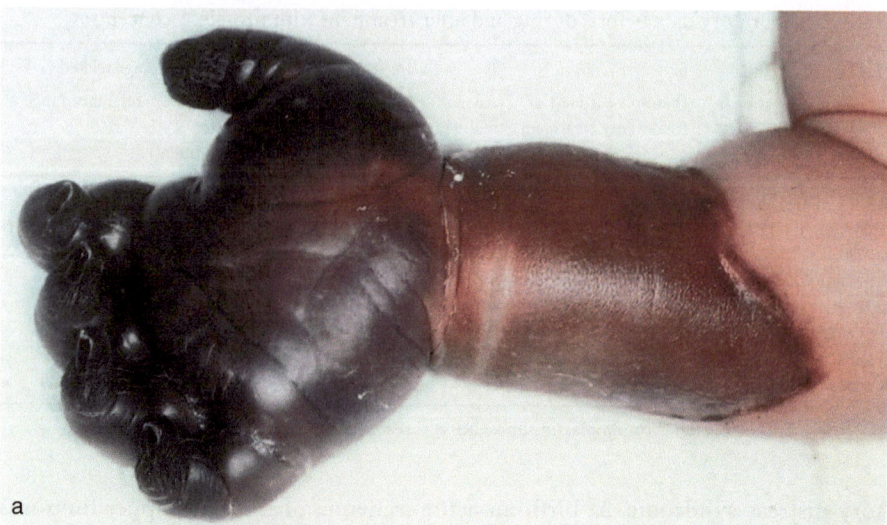

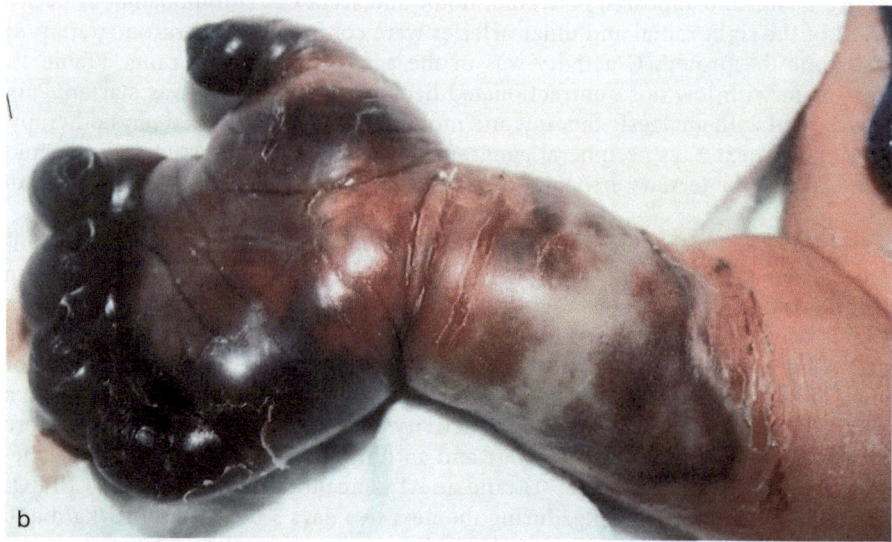

Fig. 1 a–d. Photographs of skin lesions on the ischemic right upper limb in the neonate before the start of treatment with protein C concentrate (a): Ecchymotic dislocation, edema, hemorrhage lesions and necrotic areas; 14 days later at the end of protein C substitution (b) and one (c) and 3 months (d) later: Complete healing of skin lesions and digital gangrene before and after surgical necrectomy.

improved (Fig. 1). The Doppler ultrasonography examinations during treatment showed an increased arterial flow and after one week a normal flow in the right radial and ulnar arteries was detected. Furthermore complete revascularization of both renal veins and of the inferior caval vein was obtained.

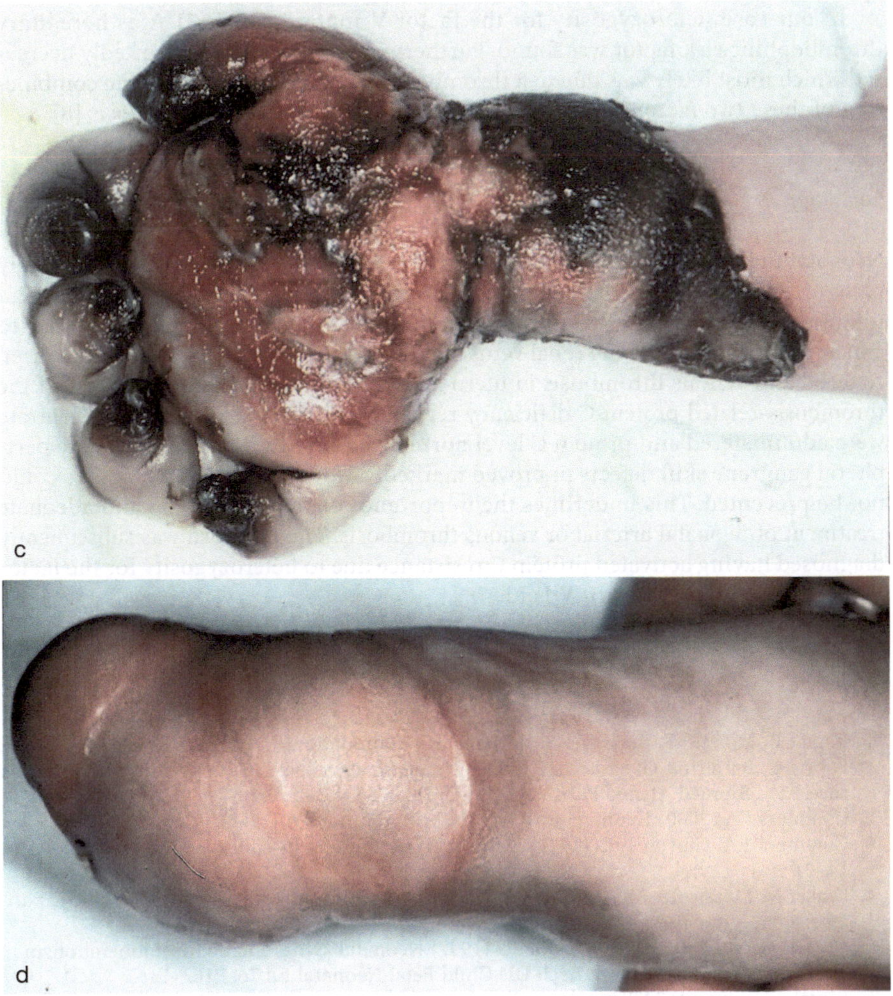

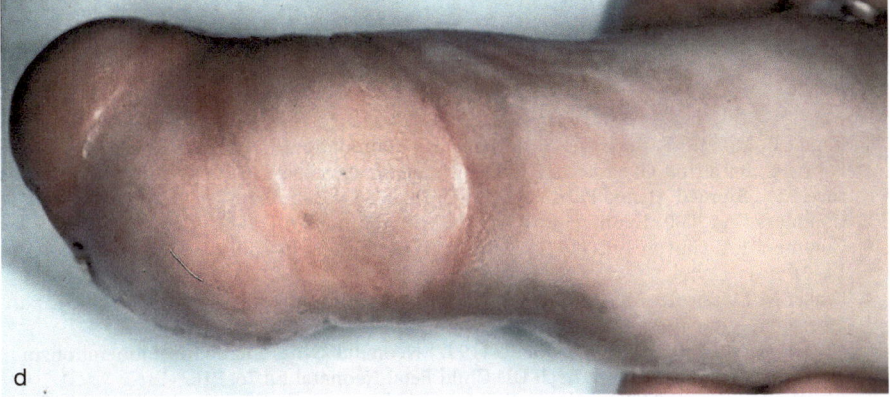

Fig. 1 c–d

Conclusions

Limb vascular occlusions are serious events in newborns. Therefore early identification and adequate treatment are very important, as it can avoid invasive surgical procedures or loss of function.

The use of protein C concentrate should not be restricted to newborns representing a purpura fulminans [6, 9]. In newborns with extended thrombosis and low protein C levels the application of protein C concentrate might also be of advantage which most likely is due to its fibrinolytic effect.

In our case heterozygosity for the factor V mutation G 1691 A as hereditary thrombophilic risk factor was found. Furthermore, protein C was markedly decreased which most likely was due to a thrombosis-related consumption. The combination of these two factors bears an increased risk of developing thrombosis [8].

Summary

Neonatal thromboembolic events, both arterial or venous, are rare but increasingly recognized in tertiary care neonatology. We report the presentation, treatment and follow up of a newborn with a thromboembolic event of the right upper limb due to a massive thrombosis of the renal veins and the inferior caval vein of prenatal onset. Arterial and venous thrombosis in utero may result in fetal distress. Because of the thrombosis-related protein C deficiency repeated infusions of protein C concentrate were administered and protein C level normalized rapidly. Despite the severe peripheral gangrene skin defects improved markedly. However, the loss of fingers could not be prevented. This underlines the importance of rapid detection and adequate treatment of neonatal arterial or venous thrombosis. The newborn was subsequently diagnosed having activated protein C resistance due to heterozygosity for the factor V G 1691 A mutation (factor V Leiden).

References

1. Bagna R, Tonetto P, Borgione S, Garbarini S, Mammano A, Bertino E, Murru P, Cavo L, Fabris C, Barattina G, Saracco P (2000) Neonatal arteriovenous thrombosis: report of a case. Acta Biomed Ateneo Parmense 71 (1): 781–783
2. Chalmers EA (2000) Neonatal thrombosis. J Clin Pathol 53: 419–423
3. Chalmers EA, Gibson BES (1999) Thrombolytic therapy in children. Br J Haematol 104: 14–21
4. Leaker M, Massicotte MP, Brooker LA et al. (1996) Thrombolytic therapy in paediatric patients: a comprehensive review of the literature. Thromb Haemost 76: 132–134
5. Nowak-Göttl U, von Kries R, Göbel U (1997) Neonatal symptomatic thromboembolism in Germany: two years survey. Arch Dis Child Fetal Neonatal Ed 76: F163–F167
6. Rintala E, Kauppila M, Seppälä OP, Voipio-Pulkki LM, Pettilä V, Rasi V, Kotilainen P (2000) Protein C substitution in sepsis-associated purpura fulminans. Crit Care Med 28: 2373–2378
7. Schmidt B, Andrew M (1995) Neonatal thrombosis: report of a prospective Canadian and international registry. Pediatrics 96: 939–943
8. Seligsohn U, Zivelin A (1997) Thrombophilia as a multigenic disorder. Thromb Haemostas 78: 297–301
9. White B, Livingstone W, Murphy C, Hodgson A, Rafferty M, Smith OP (2000) An open-label study of the role of adjuvant hemostatic support with protein C replacement therapy in purpura fulminans-associated meningococcemia. Blood 96: 3719–3724
10. Zenker M, Ries M, Vetter V, Rauch R, Harms D (1999) Non-catheter-related aortic thrombosis and resistance to activated protein C in a premature newborn. Acta Paediatr 88: 1035–1043

VI. Free Lectures

Chairmen:

I. SCHARRER (Frankfurt/Main)
M. VON DEPKA PRONDZINSKI (Hanover)

IMMUNATE S/D – A new Factor VIII – von-Willebrand Factor Complex Concentrate

P.L. Turecek, W. Schönhofer, T.R. Kreil, A. Weber, K. Váradi, H. Gritsch, J. Siekmann, L. Pichler, B.M. Reipert, B. Abbühl, and H.P. Schwarz

Introduction

IMMUNATE is a human plasma-derived coagulation factor VIII concentrate containing both factor VIII (FVIII) and von-Willebrand Factor (vWF) produced by Baxter AG and currently approved in a large number of countries in Europe and overseas. The complex is purified by anion-exchange chromatography. IMMUNATE's manufacturing process also includes two virus inactivation steps:
1. treatment with polysorbate 80, and
2. vapor heat treatment.

No confirmed case of possible, probable, or definite IMMUNATE-related virus transmission has been reported over the 10 years of IMMUNATE's clinical use. For the production of its plasma-derived products, Baxter AG has established a stringent plasma safety program, which goes beyond the requirements laid down in the respective regulations and comprises in addition PCR testing for HIV-1/HIV-2, HCV, HBV, HAV, and PVB19. Current virus inactivation techniques include solvent detergent (S/D) treatment, treatment with polysorbate 80, dry heat treatment and vapor heat treatment [1, 2, 3]. S/D treatment is effective in inactivating lipid-enveloped viruses [4]. Vapor heat treatment is effective against a broad spectrum of viruses, including non-enveloped viruses such as hepatitis A that are not affected by the S/D treatment [5, 6, 7, 8, 9]. To further increase the viral safety margin of the product, the polysorbate 80 step has been replaced with S/D treatment. The resulting product, IMMUNATE S/D, is manufactured by a process otherwise identical to that of IMMUNATE.

General Properties and Product Profile

The product profile is summarized in Table 1. IMMUNATE S/D is a sterile, lyophilized, high-purity human FVIII concentrate that complies with the requirements of the current edition of the European Pharmacopoeia (Ph. Eur.). IMMUNATE S/D is filled in portions of 250 IU, 500 IU, and 1000 IU (nominal potency). The FVIII concentration in both the 500 IU and 1000 IU filling sizes is 100 IU/mL. The FVIII concentration in the 250 IU filling size is 50 IU/mL. For all filling sizes, the specific activity is approx. 75 IU/mg protein without stabilizer. IMMUNATE S/D is a lyo-

I. Scharrer/W. Schramm (Ed.)
33rd Hemophilia Symposion Hamburg 2002
© Springer-Verlag Berlin Heidelberg 2004

Table 1. IMMUNATE S/D product profile

Active ingredient	Factor VIII – von-Willebrand Factor Complex Concentrate	
Indication	Hemophilia A Hemophilia A with FVIII inhibitor, acquired hemophilia von-Willebrand's Disease with FVIII deficiency	
Purification	Ion-exchange chromatography	
Viral safety measures	BAXTER Quality – QSEAL certified PCR screening Dual virus inactivation: – S/D treatment 　　　　　　　　　　　　　– Vapor heating (TIM 3) Virus removal steps	
Presentations	250 IU / 500 IU in 5 ml 1000 IU in 10 ml	
Stabilizers	Albumin von-Willebrand Factor	
Composition	FVIII conc. Ratio vWF/FVIII:C vWF multimers Spec. activity (before albumin) Albumin	50 IU/ml or 100 IU/ml plasma-like ~ 14 ~ 75 IU/mg protein 65–85%

philized, white or pale yellow powder or friable solid, which is supplied together with the required volume for reconstitution of sterilized water for injection as solvent.

Method of Manufacture

IMMUNATE S/D is manufactured from pooled human plasma. Each individual plasma donation is screened with approved tests for HBsAg and for antibodies to HIV-1/HIV-2, and HCV. The alanine transaminase (ALT) value of each single donation must not exceed twice the upper limit of normal.

The inventory hold program introduced by Baxter assures that single plasma units are only released for pooling after inventory hold for at least 60 days from the time of donation. The inventory hold and look back reports allow efficient plasma unit retrieval and the elimination of the so-called »window-period donations« of donors disqualifying at a later stage.

Prior to manufacturing, each plasma production pool is tested serologically for the presence of HBsAg and antibodies to HIV-1/HIV-2, and HCV, and by PCR for the presence of viral nucleic acids of HCV, HIV-1/HIV-2, HAV, HBV and PVB19. Only production pools non-reactive in serological testing and PCR testing for HCV, HIV-1/HIV-2, HAV and HBV and that do not contain more than 10^5 IU PVB19 DNA/mL are released for further manufacture.

The FVIII bulk powder manufacturing process can be divided into four subprocesses:
1. Fractionation and purification of FVIII-vWF intermediate from human plasma
2. Virus inactivation by solvent detergent treatment (S/D treatment)
3. Isolation of high purity FVIII-vWF complex by chromatography
4. Virus inactivation by vapor heat treatment

The process flow chart is presented in Figure 1. Crude FVIII is separated by cryoprecipitation. The coagulation factors of the prothrombin complex (PC) are removed by adsorption onto aluminum hydroxide gel. For the S/D treatment, the filtrate is treated with a mixture of 1% Triton X-100, 0.3% polysorbate 80, 0.3% TNBP for 60–65 minutes at 24°C to 28°C. Subsequently, the S/D reagents and the majority of the non-FVIII-proteins are removed by ion exchange chromatography, resulting in a high purity FVIII fraction (specific activity, approx. 75 IU/mg protein). Human albumin is added to this fraction as a stabilizer and the product is subjected to ultra- and diafiltration, freeze-drying and vapor heat treatment, in which the FVIII bulk powder is vapor heat treated for 600–700 minutes at a temperature of 60°C ± 0.5°C and a pressure of 190 mbar ± 20 mbar over ambient.

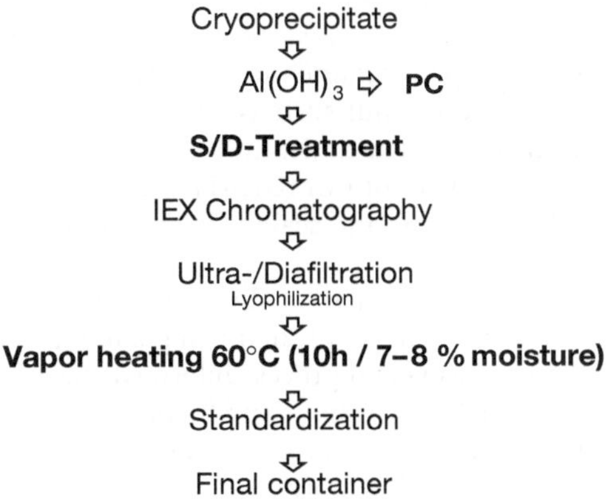

Cryoprecipitate
⇩
$Al(OH)_3$ ⇨ **PC**
⇩
S/D-Treatment
⇩
IEX Chromatography
⇩
Ultra-/Diafiltration
Lyophilization
⇩
Vapor heating 60°C (10h / 7–8 % moisture)
⇩
Standardization
⇩
Final container

Fig. 1. Manufacturing process of IMMUNATE S/D

Product Stability

IMMUNATE S/D is shown to be stable for two years when stored cool at temperatures between +2°C and +8°C. Comprehensive data from the non-S/D treated product are available that prove the stability of the non-S/D treated product. As the modification in the virus inactivation procedure is only minimal, the change is not expected to influence the stability of the product. Therefore it can be assumed that also IMMUNATE S/D can be stored at room temperature for a period of up to 1 year or more.

Following reconstitution with sterilized water for injection, the preparation remains stable for at least 3 hours at 20 to 25°C. Because the preparation does not contain preservatives, the product should be used immediately unless the method of reconstitution precludes the risk of microbial contamination. Reconstituted product must not be returned to the refrigerator.

Nonclinical Study Program

The objective of the extensive non-clinical study program was the assessment of tolerability of IMMUNATE S/D and the proof of bio-equivalence of IMMUNATE S/D and IMMUNATE in in vitro and in vivo studies, in regard to their biochemical and biophysical characteristics, FVIII structural and functional properties, in vivo safety, immunogenicity, tolerability, and pharmacokinetics (used as a surrogate for efficacy).

In Vitro Studies

Viral Safety Studies

Validation of the virus inactivation/removal capacity of the IMMUNATE S/D manufacturing process was conducted using a scaled-down laboratory version of the manufacturing process. Scaling-down procedures were carried out in accordance with the COMP guidelines to maintain the integrity of the production process in relation to the full-scale version [10]. The critical parameters chosen were identical in the scaled-down and the full-scale manufacturing processes. Biochemical characteristics of IMMUNATE S/D were measured and compared for the products of the full-scale and scaled-down manufacturing processes to verify that they were in conformity.

The effectiveness of the scaled-down process in removing and/or inactivating viral pathogens was tested using spiking experiments. In these experiments, samples of plasma and process intermediates were spiked with known concentrations of virus stock suspensions and further processed under conditions equivalent to those used in the particular manufacturing step. The virus titer of all fractions obtained in the scaled-down process was determined. In addition, the biochemical parameters of IMMUNATE S/D were measured for products of both the scaled-down and full-scale processes to confirm that they were in conformity.

HIV and HAV were tested directly as target human pathogens and three other model viruses were employed. Model viruses were used in cases where actual human pathogens could not be tested. Bovine viral diarrhea virus (BVDV) was used as a model for HCV, a lipid enveloped RNA virus. Pseudorabies virus (PRV) was used as a model for lipid-enveloped DNA viruses like HBV. Mice minute virus (MMV) was used as a model for PVB19, a non-enveloped small DNA virus.

The titers of HIV-1, BVDV, PRV, HAV, and MMV were determined based on observed virus-induced cytopathic and fusogenic effects in a tissue culture infectious dose fifty ($TCID_{50}$) assay. Results from the $TCID_{50}$ assay were, in turn, used to calculate the virus reduction factor. The virus reduction factor R represents the capacity of the process to remove and/or inactivate viruses, and is calculated using the formula below. This formula takes into consideration the volumes and titers of the samples before and after each virus inactivation or removal step, according to the Guidelines of the Committee for Proprietary Medicinal Products (CPMP) [10]:

$$R = \log \frac{V_1 \times T_1}{V_2 \times T_2}$$

where
R = log virus reduction factor
V_1 = volume of starting material, [ml]
T_1 = concentration of virus in starting material, [$TCID_{50}$/ml]
V_2 = volume of material after the step, [ml]
T_2 = concentration of virus after the step, [$TCID_{50}$/ml]

The particular virus reduction procedure at issue was considered successful if the individual virus reduction factor was greater than 4.

Solvent/Detergent Treatment
The validation procedure was used to evaluate the efficacy and robustness of the S/D treatment with respect to virus inactivation. Specifically, the virus inactivation capacity of the process was determined at the upper and lower limits specified for the total nitrogen content (a measure for protein concentration). In addition, the effectiveness of virus inactivation was also investigated at an S/D-reagent concentration far below the concentration specified for the manufacturing process.
    As S/D treatment is not effective against non-lipid-enveloped viruses, the investigation was carried out only with the following lipid-enveloped viruses:
– Human Immunodeficiency Virus 1 (HIV-1)
– Bovine Viral Diarrhea Virus (BVDV; model virus for HCV)
– Pseudorabies Virus (PRV, model virus for HBV)

The parameters critical to virus inactivation by S/D treatment are the total incubation time, the temperature and the concentration of S/D-reagents. Therefore, to investigate the efficacy of the S/D treatment under conditions least favorable for virus inactivation, two runs for each virus (runs 1 and 2) were performed at the lower limits of incubation time, temperature and concentration of S/D-reagents. To investigate the robustness of the virus inactivation, these two runs were also performed at the lower and upper limits of the manufacturing process specification for total nitrogen content (a measure of protein concentration). A third assay (run 3) was performed for each virus, using only 5% of the concentration of S/D-reagent normally used in the manufacturing process. Individual virus reduction factors were determined for each run (see Table 2). Complete virus inactivation of HIV-1, BVDV, and PRV was achieved rapidly (details on inactivation kinetics included in the respective validation report).
    The results of this study show that even under conditions deemed less favorable with respect to virus inactivation – i.e. temperature, time and concentration of S/D-reagent that were set to the lower limits specified for the manufacturing process – the lipid-enveloped viruses HIV-1, BVDV and PRV were rapidly and completely inactiva-

Table 2. Overall virus reduction factors achieved at different levels of critical S/D treatment parameters

	Run 1	Run 2	Run 3
Incubation time, temperature, and concentration	Lower limit	Lower limit	
Nitrogen content	Lower limit	Upper limit	
S/D reagent amount	100% of process specification	100% of process specification	5% of process specification
HIV-1	>3.0	>5.0	>5.4
BVDV (model virus for HCV)	>4.0	>6.4	>4.8
PRV (model virus for HBV)	>6.1	>5.9	>5.8

ted by S/D treatment. The robustness of S/D treatment with respect to inactivation of lipid-enveloped viruses is further demonstrated by the fact that complete inactivation of the three viruses tested was observed after adding only 5% of the specified amount of S/D-reagent.

Vapor Heat Treatment
The second virus inactivation step in the manufacture of IMMUNATE S/D is a well-established vapor heat treatment step. Vapor heat treatment has recently been validated for IMMUNATE S/D in order to demonstrate the robustness of this step, apart from its virus inactivation capacity.

The following viruses were used for this study:
– HIV-1
– HAV
– BVDV (model virus for HCV)
– PRV (model virus for large lipid-enveloped DNA viruses including HBV)
– Mice Minute Virus (MMV; model virus for Parvovirus B19)

In order to investigate the robustness of virus inactivation, critical process parameters were chosen to simulate a worst-case scenario. The individual virus reduction factors ($\log_{10}$) shown in Table 3 represent the minimum reductions achieved under these worst-case conditions.

Additional process and product parameters were measured to determine whether the products of the scaled-down and the full-scale manufacturing processes were equivalent. In general, all parameters measured during the process were within the ranges specified for the large-scale process or within the internal warning limits for process monitoring, except for those deliberately set outside the range specified for the large scale process. In addition to the virus inactivation capacity, the results further demonstrate the robustness of this step for HIV-1, HAV, BVDV, and PRV.

Table 3. Virus reduction factors achieved under worst-case vapor heat treatment conditions

	Run 1	Run 2
HIV-1	> 5.4	> 5.5
HAV	> 4.4	> 4.4
	> 5.7	> 5.7
BVDV (model for HCV)	> 6.5	> 6.2
PRV (model for HBV)	5.1	5.8
MMV (model for PVB19)	0.5	0.4

Biochemical Characterization of IMMUNATE S/D

In order to verify that S/D treatment had not caused significant structural or quantitative alteration to the FVIII molecule, the protein profiles of IMMUNATE S/D and IMMUNATE were compared biochemically as described below.

Protein Composition of Process Intermediates Before Heat Treatment
In order to determine whether any modification of the FVIII protein composition had occurred, process intermediates derived from the manufacture of IMMUNATE S/D and IMMUNATE before the heat treatment step were compared in terms of protein composition. Protein composition was measured using cellulose acetate electrophoresis (CAE). The study demonstrated that there was no difference between the protein composition of the IMMUNATE S/D and IMMUNATE process intermediates before heat treatment.

Profile of Protein Composition in the Final Product
The goal of this study was to compare the protein composition of IMMUNATE S/D with IMMUNATE. The protein composition of six batches of final containers of IMMUNATE S/D, derived from three different final process intermediates, were compared with the protein composition of 46 IMMUNATE batches produced in 2001. Protein composition was measured using CAE. The study showed that there was no difference between the protein composition in IMMUNATE S/D and IMMUNATE.

Chromatographic Analysis
IMMUNATE S/D and IMMUNATE were profiled on the basis of their molecular weights and the quantities of protein in each weight-separated fraction. High-performance size exclusion chromatography (HP-SEC) was performed under isocratic conditions in order to allow the simultaneous determination of the molecular weights and quantities of the separated components. Four batches each of IMMUNATE S/D and IMMUNATE were compared. Neither quantitative nor qualitative differences were observed.

Product Comparison by 2D-Electrophoresis
IMMUNATE S/D and IMMUNATE were compared based on structure and electrical charge using 2D-electrophoresis. Three batches each of IMMUNATE S/D and IMMUNATE were analyzed. A computational comparison showed no difference between

the spot patterns of IMMUNATE S/D and IMMUNATE, indicating that the two did not differ in terms of protein composition.

To verify that S/D treatment did not alter FVIII potency and functional integrity, several studies were used to characterize and compare these properties for IMMUNATE S/D and IMMUNATE.

Potency and Structure of Active Ingredients
The structural integrity of the active ingredients of IMMUNATE S/D, FVIII and vWF, was examined using several methods:
1. electrophoretic techniques and immunoblotting;
2. measurement of FVIII and vWF antigen content;
3. functional assays of FVIII;
4. functional assays of vWF activity, using the collagen-binding (vWF:CB) and ristocetin cofactor (vWF:RCo) methods, and
5. vWF multimer analyses. Six batches of IMMUNATE S/D were compared with eleven batches of IMMUNATE.

Electrophoretic separation, immunoblotting and detection of FVIII with polyclonal and with monoclonal antibodies (directed against the heavy chain of FVIII) allowed visual comparison of the FVIII-specific polypeptide bands present in IMMUNATE S/D and IMMUNATE. All major FVIII-specific bands were similar for IMMUNATE S/D and IMMUNATE.

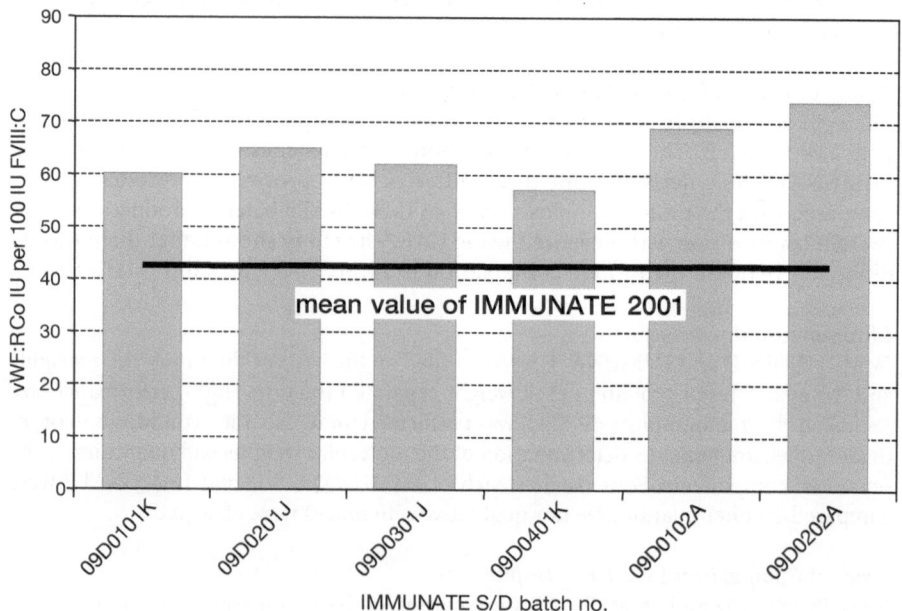

Fig. 2. Content of vWF:RCo activity of IMMUNATE S/D in comparison to IMMUNATE. The bar represents the mean of vWF:RCo activity of IMMUNATE manufactured in 2001.

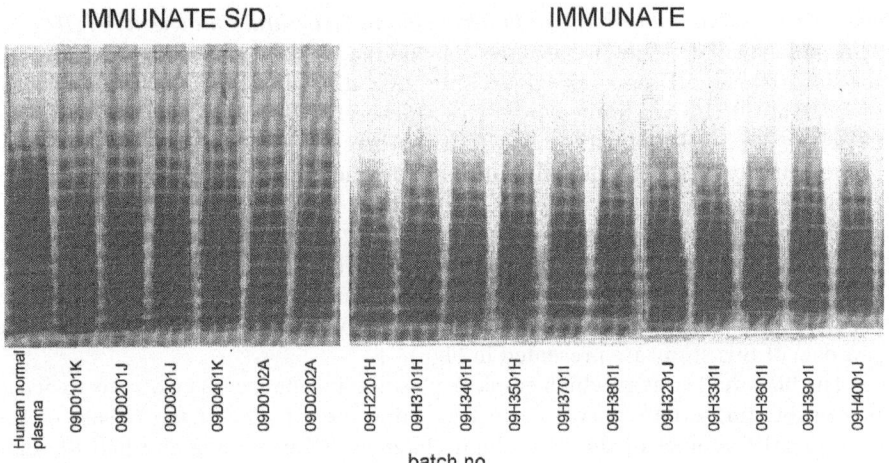

IMMUNATE S/D   IMMUNATE

batch no.

Fig. 3. IMMUNATE S/D (09D) multimer analysis (1% agarose) in comparison to randomly chosen batches of IMMUNATE (09H).

Factor VIII:C activities and factor VIII antigen levels did not differ between IMMUNATE S/D and IMMUNATE. In addition, the ratio of factor VIII antigen to FVIII:C activity was indistinguishable for the two products. VWF antigen potency, ristocetin cofactor activity and collagen binding activity were measured. For the collagen-binding test, two different assays were used: one applying type III collagen from human placenta and one using type I collagen from an equine source. The vWF:RCo assay results are shown in Figure 2.

When compared to the current IMMUNATE product vWF activity, parameters were higher than the mean value observed in 46 batches of IMMUNATE. However, all results were not above the maximum level measured in the 46 batches of the IMMUNATE product indicating a trend towards increased vWF activity in IMMU-NATE S/D within the range of the current product.

These results were also reflected by the multimer analyses, where the six batches of IMMUNATE S/D investigated showed a relatively constant level of vWF multimers with more bands in the higher molecular mass range of multimers when compared to randomly chosen IMMUNATE batches (Fig. 3).

Characterization of FVIII Function as a Cofactor of Factor IXa
IMMUNATE S/D and IMMUNATE were compared in terms of the functional competency of FVIII to serve as a cofactor of factor IXa and thereby to participate in the Xase complex. The time course of factor X activation was studied both with and without FVIII activation by thrombin.

No differences were observed in the kinetic parameters of Xase-complex formation for IMMUNATE S/D versus IMMUNATE, showing that S/D treatment did not affect FVIII's ability to participate in the assembly of the Xase complex.

Assessment of Thrombin-induced Functional and Structural Changes in FVIII
Thrombin-mediated functional activation and inactivation of FVIII were compared
for IMMUNATE S/D and IMMUNATE. In vivo, thrombin mediates the activation
of FVIII to FVIIIa via limited proteolysis. Several proteolytic cleavage events are
necessary for FVIII activation, in which the inactive FVIII dimer converts to an
active heterotrimer. Subsequently, thrombin degrades activated FVIII further, inactivating it.

Electrophoretic analysis and immunoblotting with specific antibodies against
FVIII were used to analyze 3 batches each of IMMUNATE S/D and IMMUNATE.
Immunoblots were scanned using a calibrated scanner and analyzed using image
processing software to perform a quantitative analysis of the cleavage products. The
raw data of this study are presented in Figure 4.

The Biacore™ system, which employs plasmon resonance spectroscopy to detect
protein-binding events, was used to determine the kinetics of the release of the
N-terminal fragment of the FVIII light chain. The time course and half-life data
were equivalent for IMMUNATE S/D and IMMUNATE, supporting the conclusion
that the conformational structures of FVIII for the two products are equivalent
throughout the activation process. In addition, no differences were found in the time
course of activation and inactivation of FVIII, nor in the kinetic parameters of the
thrombin-catalyzed proteolysis of FVIII.

Biomolecular Interaction Studies Using FVIII Specific Antibodies
The Biacore™ system was used to characterize the FVIII affinity of 3 batches of
IMMUNATE S/D and IMMUNATE, by measuring the binding kinetics of 4 domain-
specific monoclonal antibodies to the FVIII molecule. The results of this study are
presented in Table 4.
The two products did not differ in terms of their rates of association or dissociation, nor the affinity constants and dissociation constants of the FVIII-antibody
interaction. These data further support the conclusion that S/D treatment did not
affect the structural integrity of the FVIII.

Table 4. IMMUNATE S/D – Biomolecular interaction studies using monoclonal antibodies
(Biacore)

	Product	ka (1/Ms)	Kinetic Parameters kd (1/s)	KA (1/M)	KD (M)
MoAb-530	IMMUNATE	5.66E+05	2.84E-03	2.02E+08	5.24E-09
(A2 domain)	IMMUNATE S/D	5.32E+05	2.35E-03	2.59E+08	4.55E-09
MoAb-8860	IMMUNATE	4.04E+05	1.51E-04	7.99E+09	3.34E-10
(A2 domain)	IMMUNATE S/D	4.19E+05	3.09E-04	3.33E+09	7.83E-10
MoAb-532	IMMUNATE	3.09E+05	1.84E-04	7.54E+09	5.63E-10
(A2 domain)	IMMUNATE S/D	3.45E+05	4.04E-04	9.64E+08	1.04E-09
MoAb-10104	IMMUNATE	7.13E+05	2.83E-04	2.83E+09	3.91E-10
(A2 domain)	IMMUNATE S/D	7.31E+05	2.28E-04	1.87E+11	2.66E-10

→ *No relevant differences between IMMUNATE and IMMUNATE S/D*

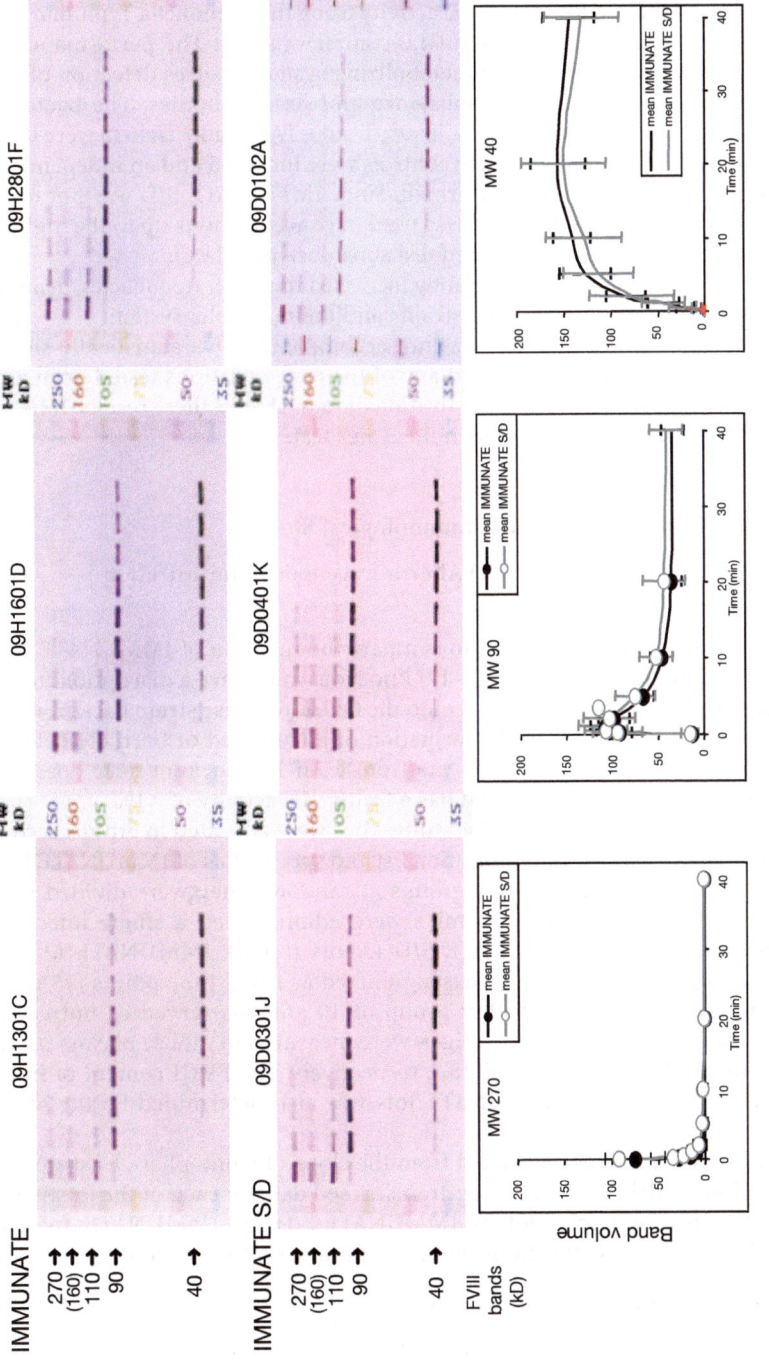

Time course: 0 (before thrombin) and 0.25, 0.5, 1, 2, 5, 10, 20 40 minutes

Fig. 4. IMMUNATE S/D – Assessment of thrombin-induced functional and structural changes of FVIII. Kinetics of thrombin (1 nM) cleavage of FVIII heavy chain detected by anti-human FVIII A2 mab.

Mutagenicity

IMMUNATE S/D was tested for mutagenic activity using the Salmonella Typhimurium Reverse Mutation Test (Ames test) in a GLP-compliant study. The performance of the test with and without an external metabolizing system ensures detection of the mutagenic activity of both the test substance and its metabolites. The bacterial strains Salmonella typhimurium TA 97a, TA98, TA100, TA102 and TA1535 were used as the test system. Negative and positive controls were included and an independent repetition of the experiment was performed. Since IMMUNATE S/D was not toxic to any of the bacterial strains tested, it was used in concentrations up to the highest possible amount (100 μl of the undiluted test substance per plate).

All positive controls showed significantly increased mutation frequencies, demonstrating the sensitivity of the bacterial strains and the metabolic system.

IMMUNATE S/D administration was not accompanied by a statistically significant increase in mutation frequency at any of the concentrations tested or in any of the bacteria strains used. Metabolic activation did not change these results. IMMUNATE S/D is therefore non-mutagenic in the Ames test.

Pharmacological, Toxicological and Immunological Studies

Pharmacokinetics of IMMUNATE S/D After Intravenous Administration in Factor VIII (E-17) Knockout Mice

A hemophilic mouse model was used to compare the function of IMMUNATE S/D and IMMUNATE in vivo. Factor VIII (E-17) knockout mice have a disruption in the exon-17 portion of the FVIII gene (bred onto the C57/Bl6 mouse strain background) [11]. This disrupted gene leads to the formation of a truncated or partially deleted protein, causing a FVIII deficiency. Plasma from exon-17 knockout mice does not contain detectable FVIII light chain and has a factor VIII activity of <1%.

A total of 360 mice were used in this study. Mice were allocated to groups according to a computer generated randomization list and specific lots of IMMUNATE S/D or IMMUNATE were assigned to the groups at random. They were divided into 5 groups of 70 mice each. These 70 mice were administered a single injection of 500 IU/kg i.v. of either IMMUNATE S/D (3 lots tested), IMMUNATE (2 lots tested). 10 out of these 70 mice were exsanguinated at 1 of 7 time points (15 min, 1 h, 2 h, 3 h, 6 h, 9 h, 24 h). Another group of 10 animals served as untreated controls. Human FVIII activity and antigen were measured in mouse plasma using a chromogenic FVIII assay and an ELISA, respectively. The FVIII content of individual IMMUNATE S/D and IMMUNATE lots was also determined by the same methods.

The half-life of FVIII was calculated from the slope of a one-phase least square linear regression model, fitted to the log-transformed data for each of the lots separately, as well as for the pooled lots of IMMUNATE S/D and IMMUNATE. In vivo recovery (IVR [%]) was calculated using the 15-minute samples as follows:

$$\text{IVR } [\%] = \frac{(C_{max}\,[\text{IU/dl}] - C_{pre}\,[\text{IU/dl}]) \times PV\,[\text{dl}]}{\text{dose}\,[\text{IU}]} \times 100$$

Table 5. Pharmacokinetics of IMMUNATE S/D. Half-life (h) and in vivo recovery (%) for factor VIII antigen

	Half-life (h)	95% CI*	IVR (%)	95% CI*
IMMUNATE S/D	6.6	5.7–7.5	43.8	41.6–48.1
IMMUNATE	6.2	5.3–7.1	41.5	37.1–49.9
Difference	0.4	−0.8–1.5	2.3	−3.3– 8.5

* Confidence Interval

The pharmacokinetic parameters of IMMUNATE S/D and IMMUNATE were statistically not significantly different (Table 5).

Acute Toxicity in Mice

Acute toxicity levels of IMMUNATE S/D and IMMUNATE were assessed in male and female mice. Mice were assigned to 16 experimental groups of 10 mice (5 males and 5 females) per group (total n = 160). Mice in each group received a single intravenous injection of one of the following: IMMUNATE S/D (from 1 of 3 lots); IMMUNATE (from 1 lot); formulation buffer; or isotonic saline. IMMUNATE S/D and IMMUNATE were administered at doses of 2000, 5000, and 10000 IU/kg. Formulation buffer was administered at volumes of 20, 50, and 100 ml/kg (equivalent to the amount of buffer present in 2000, 5000, and 10000 IU/kg doses of drug product, respectively). Isotonic saline was administered at a volume of 100 ml/kg.

The mice were observed for 14 days for clinical symptoms including unusual behavior. The animals were weighed at days 0, 7, and 14 to provide an indication of general health, and the numbers of deaths were recorded. At the end of the observation period the surviving animals were killed by CO_2 inhalation and examined for pathological findings.

There was no difference in body mass development between mice treated with IMMUNATE S/D versus IMMUNATE. 2 of 30 animals that died after injection of 10000 IU/kg IMMUNATE S/D showed edema of the lungs and cardiac dilatation. Although lung hemorrhages were frequently found in animals killed at the end of the study, they were assumed not to be related to the injection of the test article because such hemorrhages frequently occur in animals killed by CO_2 inhalation. The »No Observed Adverse Effect Level« (NOAEL) for this study in mice was ≥ 2000 IU/kg for IMMUNATE S/D as well as for the IMMUNATE lot tested.

Acute Toxicity in Rats

Acute toxicity levels of IMMUNATE S/D and IMMUNATE were assessed in male and female rats. Rats were assigned to 6 experimental groups of 10 rats (5 males and 5 females) per group (n = 60). Rats in each group received a single intravenous injection of one of the following: IMMUNATE S/D (from 1 of 3 lots); IMMUNATE (from 1 lot); formulation buffer; or isotonic saline. IMMUNATE S/D and IMMUNATE were administered at a dose of 2000 IU/kg. Formulation buffer and isotonic saline were administered at a volume equivalent to that contained in a dose of 2000 IU/kg of

IMMUNATE. (Based on the limit test, 20 mL/kg was the maximum volume feasible as a bolus injection in rats.)

The rats were observed for 14 days for clinical symptoms including unusual behavior. The animals were weighed at days 0, 7, and 14 to provide an indication of general health. At the end of the observation period the animals were killed by CO_2 inhalation and examined for pathological findings.

No statistically significant influence of IMMUNATE S/D, IMMUNATE, or the formulation buffer on the growth rate could be detected during the 14 days of observation after injection. The only pathological findings were frequent lung hemorrhages distributed equally over all groups, but these were assumed not to be related to the test article because such lung hemorrhages frequently occur in animals killed by CO_2 inhalation. The »No Observed Adverse Effect Level« (NOAEL) in this study was equal or greater than 2000 IU/kg for both IMMUNATE S/D and IMMUNATE.

Local Tolerance in Rabbits

The local tolerance of IMMUNATE S/D was tested after intra-arterial, intravenous and paravenous application in rabbits. Three lots of IMMUNATE S/D were compared with one lot of IMMUNATE, or formulation buffer. Each of the five items was either infused (2 minutes) intra-arterially or intravenously both at a volume of 10 ml, or injected paravenously at a volume of 0.5 ml into the right ear of each of 4 rabbits (2 males and 2 females), resulting in a total of 60 rabbits. An equivalent volume of isotonic saline was given as a negative control to the left ear by the same route. The target concentration of the drugs was 100 IU/ml.

The behavior of the animals was observed and the injection sites examined macroscopically for changes for the first 30 minutes after treatment, intermittently thereafter up to 6 h, and again at 24 h, 48 h, and 72 h.

For histopathological examination, tissue sections were collected from the following areas: a site distal to the injection site and one at the tip of the ear supplied by the artery after intra-arterial application; a site proximal to the injection site after intravenous application; and the injection site after paravenous application. After sectioning and staining, the sections were examined microscopically. Histopathological evaluation focused on damage to the endothelium for intra-arterial and intravenous routes of administration. Perivascular inflammation of connective tissue was evaluated for all three routes of administration. For the intra-arterial infusion route, both the artery itself and the supply area (tip of the ear) were examined. Each observation was quantified according to a scoring system.

No alterations in behavior were seen in the animals during the observation period. Macroscopic and microscopic examinations of the injection sites showed virtually no pathological alterations in any group, demonstrating that local tolerance was equivalent for IMMUNATE S/D and IMMUNATE.

Immunogenicity in Hemophilic Mice

This study compared the immunogenicity of IMMUNATE S/D and IMMUNATE in FVIII (E-17) knockout mice [12, 13, 14] as outlined in Figure 5.

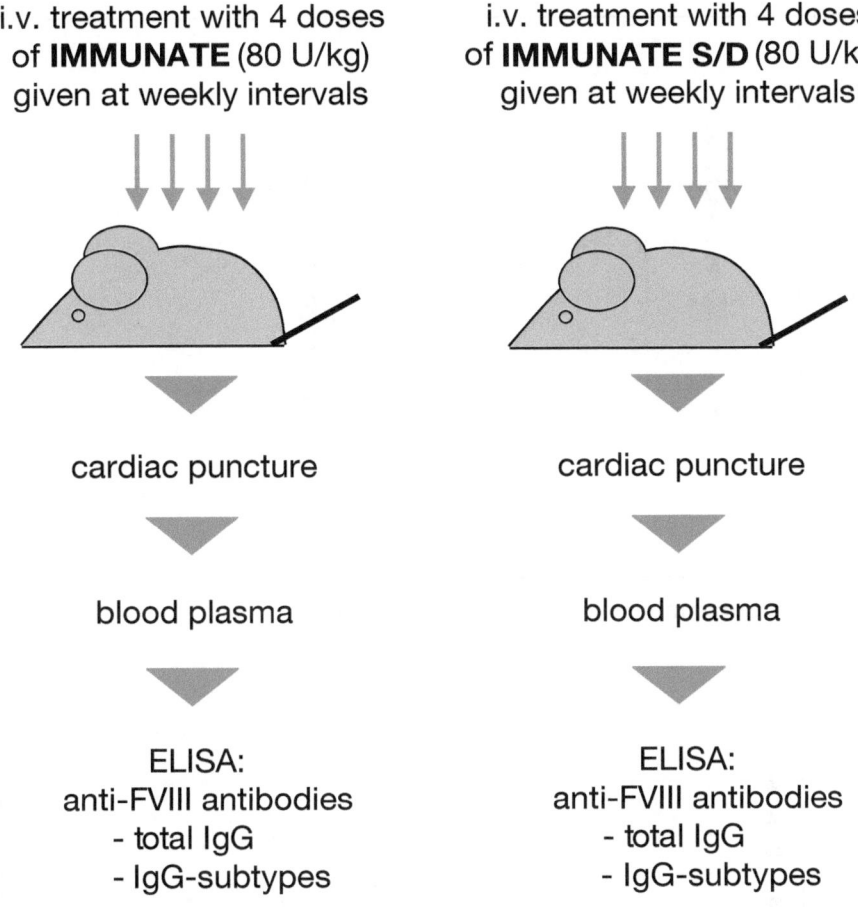

i.v. treatment with 4 doses
of **IMMUNATE** (80 U/kg)
given at weekly intervals

i.v. treatment with 4 doses
of **IMMUNATE S/D** (80 U/kg)
given at weekly intervals

cardiac puncture

cardiac puncture

blood plasma

blood plasma

ELISA:
anti-FVIII antibodies
- total IgG
- IgG-subtypes

ELISA:
anti-FVIII antibodies
- total IgG
- IgG-subtypes

Fig. 5. Immunogenicity model for IMMUNATE S/D. Methods for immunization and analyses.

The study compared three lots of IMMUNATE S/D (n = 20 per group) and three lots of IMMUNATE (n = 20 per group), in a total of 120 mice.

Each item was injected intravenously at 80 IU/kg once weekly for four weeks. One week after the last treatment, mice were exsanguinated by heart puncture. From the plasma samples obtained, five variables were measured using ELISA assays: the total anti-FVIII antibody titer and that of four IgG subclasses, IgG1, IgG2a, IgG2b and IgG3. The results of the immunological studies are shown in Figures 6A, B.

Statistical analysis of all data was performed. No significant differences were observed between the three lots of IMMUNATE S/D and the three lots of IMMUN-ATE. Both the total anti-FVIII antibody titers and the IgG-subclass distribution of anti-FVIII antibodies were equivalent for IMMUNATE S/D and IMMUNATE. In summary, IMMUNATE S/D and IMMUNATE did not differ regarding their immunogenicity in knockout mice.

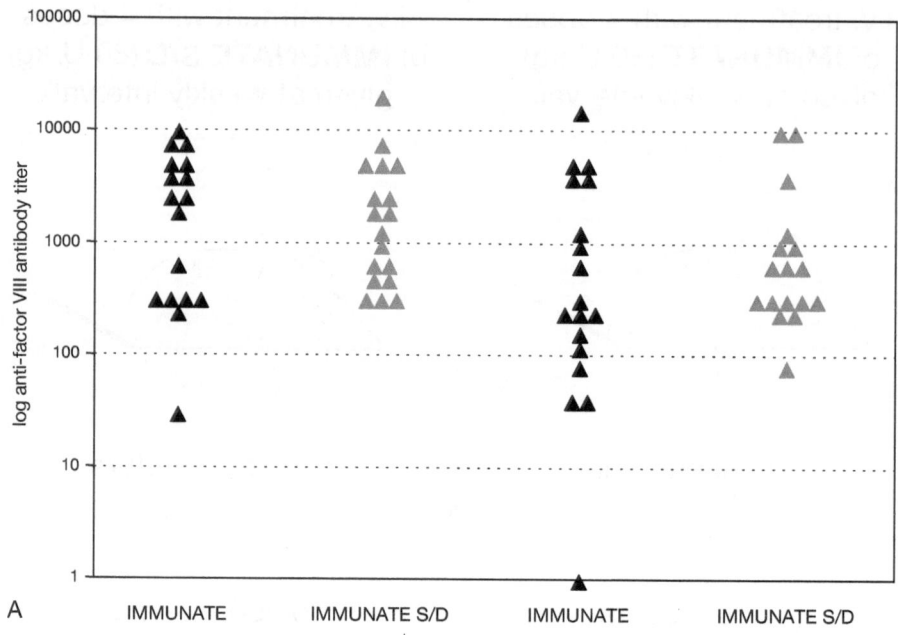

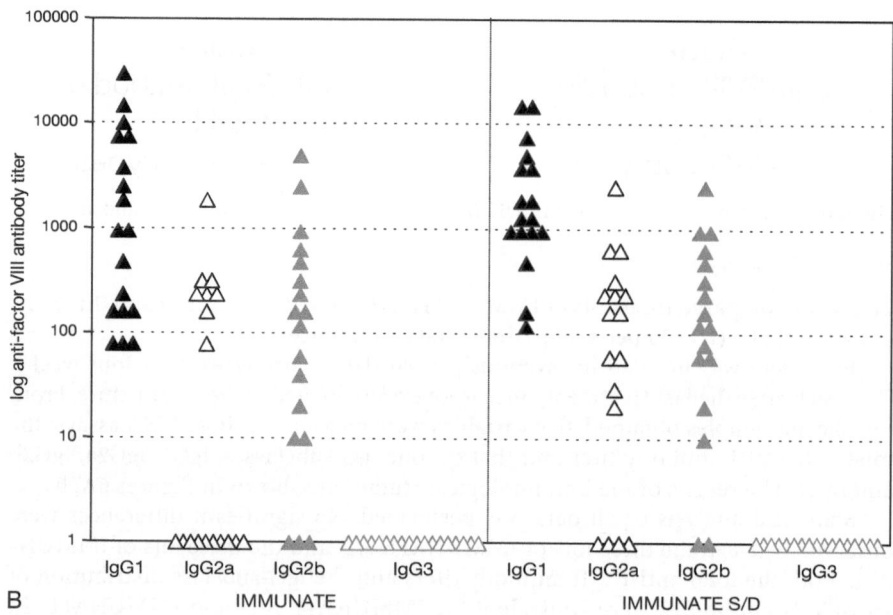

Fig. 6. Immunogenicity of IMMUNATE S/D and IMMUNATE (each 4 doses of 80 U FVIII/kg).
A) Comparison of antibody titers B) Comparison of IgG subclass titers.

Summary

Ongoing concerns about the potential for viral contamination of plasma-derived coagulation FVIII concentrates have been the impetus for continual increases in the level of plasma screening and virus inactivation of Baxter's plasma-derived FVIII concentrates. These improvements go beyond the requirements laid down in the respective regulations by including, in addition, PCR testing for HIV-1/HIV-2, HCV, HBV, HAV, and PVB19 (vWF complex). Thus, for its next generation coagulation FVIII-vWF complex concentrate product, IMMUNATE S/D, Baxter has replaced the polysorbate 80-virus inactivation step with a more robust solvent-detergent (S/D) virus inactivation step. The complete purification process for IMMUNATE S/D includes purification by ion exchange chromatography, S/D treatment and vapor heat treatment. These treatments are used to decrease the risk of transmission of lipid-enveloped and non-enveloped, blood-borne viruses. The final product is a lyophilized formulation of plasma-derived FVIII concentrate provided in 250, 500, and 1000 IU/vial.

In vitro studies demonstrated that the introduction of conventional S/D reagents does not alter the structure or function of the FVIII molecule. In addition, characterization of the vWF content in IMMUNATE S/D demonstrated an increase in vWF content and activity.

Additional in vitro and in vivo nonclinical studies demonstrated the safety profile of IMMUNATE S/D. None of the product lots of IMMUNATE S/D differed from IMMUNATE with regard to immunogenicity, mutagenicity, acute toxicity, or local tolerance. Virus safety studies have demonstrated a significant (four-log reduction, or greater) clearance of HIV and HAV, as well as of model viruses for HCV and PRV and thus an excellent safety record against lipid- and non-lipid enveloped viruses.

Previous human experience with Baxter's currently licensed product, IMMUNATE, and the bioequivalence of IMMUNATE S/D and IMMUNATE in preclinical, biochemical, immunological, pharmacological and toxicological studies demonstrated that safety and efficacy profiles of IMMUNATE S/D are consistent with those reported in the medical literature and supports conductance of a phase III clinical trial for treatment of patients with hemophilia A.

References

1. Brettler DB, Levine PH. Factor concentrates for treatment of hemophilia: which one to choose? Blood 1989; 73: 2067–2073
2. Mannucci PM. The choice of plasma-derived clotting factor concentrates. Baillieres Clin Haematol 1996; 9: 273–290
3. Rodgers GM, Greenberg CS. Inherited coagulation disorders. In: Lee GR, Foerster J, Lukens J, Paraskevas F, Greer JP, Rodgers GM, eds. Vol. 2: Wintrobe's Clinical Hematology. Baltimore, MD: Lippincott Williams & Wilkins; 1999: 1682–1732
4. Eriksson B, Westman L, Jernberg M. Virus validation of plasma-derived products produced by Pharmacia, with particular reference to immunoglobulins. Blood Coagul Fibrinolysis 1994; 5 (Suppl 3): S37–S44
5. Barrett PN, Meyer H, Wachtel I, Eibl J, Dorner F. Determination of the inactivation kinetics of hepatitis A virus in human plasma products using a simple TCID50 assay. J Med Virol 1996; 49: 1–6

6. Mannucci PM, Schimpf K, Abe T, Aledort LM, Anderle K, Brettler DB, Hilgartner MW, Kernoff PBA, Kunschak M, McMillan CW, Preston FE, Rivard GE. Low risk of viral infection after administration of vapor-heated factor VIII concentrate. Transfusion 1992; 32: 134–138

7. Mannucci PM. Clinical evaluation of viral safety of coagulation factor VIII and IX concentrates. Vox Sang 1993; 64: 197–203

8. Shapiro A, Abe T, Aledort LM, Anderle K, Hilgartner MW, Kunschak M, Preston FE, Rivard GE, Schimpf K and The International Factor Safety Study Group. Low risk of viral infection after administration of vapor-heated factor VII concentrate or factor IX complex in first-time recipients of blood components. Transfusion 1995; 35: 204–208

9. Horowitz B, Bonomo R, Prince AM, Chin SN, Brotman B, Shulman RW. Solvent/detergent-treated plasma: a virus-inactivated substitute for fresh frozen plasma. Blood 1992; 79: 826–831

10. Committee for Proprietary Medicinal Products (CPMP) Note for Guidance on Virus Validation Studies: The Design, Contribution and Interpretation of Studies Validating the Inactivation and Removal of Viruses. CPMP/BWP/268/95. 1996. London, European Agency for the Evaluation of Medicinal Products.

11. Bi L, Lawler AM, Antonarakis SE, High KA, Gearhart JD, Kazazian HH, Jr. Targeted disruption of the mouse factor VIII gene produces a model of haemophilia A. Nat Genet 1995; 10: 119–121

12. Reipert BM, Ahmad RU, Turecek PL, Schwarz HP. Characterization of antibodies induced by human factor VIII in a murine knockout model of hemophilia A. Thromb Haemost 2000; 84 (5): 826–832

13. Muchitsch EM, Pichler L, Turecek PL, Gritsch H, Richter G, Auer W, Schwarz HP. Charakterisierung der Faktor VIII-knockout-Maus für den Einsatz in der biomedizinischen Forschung (Characterization of FVIII knockout mice: A new tool in biomedical research). Wien Tierärztl Mschr 1999; 86: 339–346

14. Muchitsch EM, Auer W, Pichler L, Turecek PL, Zimmermann K, Richter G, Gritsch H, Schwarz HP. Phenotypic expression of murine haemophilia – Letter to the Editor. Thromb Haemost 1999; 82 (4): 1371–1373

Favorable Response to Protein C in Venoocclusive Disease after Allogeneous Stem Cell Transplantation

S. Eber, F. Scherer, and T. Güngör

Introduction

Hepatic venoocclusive disease (VOD; syn: sinusoidal obstruction syndrome) may be a severe, lethal early complication after stem cell transplantation (SCT) (Table 1; frequency of 24% in our patient cohort [see also 2, 8]. VOD-»Baltimore« criteria include an increase of bilirubin >2 mg/dl (34 mmol/l) and 2 of the following criteria: hepatomegaly, ascites and gain of weight of >5% (Table 2). In confounding cases the demonstration of hepatofugal portal vein blood flow by abdominal ultrasound with doppler may prove the diagnosis. The underlying pathomechanism is an endothelial damage of small liver sinusoids and the surrounding centrilobular hepatocytes due to alkylating chemotherapeutics e.g. busulfan and cyclophosphamide. The primary lesion is deformation of sinusoidal endothelial cells which are detached from the basement membrane and disappear from the liver sinusoids. As damage progresses, most of the obstruction of sinusoidal blood flow is from extracellular matrix generated by Kupffer cells [4].

Table 1. Sinusoidal obstruction syndrome (VOD) after stem cell transplantation (SCT)

- Frequency in children: 24% (BMT Unit, Children's Hosp. Zurich; n = 45, 1998–2002)
- Pathophysiology:
  Primary: Damage of sinusoidal endothelial cells and surrounding liver cells, stasis by edema.
  Secondary: Microthrombi, ischemia, portal hypertension, hepatorenal syndrome, multisystem organ failure
- Risk factors: preexisting liver disease (hepatitis, fibrosis); irradiation, busulfan

Table 2. Symptoms: modified Baltimore criteria

- Unexplained Icterus, bilirubin > 2mg/dl
- Rapid gain of weight of 5%
- Ascites
- Hepatomegaly, in US: hepatofugal flow
- Renal dysfunction, oliguria
- Fulminant liver failure, liver capsule pain
- Encephalopathy
- Letality 5% (up to 100% for severe VOD)

I. Scharrer/W. Schramm (Ed.)
33rd Hemophilia Symposion Hamburg 2002
© Springer-Verlag Berlin Heidelberg 2004

There is little evidence that VOD is primarily a thrombotic process; in an animal model of this disease, there were no ultrastructure findings of a thrombotic process. Remarkably, in more advanced disease fibrinolytic therapy has resolved the obstruction [5, 7], indicating that in those severe cases thrombosis of small liver veins may play a role (Table 1).

Roughly 80% of patients with VOD have complete resolution of signs and symptoms without requiring any specific therapy. However mortality comes up to 100% at day +100 after SCT in severe cases [9]. Recently, trials with defibrotide showed promising results in severe VOD and multi-system organ failure [3, 10]. We report the results of protein C (PC) addition in two patients with moderate and severe VOD that did not resolve by defibrotide therapy.

Drug description and application device

We used protein C concentrate (Ceprotin; Baxter BioScience) produced from human source plasma via different chromatographical procedures including an immunoaffinity step, the production process including two viral inactivation procedures with independent mode of action (tween 80, vapour heat treatment). Source plasma has been PCR tested for HIV, HAV, HBV, HCV and parvovirus B 19. Stability of the protein after dissolution has been demonstrated for 4 days making it suitable to be used for continuous infusion [11]. Protein C was administered as a bolus of 100 IU/kg initially, followed by continuous infusion of 200 IU/kg/day (divided in four equal doses) (Table 3).

Table 3. Protein C substitution for VOD after BMT

- Highly purified plasmatic non activated Protein C concentrate (Ceprotin®, Baxter)
- Initial bolus 100 IU/kg
- Continuous infusion 200 IU/kg/day in 4 x until stop of symptoms

Results

Patient 1 (E.G, Swiss, now 1.75 y) (Table 4) suffered from an acute myelogenous leukemia of early infancy [megakaryoblastic form, M7 according to international FAB classification with translocation [t (1; 22)]. After complete first remission by conventional chemotherapy (BFM-AML Protocol) an allogeneic stem cell transplantation with a matched unrelated donor was performed. Conditioning comprised liposomal busulfan i.v. (total dose 20 mg/kg, delivered on days – 12 to – 8), etoposide with 45 mg/kg (on day – 7) and cyclophosphamide (2 x 60 mg/kg; day – 6 and – 5). As VOD prophylaxis the patient received a low dose heparin (100 IU/kg) and antithrombin (AT) substitution (if levels below 70%). Two weeks after delivering the transplant the patient got a CMV infection with early antigen being detected in blood and increased transaminases, leading to grade 3–4 severe skin and probably liver graft vs host disease. At that time he also developed severe VOD with weight gain (25%), hepatomegaly, mas-

Table 4. Patient 1 (AML; 1,75 y.)

Postnatal	AML M7 [t (1; 22)]; full remission after chemotherapy (AML-BFM 98)
1 year	MUD-BMT (liposomal busulfan i.v., 20 mg/kg; VP 16; 45 mg/kg); cyclophosphamide 120 mg/kg
Days post Transplant + 14	Primary CMV-Hepato- infection, liver transaminases ↑; severe skin Graft vs host disease (3°–4°)
	VOD: Weight ↑ (25%); hepatomegaly; consumption of thrombocytes ↑↑

sive ascites and severe thrombocytopenia requiring up to twice daily transfusion. Bilirubin was elevated to 300 mmol/l (Fig. 1). Doppler ultrasound showed a reversed hepatoportal venous blood flow. Therapy with defibrotide (60 mg/kg) was started immediately. Nevertheless, the pulmonary situation deteriorated rapidly with an oxygen demand. Defibrotide was stopped after 5 days. Thrombolytic therapy using rTPA and a continuous PC substitution (initial PC level 16%) were started. Lysis therapy had to be abandoned due to respiratory tract bleeding. Global coagulation (PT 34%, aPTT 250 sec) and PC level normalized within hours after PC application (Table 7). A normal hepatopetal portal flow could be achieved by high dose defibrotide (120 mg/kg) and continued PC substitution over several weeks (Fig. 1).

Patient 2 (M.K, Iraqi, 11 y) (Table 4) suffered from beta-thalassemia major with secondary severe hemosiderosis, as well as chronic persisting hepatitis C infection with liver fibrosis. He received a matched related bone marrow alloSCT, using liposomal busulfan i.v., reduced cyclophosphamide dose and fludarabine. VOD prophylaxis comprised heparin and AT as in patient 1; in addition, he got prophylactical defibrotide (20 mg/kg) and N-acetylcysteine (100 mg/kg i.v., 3 h after end of each busulfan infusion). Two weeks after transplantation he developed moderate to severe VOD (weight gain of 10%; maximal bilirubin level of 30 mmol/l and reversed portal venous blood flow proven by Doppler ultrasound. He showed a temporary improvement under defibrotide treatment. Due to clinical deterioration (hepatic pain, increased ascites) and low PC level (38%; see Table 6) a continuous PC substitution (50 IU/kg

Table 5. Patient 2 (Thalassaemia major; 11 y.)

2¹/₂ y.	Iraqi; diagnosis of thalassemia major; since then regularly transfusions
7 y.	Severe hemosiderosis, chronic hepatitis C with transaminases ↑ and liver fibrosis, start of desferal
11 y.	HLA genoidentical sc BMT (from father), busulfan i.v. (14 mg/kg); fludarabine (100 mg/sqm); cyclophosphamide (90 mg/kg in 4 doses)
Day +6 post transplant	VOD: Weight ↑; hepatomegaly; ascites; consumption of thrombocytes ↑↑; Defibrotide ↑ (60–80 mg/kg); Solumedrol;
Day +13	ascites ↑; general state of health ↓ ; coagulation ↓ : application of Protein C

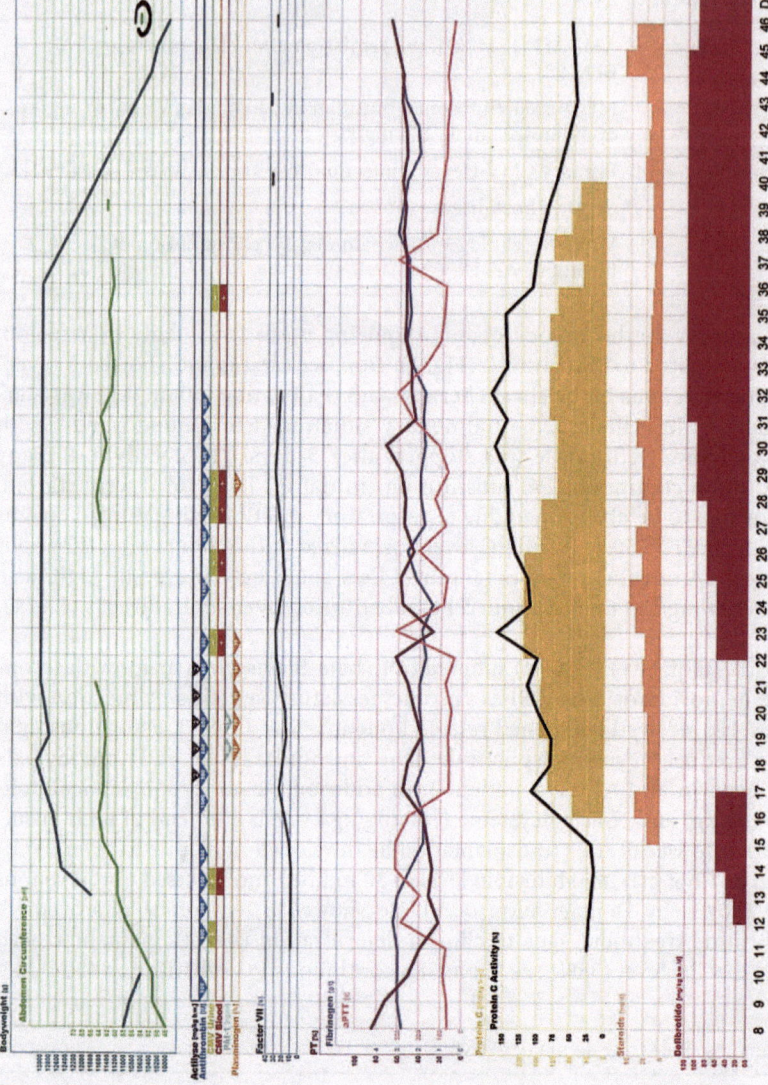

Fig. 1. Severe VOD after SCT for AML (patient 1): body measures, global coagulation parameters [prothrombin time (PT; after Quick), activated partial thromboplastin time (aPTT) and fibrinogen level], coagulation factors (factor VII, plasminogen and plasminogen activator inhibitor (PAI-1); and data on therapy with protein C, defibrotide (given as I.U per kg and day) as well as tissue plasminogen activator (actilyse). Note the inital low levels of protein C and the rise of plasminogen, factor VII and prothrombin time under protein C substitution. Antithrombin levels were kept above 100% by repeated substitution. Steroids had to be added because of severe graft vs host disease. VOD and GVHD were probably triggered by severe cytomegaly infection in this patient with CMV virus being proven in urine on day 11 after transplantation. Days after transplant are given on X – axis.

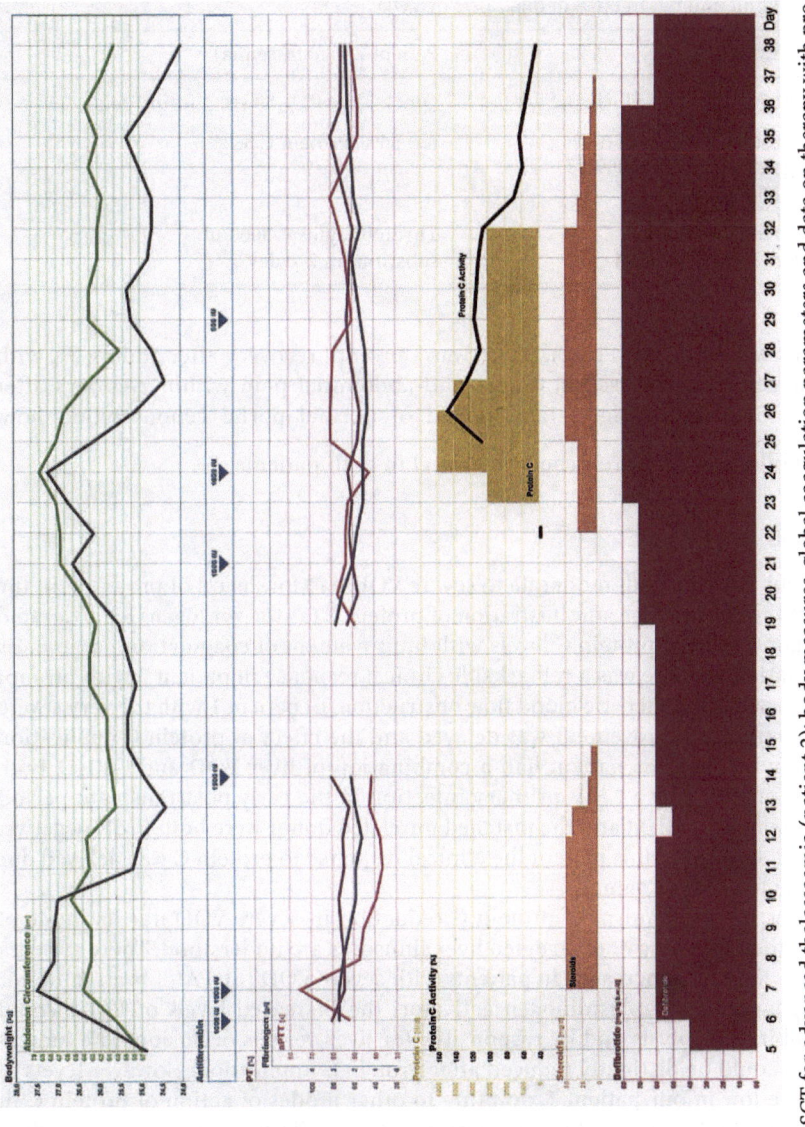

Fig. 2. Moderate VOD after SCT for advanced thalassaemia (patient 2): body measures, global coagulation parameters and data on therapy with protein C (given as total dose of I.U. per day) and defibrotide. Note the immediate decrease of abdominal circumference and body weight after start of protein C therapy. Protein C levels were low before the treatment and distintly rose afterwards. Steroids were added for treatment of the inflammatory reaction in liver VOD. Antithrombin levels were kept above 100% by repeated substitution. Days after transplant are given on X-axis.

Table 6. Coagulation parameters at diagnosis of VOD

Patient 1 (AML)	Patient 2 (Thalassemia)
Quick 21%; PTT 283 sec; Fibrin 3,2 g/l	Quick 53%; PTT 52 sec; Fibrin 1,5 g/l
AT: 71%; Protein C 16%; F VII 9% Plasminogen 23%, PAI-1: 208%; D-dimer 1,88 µg/l	AT: 56%, Protein C 38%
Thrombocytes < 5000/µl; substitution 2 x/day	Thrombocytes < 3000/µl; substitution 2 x/day

every 6 h) was initiated (Fig. 2). There was a prompt recovery after adding PC with dramatic reduction of ascites, weight and abdominal pain within 2–3 days after start of PC infusion (Fig. 2) and return of normal portal venous blood flow.

Elevated bilirubin levels returned to normal in both patients.

Discussion

Both of our patients with moderate to severe VOD had low levels of protein C in the course of the disease. The administration of protein C (as the zymogen) led to a rapid and sustained rise of protein C levels with improvement of coagulation parameters in both patients. There was a remarkable clinical response in patient 2 with prompt resolution of signs of hepatic blood flow obstruction. In patient 1 with the very severe form the clinical improvement was delayed and the effect of protein C application is less convincing. This patient had a combination of liver VOD and GVHD, both triggered probably by a CMV primary infection in the early posttransplant period since initially the patient and the matched unrelated donor were both CMV negative. It may well be, that in this patient the clinical response to protein C was delayed due to multifactorial liver damage.

Neither the mechanism of protein C reduction in severe VOD nor its mode of action in the reopening of obstructed liver sinusoids are understood. There are data that PAI-1 levels are increased in patients with severe VOD [6]. PAI-1 is an inhibitor of endogenous tissue plasminogen activator: the increased levels of PAI-1 could thus inhibit fibrinolysis and be responsible for liver venous occlusion. The increased levels could be distinctly reduced after protein C application. However levels of PAI-1 were low in our patient 1, pointing to other modes of action of protein C in this patient. Another mode of action of protein C is inhibition of coagulation leading to decreased levels of thrombin. As a consequence thrombin activatable fibrinolysis inhibitor (TAFI) cannot be activated any longer leading to a sustained endogenous fibrinolysis. TAFI is a PAI-1 independent inhibitor of fibrinolysis. We did not measure TAFI levels in our patients and hence cannot argue for a disturbance of TAFI pathway in our patients.

Furthermore in view of the observations with protein C in septic shock the beneficial effect on the liver seen in our patient may be due to an effect of PC on IL-6 related downregulation of the ABCC2 anion transporter in the liver leading to an improvement in bilirubin export into the biliary system. However such a mechanism would be very difficult to investigate in human beings.

Until now, data trying to prove the efficacy of VOD-prophylactic measures with prostaglandin E1 and ursodesoxycholic acid are contradictory [1].

Our data indicate that PC substitution may be an useful adjunctive treatment in severe VOD. The use of protein C has not been evaluated thoroughly. However it may turn out very difficult to prove the clinical effect for any treatment in VOD when the spontaneous resolution rate is so high. A prospective study showing the efficacy of protein C in VOD will therefore be rather difficult to conduct. In view of the difficulty in conducting placebo-controlled treatment trials in this patient population, it would seem useful to consider a PC prophylaxis trial in patients at very high risk for fatal sinusoidal obstruction syndrome/VOD. The danger of bleedings under PC administration is neglectable.

Conclusion

In our 2 patients neither prophylactic nor therapeutic administration of AT and of defibrotide were able to prevent moderate to severe VOD, proven by Doppler ultrasound reversed portal venous blood flow. Our data indicate that PC substitution may be a useful adjunctive treatment in severe VOD. Until controlled studies will be initiated we recommend a stratified treatment in VOD, starting with defibroide, and adding PC in unresponsive cases.

References

1. Carreras E (2000) Veno-occlusive disease of the liver after hemopoietic cell transplantation. Eur H Haematol 64: 281–291
2. Carreras E, Bertz H, Arcese W, et al. (1998) Incidence and outcome of hepatic veno-occlusive disease after blood and marrow transplantation (SCT); a prospective cohort study of the European Group for Blood and Bone marrow transplantation chronic leukaemia working party. Blood 92: 3599–3604
3. Chopra R, Eaton JD, Grassi A, et al. (2000) Defibrotide for the treatment of hepatic veno-occlusive disease: results of the European compassionate – use study. Brit J Haematol 111: 1122–1129
4. DeLeve LD, Shulman HM, McDonald GB (2002) Toxic injury to hepatic sinusoids: Sinusoidal obstruction syndrome (veno-occlusive disease). Seminars in Liver Disease 22: 27–41
5. Jenner MJ, Micallef IN, Rohatiner AZ, et al. (2000) Successful therapy of transplant-associated veno-occlusive disease with a combination of tissue plasminogen activator and defibrotide. Med Oncol 17: 333–336
6. Kreuz W, Veldman A, Pötsch B, Scharrer I, Martin H, Hoelzer D (1998) Treatment of veno-occlusive disease after bone marrow transplantation: Continuous infusion of recombinant tissue plasminogen activator and simultaneous infusion of protein C. Annal Hematol 76 (Suppl I): A 85
7. Kulkarni S, Powles R, Sirohi B, et al. (2001) Combination of tissue plasminogen activator (rt-PA) and low dose heparin with or without defibrotide for the treatment of clinically suspected hepatic veno-occlusive disease (HVOD) following allogeneic hematopoetic stem cell transplant (AHSCT) form hematological malignancies. Blood 98-1: 853a

8. Mc Donald GB, Hinds MS, Fischer LD, et al. (1993) Veno-occlusive disease of the liver and multiorgan failure after bone marrow transplantation: a cohort study of 355 patients. Ann Intern Med 118: 255–267
9. Richardson PG, Elias AD, Krishnan A, et al. (1998) Treatment of severe veno-occlusive disease with defibrotide: compassionate use results in response without significant toxicity in a high-risk population. Blood 92: 737–744
10. Richardson PG, Warren DL, Momtaz P, et al. (2001) Multi-institutional phase II, randomized dose finding study of defibrotide (DF) in patients with severe veno-occlusive disease and multi-system organ failure post stem cell transplantation: promising response rate without significant toxicity in a high-risk population. Blood 98–1: 853a
11. Weber A, Nikolic N, Hondl F, et al. In vitro evaluation of stability of protein C concentrate for continuous infusion. XVII congr Int soc Thromb Hemost, Washington, Aug 14–21, 1999

Phase III Clinical Evaluation of rAHF-PFM Prepared Using a Plasma/Albumin Free Method

M. von Depka Prondzinski, and A. Tiede

Introduction

rAHF-PFM, the first third-generation recombinant Factor VIII concentrate, has been under clinical evaluation since November, 2000. No materials of human or animal origin are used in the production and final formulation of rAHF-PFM. To achieve this, the cell culture used to produce Recombinate, a preparation that has proven safety and efficacy for more than a decade, has been adapted to a protein-free medium. The monoclonal antibodies employed for immunoaffinity chromatography are produced in a protein-free medium, i.e. without the addition of any human- or animal-derived materials as well.

Factor VIII is stabilized in the finished product by means of a mixture of sugars, salts and amino acids. The above described process which is entirely without the addition of any human or animal derived material is expressed in the preliminary product name »rFVIII **PFM**« (for **p**lasma-free/albumin-free **m**ethod) which is used during the clinical trials.

A dedicated solvent/detergent viral inactivation step has been included. The reconstitution volume of the new concentrate is 5 ml, and an additional product potency of 1,500 IU has been added to the three usual package sizes.

The shelf life of the new concentrate at 2–8 °C is at least 18 months. Simulated continuous infusion studies have shown stability over at least 48 hours.

State-of-the-art methods have been employed to show that the physicochemical properties of rAHF-PFM are comparable to those of Recombinate. These methods

Table 1. rAHF-PFM: a third generation rFVIII

Fermentation technology	Continuous chemostat perfusion
Medium	Protein-free medium
Purification	• Immunoaffinity chromatography • Cation exchange chromatography • Anion exchange chromatography
Viral inactivation	Solvent detergent treatment S/D
Formulation	Sugars, salts and amino acids
Volume	5 ml
Potencies	250, 500, 1000 + 1500 IU/vial

I. Scharrer/W. Schramm (Ed.)
33rd Hemophilia Symposion Hamburg 2002
© Springer-Verlag Berlin Heidelberg 2004

comprise an evaluation of the protein primary structure, post-translational modifications, secondary structure, tertiary structure, protein integrity and functional properties.

The preclinical evaluation in rats and rabbits demonstrated that the rAHF-PFM process retained the physicochemical and biochemical characteristics of Recombinate. On the basis of these results, a level of safety, tolerability and hemostatic efficacy of rAHF-PFM comparable to that of Recombinate can be predicted.

Clinical Study Program

The clinical program comprises seven separate studies for which patients from the U.S., E.U., Canada and Japan have been or are being recruited (Table 2). The pivotal study involving 111 previously treated patients (PTPs) to determine the pharmacokinetics, safety, efficacy and immunogenicity of rAHF-PFM has been completed in the meantime. Eighty study subjects continue to be evaluated in a continuation study. While a surgery study and a pediatric study have already been initiated, the study involving previously untreated patients (PUPs) is still in the planning stage. Following the licensure a phase IV study will be initiated.

Table 2. Clinical study program (U.S., Canada, E.U., and Japan)

- Pivotal, phase II-III study (n=111)
- Continuation study (n = 80)
- Surgery study (study initiated, n=25 planned)
- Pediatric previously treated patients (study initiated, n=50 planned)
- PUP study (n=25 planned)
- Phase IV study (n=60 planned)
- Japanese clinical study (study initiated, n=15 planned)

rAHF-PFM Manufacturing Strategy

rAHF-PFM was originally produced on a pilot scale at Baxter's Biomedical Research Center in Orth, Austria, using a 1,200 l bioreactor. This product was used for the pivotal and surgery studies. Commercial-scale production is carried out at a new facility in Neuchâtel, Switzerland, using a 2,500 l bioreactor. This product has been available since October, 2001, and was used in the final part of the pivotal study. It is also used in the surgery study and will be used for all other studies (continuation, pediatric, PUP and phase IV studies).

Pivotal Phase III Study Design

A total of 111 PTPs with a baseline FVIII activity of ≤ 2% from 13 U.S. and 10 E.U. centers were enrolled in the pivotal study, which is a prerequisite for the rAHF-PFM licensure. All patients were more than 10 years of age, immunocompetent and had at least 150 exposure days. 108 patients were treated, the last of them on March 31st, 2002. The study's objective was to determine the basic clinical properties of rAHF-PFM and to demonstrate the equivalence of the products from both pilot and commercial production facilities. The study was designed in three parts:

The first part, involving half of the enrolled subjects, was a randomized, cross-over pharmacokinetic comparison of Recombinate and pilot-scale rAHF-PFM.

The second part, involving all study subjects, was an assessment of safety, efficacy and neoantigenicity over a minimum of 75 exposure days each.

The last part was a cross-over and, additionally, double-blind comparison of rAHF-PFM from pilot-scale production and rAHF-PFM from commercial production. This study involved all subjects not assigned to part one.

Pivotal Study Part 1: Pharmacokinetic comparison

The results of the first pharmacokinetics study involving 30 patients demonstrated the bioequivalence of Recombinate and pilot-scale rAHF-PFM. AUC (area under the curve), recovery and half-life of both concentrates reveal no differences (see Fig. 1 and Table 3).

Pivotal Study Part 2: Efficacy

A total of 510 bleeding episodes were treated with a median dose of 32.9 IU rAHF-PFM/kg (8.7–225.8 IU/kg). Ninety-three % of the bleedings could be resolved with a maximum of 2 infusions. The hemostatic efficacy of rAHF-PFM was rated as excellent or good in 86% of the treated bleeding episodes.

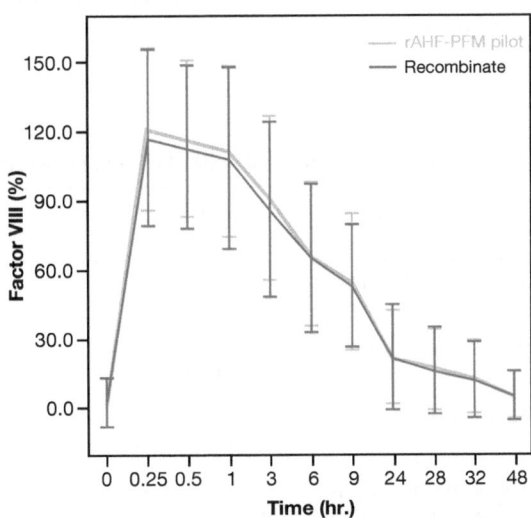

Fig. 1. Pharmacokinetic studies suggest rAHF-PFM and Recombinate rAHF are bio-equivalent

Table 3. Pharmacokinetic parameters of rAHF-PFM and Recombinate

Parameter	Recombinate rAHF (n=30)	rAHF-PFM pilot (n=30)
$AUC_{(0-48 hr)}$ (IU·hr/dl)	1515 (970–2205)	1533 (876–2642)
Adjusted recovery[a]	2.55 (1.47–3.89)	2.40 (1.54–3.88)
Half-life (hrs)	11.39 (7.89–18.12)	11.98 (6.74–24.70)

* all pharmacokinetic parameters expressed as means (min-max)
[a] adjusted recovery = FVIII IU/dl plasma per FVIII IU/kg BW infused

The study also assessed the efficacy of rAHF-PFM in prophylaxis. The regimen included 3–4 infusions per week with a dose of 25–40 IU each over the first 75 exposure days.

The median dose was 30.7 IU/kg (9.4–110.7 IU/kg). A mean new bleeding rate of 6.2 bleedings per patient and year was observed during this treatment. Patients who were compliant (n=70) experienced a mean of 4.3 bleeds per year, while patients who were less compliant (n=37) showed a mean of 9.8 bleedings per year.

Pivotal Study Part 3: Pharmacokinetic Results

The pharmacokinetic comparison of pilot-scale rAHF-PFM and rAHF-PFM from Neuchâtel also revealed no differences (see Table 4). The AUC, recovery and half-life parameters in 37 patients do not differ from those of the previous pharmacokinetics study.

Table 4. Pilot and commercial scale rAHF-PFM have equivalent pharmacokinetic properties

Parameter	rAHF-PFM pilot (n=37)	rAHF-PFM commercial (n=37)
$AUC_{(0-48 hr)}$ (IU·hr/dl)	1544 (856–2216)	1494 (767–2392)
Adjusted recovery[a]	2.55 (1.73–4.05)	2.46 (1.71–3.41)
Half-life (hrs)	11.60 (7.59–15.03)	11.72 (8.14–17.34)

* all pharmacokinetic parameters expressed as means (min-max)
[a] adjusted recovery = FVIII IU/dl plasma per FVIII IU/kg BW infused

Pivotal Study Parts 1–3: Safety

No serious adverse event (SAE) related to rAHF-PFM was reported during the pivotal study. Seven patients developed 19 adverse events (AE) possibly or probably related to rAHF-PFM administration. Seventeen adverse events were classified as mild and one patient reported 2 severe events (high fever, headache).

Pivotal Study Parts 1–3: Inhibitors

One patient developed a low titer inhibitor (2 BU). This inhibitor occurred after 30 exposure days. The inhibitor was transient and could no longer be detected after 8 weeks.

Continuation Study

This study was designed to provide additional pharmacokinetics, immunogenicity, safety and efficacy data on commercial-scale rAHF-PFM in long-term use. This study was open for 80 subjects who completed the pivotal study. Patients will remain on rAHF-PFM until licensure. The pharmacokinetic parameters before and after 75 exposure days are compared.

Surgery Study

This study will evaluate the efficacy and safety of rAHF-PFM when used for bleeding phrophylaxis in invasive or surgical procedures. rAHF-PFM may either be administered as a bolus or as continuous infusion (CI), with up to 2 weeks of study drug treatment for non-orthopedic procedures and up to 6 weeks of study drug treatment for orthopedic procedures. Twenty-five patients are anticipated to be enrolled for this purpose.

The following endpoints or parameters were established:
- Assessment of perioperative bleeding
- Total, daily weight adjusted dose of rAHF-PFM
- Changes in daily, rAHF-PFM clearance rate after 72 hours of replacement therapy (CI patients only)
- Global assessment of hemostatic efficacy on a scale of excellent, good, fair or none intra-operatively (surgeon)
  post-operatively (hemophilia treater)
- Days on treatment and total dose
- Safety parameters (AEs, toxicology measures, inhibitor screening)

Surgical procedures under rAHF-PFM have been performed in 10 patients:
- 6 major procedures
  - Transposition of left ulnar nerve

- Total hip joint replacement
- Knee joint replacement
- Knee arthrodesis
- Left elbow synovectomy
- Right knee arthroscopy/chondroplasty/synovectomy*
● 4 minor procedures
- Insertion of Mediport*
- Dental extraction
- Teeth extraction
- Wisdom teeth extraction

---

* CI procedures

Intra- and post-operative hemostatic efficacy of rAHF-PFM were rated as excellent or good in all patients. No supplemental loading doses were required for any patient. The extent of intra-operative blood loss was as expected in 9 out of 10 patients. In addition, neither serious adverse events nor non-serious adverse events related to rAHF-PFM treatment were reported. No inhibitors were observed.

Pediatric Study

In this study, rAHF-PFM is being evaluated in previously treated patients (PTPs) younger than 6 years of age and a baseline FVIII activity of $\leq 2\%$ in order to assess its immunogenicity, safety, efficacy and pharmacokinetics. These pediatric patients must have a minimum of 50 exposure days and no history of inhibitors. Fourteen European and 16 North American centers were selected to participate in the study.

The pharmacokinetic parameters were determined in 11 out of the 16 children treated thus far (as of September 30, 2002). As expected, the results obtained are slightly lower than those in adults (see Table 5).

Table 5. rAHF-PFM pharmacokinetic properties in pediatric patients

Parameter	rAHF-PFM (n=11)
$AUC_{(0-48\,hr)}$ (IU·hr/dl)	1521 (792–2285)
Adjusted recovery[a]	2.06 (1.50–3.39)
Half-life (hrs)	10.48 (8.31–13.87)

* all pharmacokinetic parameters expressed as means (min-max)
[a] adjusted recovery = FVIII IU/dl plasma per FVIII IU/kg BW infused

PUP Study

This study will investigate the hemostatic efficacy and safety of rAHF-PFM in previously untreated patients (PUPs). A total of 25 PUPs of any age with a baseline FVIII activity of ≤2% are anticipated to be enrolled.

Conclusions

rAHF-PFM is the first Factor VIII recombinant therapy to be clinically developed and prepared without the addition of any human or animal raw materials in the cell culture process, purification or final formulation.

The physicochemical characterization of the rAHF-PFM FVIII molecule demonstrated structural equivalence with the Recombinate molecule. The preclinical evaluations suggested the comparability of hemostatic efficacy, safety and tolerability of rAHF-PFM and Recombinate.

The clinical trials program for rAHF-PFM began in November, 2000, with initiation of the pivotal study in order to evaluate pharmacokinetics (PK), safety, efficacy and immunogenicity in previously treated study subjects with baseline factor VIII levels ≤2%. Study subjects who completed the pivotal trial had the option to enroll in a continuation study of rAHF-PFM, which will extend the period of observation in this study cohort. Additional open-label studies, either ongoing or planned, will evaluate the safety, efficacy and immunogenicity of rAHF-PFM when used as hemostatic cover for subjects undergoing surgery, in previously treated pediatric subjects under six years of age, and PUPs. A phase IV, post-licensure study is planned, too.

Although the full clinical development program has not yet been completed, the current study results suggest the pharmacokinetic bioequivalence of Recombinate and rAHF-PFM and demonstrate the expected hemostatic efficacy of the new concentrate. Inhibitor results derived from adolescent and adult previously treated study subjects demonstrate that it is non-neoantigenic.

Based on these positive results, the application for U.S. licensure was submitted in June, 2002, and the application for E.U. and Canadian licensure was submitted in September, 2002.

rAHF-PFM is a new category of full-length FVIII concentrate produced without the addition of animal or human materials and does, besides factor VIII, contain salts, sugars and amino acids only. It therefore complies with the physicians' and patients' strictest safety requirements.

Table 6. Summary of rAHF-PFM product characteristics

- Cell cultures for production of full-length rFVIII molecule and anti-FVIII Mab adapted to protein-free media without the addition of human- or animal-derived raw materials
- rAHF-PFM is purified, formulated and stabilized without any added raw materials of human or animal origin
- Dedicated (S/D) viral-inactivation step
- Wider range of nominal product potencies: 250, 500, 1000, 1500 IU
- Smaller reconstitution volume (5 ml) for enhanced convenience

Anti-Prionin IgG, Possible new Serum Markers for Contact and Infection with Transmissible Spongiform Encephalopathies: Preliminary Results from Screening 100 Blood Donors

A. Schön, J. Bergmann, P. Kühnl, and K. Gutensohn

Introduction

Transmissible spongiform encephalopathies (TSE) are a group of rare neurodegenerative diseases that affect humans and animals. There is compelling evidence that variant Creutzfeldt-Jakob disease (vCJD) in humans results from the consumption of cattle affected by bovine spongiform encephalopathy (BSE) [2]. Although there is no reported case of transmittance of vCJD by blood or blood products, this theoretical risk has not yet been ruled out. A pre-symptomatic test, which would assess the potential threat to public health, is still lacking. In this study we used a new ELISA which detects IgG against prionins, a possible new serum marker for TSEs. Prionins are species-specific proteins, encoded from genes within the prion genes (Fig.1).

Because of their predicted biochemical features prionins are possible candidates for the as yet unidentified protein X, which should be a key-factor for onset of prion diseases [3]. The disease related expression of prionins elicits an auto-immune response, as the normally not expressed protein is unknown to the immune system. Anti-prionin antibodies occur at the earliest stage of the disease and modulate the pathogenic effect of prionins successfully for many years. These antibodies are therefore perfect target molecules for the pre-symptomatic diagnosis of TSEs.

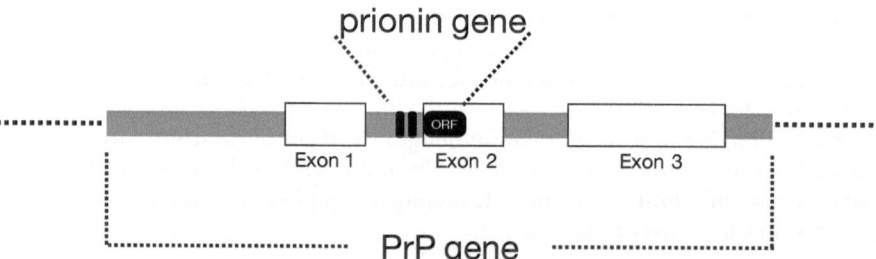

Fig 1. The prionin gene, a gene within the PrP gene

Materials and Methods

At this stage, 100 healthy donors (50 female and 50 male), fulfilling the criteria requested by the University Hospital Eppendorf and the German Society of Blood Transfusion (DGTI) for extracorporal apheresis, were included in this study. Blood

I. Scharrer/W. Schramm (Ed.)
33rd Hemophilia Symposion Hamburg 2002
© Springer-Verlag Berlin Heidelberg 2004

samples were taken during regular blood donation from antecubital venipuncture and collected into single-use tubes (S-Monovette, Sarstedt, Germany). For preparation samples were centrifuged for 15 minutes at 2800 rpm. The serum was aliquotted into cryotubes (NalgeNunc International, Denmark) and stored frozen at –20° C. The BSE Plus (hc) test (Altegen Inc., Wilmington, USA) was performed with 1.5 µl of serum thawed prior at room temperature according to the specifications of the producer. All samples were analyzed for antibodies against epitopes of three different prionins, allowing to detect, and distinguish, exposure to BSE, scrapie and presence of latent vCJD. The test results were quantified in an ELISA reader using the 492 nm filter.

Results

Our results showed that none of the tested persons was positive for exposure to BSE or scrapie. Also none of the tested samples was positive for latent vCJD.

Discussion

The predictions about the total number of vCJD cases have not been fulfilled to date. However, the theoretical risk of iatrogenic vCJD infections still exists [1]. Especially the unknown incubation period of the disease permits the discussion about possible infections. To minimize the risk for human-to-human disease transmission through blood donations, a donor policy excludes donations from anyone who lived in the UK for a continued period of 6 months or more, who received cadaver-pituitary growth hormone or a dura mater graft, and anyone who has a family history of neurodegenerative disease. Standard of diagnosing vCJD is the examination of tissue [4]. Final decision is made by post-mortem analyze of brain tissue. To date there is no test available which can detect preclinical infection. The main problem for the development of such an ante-mortem blood test is the low concentration of prions in blood and the absence of reliable surrogate markers.

The prionin hypothesis assumes that the appearance of anti-prionin auto-antibodies is characteristic for the preclinical period of TSEs. The BSE plus (hc) test we used in this study bases on a simple capture ELISA technology. It therefore might be a sensitive and repeatable test to identify preclinical infected people by blood. The prionin hypothesis has not yet been verified. To complete the research phase additional experiments with laboratory animals and cattle to control the course of the immune reaction are needed. To prove the hypothesis that expression of prionins is the initiating pathological event in TSE, scientific work which shows the infectivity of in vitro produced prionins is needed as well. To finish this work several studies in different European countries are in progress.

For a region without many cases of BSE and without suspicious cases of vCJD, the outcome of the test with 100% negative results was as expected. The study will be continued.

References

1. Budka H. Prions and transfusion medicine. Vox Sang, 2000; 78: 231–238
2. Collinge J. Variant Creutzfeldt-Jakob disease. Lancet, 1999; 354: 317–324
3. Kaneko K. et al. Evidence for protein X binding to a discontinuous epitope on the cellular prion protein during scrapie prion propagation. Proc Natl Acad Sci, 1997; 94: 10069
4. Korth C. et al. Prion (PrP^{sc})-specific epitope defined by a monoclonal antibody. Nature, 1997; 74–78

Experimental Approaches to Hemophilia Gene Therapy: Gene Transfer into Hematopoietic Stem Cells

A. Tiede, M. Eder, M. Scherr, A. Ganser,
and M. von Depka Prondzinski

Introduction

Autologous transplantation of gene-modified hematopoietic stem and progenitor cells (HPC) is currently evaluated for treatment of monogeneic hematopoietic disorders. Clinical studies have successfully used retroviral gene transfer into HPC to correct X-linked severe combined immunodeficiency (X-SCID) [1, 2]. We currently evaluate gene transfer into HPC for hemophilia A gene therapy. Transplantation of HPC transduced with a gene for coagulation factor VIII (FVIII) may potentially provide a permanent pool of FVIII-expressing hematopoietic cells. In addition, immune tolerance against neo-antigenic FVIII might be achieved as reported for other transgenes in animal models. However, it has been unclear whether cells of hematopoietic origin are capable of FVIII biosynthesis and secretion, because transplantation of FVIII-transduced bone marrow cells into conditioned mice did not result in the expression of detectable FVIII in the plasma [3, 4]. Others have found that certain myeloid cell lines were able to efficiently produce FVIII after transduction in vitro [5, 6]. We therefore studied the expression of recombinant FVIII after gene transfer into various hematopoietic cell types.

Materials and methods

A gene for canine B-domain deleted FVIII (cFVIII-BDD) was obtained from D. Lillicrap (Kingston, Ontario, Canada, [7]) and was inserted into a lentiviral vector backbone based on pRRL-CMV-EGFP-SIN [8]. Viral particles were pseudotyped with the vesicular stomatitis virus G protein (VSV.G). The number of particles was determined by transduction of 293T cells with serial dilutions of vector supernatant. Transduction rates were quantified by real-time PCR using primers and probes specific for cFVIII-BDD. The copy number of an autosomal gene, *HCK*, was determined in parallel to correct for DNA input.

Prior to transduction, cell lines and primary hematopoietic cells were seeded at 0.5 to 2×10^6/ml in serum-free medium (X-VIVO/10) supplemented with 1% human serum albumin, 200 µM dNTP, and 4 µg/ml protamine sulfate. Dilutions of vector stocks were added to give the indicated multiplicity of infection (MOI; i.e. 293T-transducing units per cell). After over-night incubation, cells were washed and seeded into RPMI1640 medium containing 10% heat-inactivated foetal calf serum (FCS)

I. Scharrer/W. Schramm (Ed.)
33rd Hemophilia Symposion Hamburg 2002
© Springer-Verlag Berlin Heidelberg 2004

and 5 mM L-glutamine. As indicated, media were supplemented with growth factors and cytokines.

Human CD34$^+$ cells were enriched from peripheral blood of a healthy donor following mobilization with G-CSF as described [9]. Transduced CD34$^+$ cells were cultured in RPMI 1640 medium containing FCS and glutamine. Methylcellulose assays were performed as described [9].

FVIII secretion into cell culture supernatant was detected by one-stage assay using FVIII-depleted human plasma and Pathromtin reagent obtained from Dade Behring (Marburg, Germany). Reference curves were established using human recombinant B-domain-deleted FVIII (ReFacto, Wyeth Pharma, Münster, Germany) diluted in cell culture medium.

Results and discussion

A lentiviral vector was constructed containing cFVIII-BDD under control of a cytomegalovirus (CMV) promoter. Due to size limitations, the vector did not contain an additional reporter gene such as green fluorescent protein. Therefore, transduction of target cells was quantified by real-time PCR (Fig. 1). Detectable transduction of 293T cells occurred up to a vector dilution of $3 \cdot 10^5$. The sensitivity of PCR was 20 copies per reaction, and approximately 1/20 of the DNA of the cells transduced were used per reaction, resulting in an estimated vector titer of $20 \times 20 \times 3 \cdot 10^5 = 1.2 \cdot 10^8$ transducing units per ml. Secretion of FVIII as detected by one-stage clotting assay correlated well with transduction and was also detectable up to a vector dilution of $3 \cdot 10^5$.

The transduction of various hematopoietic cell lines at a MOI of 10 (*i.e.* 10 transducing units per cell) resulted in a transduction rate between 520 and 7600 vector copies per 1000 cells (Fig. 2). FVIII was detected in cell culture supernatant ranging between <10 mU/ml (not detectable) and 1000 mU/ml (100% of normal plasma activity). Transduction and FVIII secretion was efficient in several myeloid (K-562, TF-1) and myelo-monocytic cell lines (Monomac-1, Mutz-3). In contrast, FVIII secretion was ineffective in other cell lines (HL-60, U-937) although efficient transduction was achieved. These data are consistent with the results by Tonn et al. [5] who observed efficient production of recombinant human FVIII-BDD in K-562 and TF-1, but not in PLB and KG-1 cells. In lymphatic cell lines (BV-173, Molt-4), we failed to detect FVIII secretion, but transduction rates were also low. Tonn et al. have found low amounts of human FVIII-BDD secreted by transduced lymphatic cell lines (Raji, Jurkat) after enrichment of reporter gene-expressing cells by flow cytometry [5]. In all hematopoietic cell lines tested here, FVIII secretion was less effective compared to the reference cell line (293T renal embryonic carcinoma).

The transduction of primary hematopoietic cells from peripheral blood was first tested using eGFP-encoding lentiviral vectors at an MOI of 10 (Fig. 3a). CD14$^+$ monocytic cells were transduced very efficiently (~75%). In contrast, other peripheral blood-derived mononuclear cells (mainly lymphocytes) were transduced less efficiently (~15%). Using FVIII-encoding lentiviral vectors, similar results were obtained (Fig. 3b). Secretion of FVIII was detected in the supernatant from FVIII-

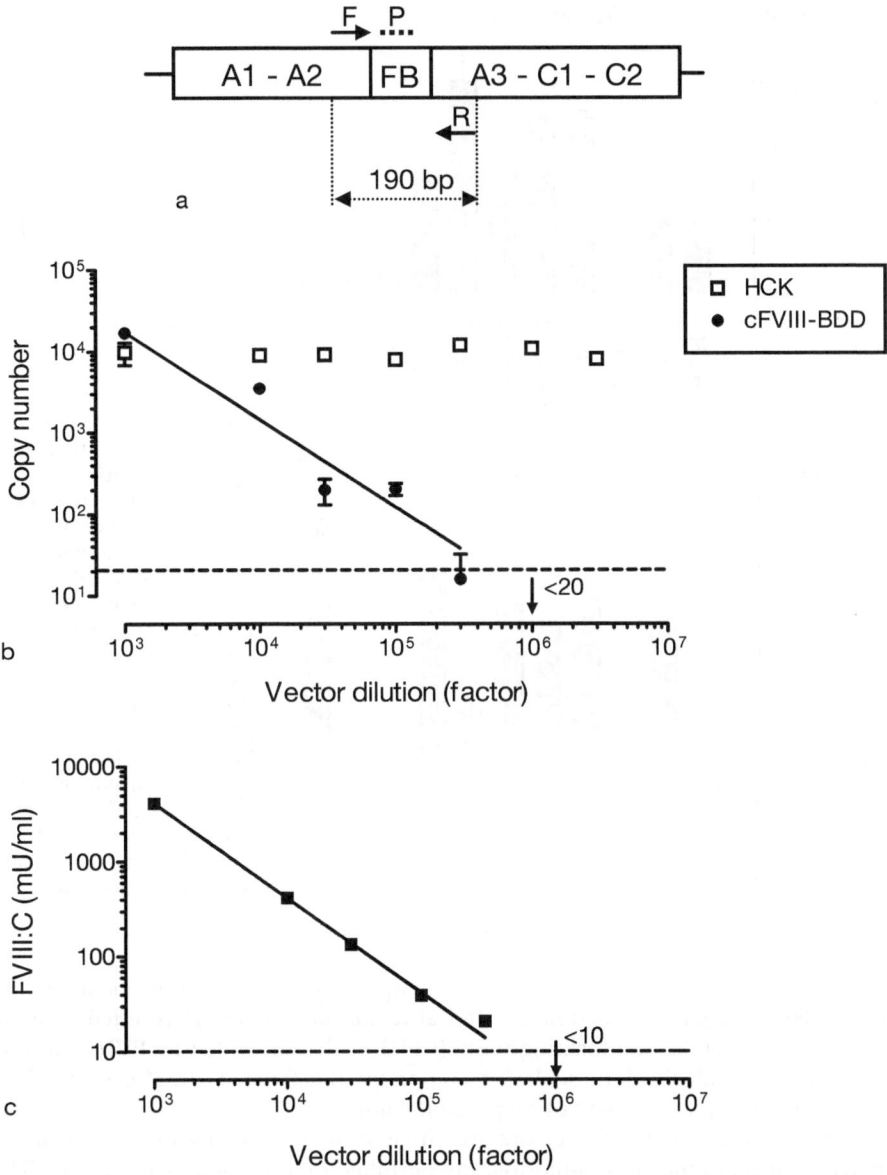

Fig. 1a–c. Quantification of transduction rates by real-time PCR specific for cFVIII-BDD. **(a)** Primers (F, forward; R, reverse) and probe (P) for real-time PCR (TaqMan PCR) spanning the B-domain deletion of cFVIII-BDD. **(b)** 293T cells were transduced with serial dilutions of lentiviral supernatant (X-axis). Genomic DNA was extracted from transduced cells and copy numbers of cFVIII-BDD were determined by real-time PCR. Copy numbers of an autosomal human gene, HCK, were determined in parallel for DNA input normalization. **(c)** Detection of recombinant cFVIII-BDD by one-stage clotting assay in the supernatant of transduced 293T cells (same experiment as in B).

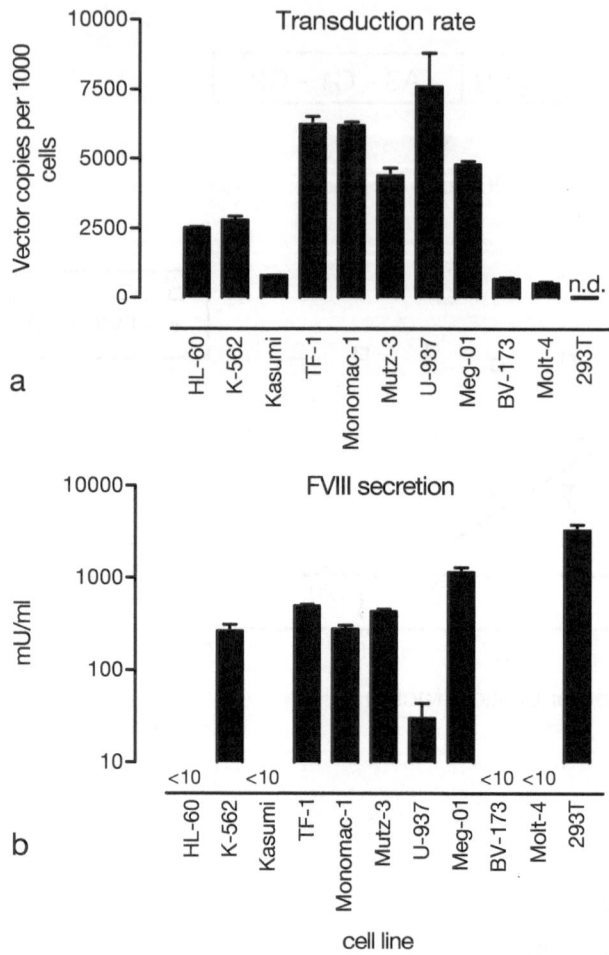

Fig. 2a, b. Secretion of recombinant cFVIII-BDD by hematopoietic cell lines. **(a)** Cells were transduced at a MOI of 10, and transduction was quantified by real-time PCR. The bars show the vector copy numbers per 2000 HCK copies (an equivalent of approximately 1000 cells). **(b)** Detection of secreted recombinant cFVIII-BDD by one-stage clotting assay in the supernatant of cell lines six days after transduction ($1\cdot10^6$ cells/ml). Untransduced cell lines did not secrete detectable FVIII (<10 mU/ml, not shown).

transduced monocytic cells, but not from lymphatic cells (Fig. 3c). Transduction of CD34[+] HPC using FVIII-encoding lentiviral vectors at a MOI of 15 resulted in up to 50% transformed colony-forming units (CFU) as demonstrated by FVIII-specific PCR from individual colonies. FVIII secretion by transformed CD34[+] cells was low (10–20 mU/ml) after six days of suspension culture.

In conclusion, lentiviral vectors are efficient in transducing various hematopoietic cell types including non-dividing peripheral blood monocytes and CD34[+] HPC. Several myelo-monocytic cell lines as well as primary peripheral-blood derived monocytes are efficient producers of FVIII. In contrast, lymphatic cells were unable to produce and/or secrete functional recombinant FVIII. CD34[+] HPC secreted low amounts of FVIII although efficient transduction was achieved. In perspective, FVIII gene transfer into CD34[+] HPC followed by transplantation into conditioned recipients may result in FVIII-transduced differentiated hematopoietic cells that are able to secrete functional recombinant FVIII.

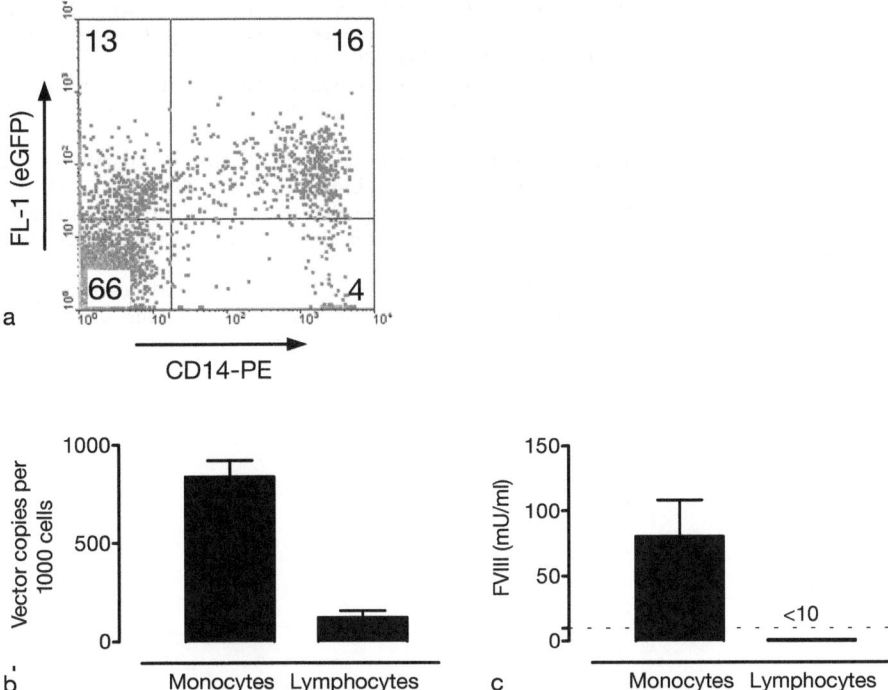

Fig. 3a–c. Secretion of recombinant cFVIII-BDD by primary hematopoietic monocytes and lymphocytes. **(a)** Peripheral blood-derived mononuclear cells (PBMNC) were transduced with eGFP-encoding lentiviral vector. CD14+ cells (mainly monocytes) were efficiently transduced as demonstrated by eGFP expression (upper versus lower right quadrant). CD14+ cells (mainly lymphocytes) were less efficiently transduced (upper versus lower left quadrant). **(b)** Adherent PBMNC (mainly monocytes) and adherent cell-depleted PBMNC (mainly lymphocytes) were transduced with cFVIII-encoding vectors. Transduction rates were determined by real-time PCR as described above. **(c)** Secretion of recombinant cFVIII-BDD was determined by one-stage clotting assay. Untransduced cells did not secrete detectable FVIII (<10 mU/ml, not shown).

References

1. Cavazzana-Calvo M, Hacein-Bey S, de Saint Basile G, Gross F, Yvon E, Nusbaum P, Selz F, Hue C, Certain S, Casanova JL, Bousso P, Deist FL, Fischer A. Gene therapy of human severe combined immunodeficiency (SCID)-X1 disease. Science 2000; 288: 669–672
2. Hacein-Bey-Abina S, Le Deist F, Carlier F, Bouneaud C, Hue C, De Villartay JP, Thrasher AJ, Wulffraat N, Sorensen R, Dupuis-Girod S, Fischer A, Davies EG, Kuis W, Leiva L, Cavazzana-Calvo M. Sustained correction of X-linked severe combined immunodeficiency by ex vivo gene therapy. N Engl J Med 2002; 346: 1185–1193
3. Hoeben RC, Einerhand MP, Briet E, van Ormondt H, Valerio D, van der Eb AJ. Toward gene therapy in hemophilia A: retrovirus-mediated transfer of a factor VIII gene into murine hematopoietic progenitor cells. Thromb Haemost 1992; 67: 341–345
4. Evans GL, Morgan RA. Genetic induction of immune tolerance to human clotting factor VIII in a mouse model for hemophilia A. Proc Natl Acad Sci U S A 1998; 95: 5734–5739

5. Tonn T, Becker S, Herder C, Grez M, Seifried E. Hematopoietic stem cells as targets for gene therapy of hemophilia A. In: Scharrer I, Schramm W, eds. *32nd Hemophilia Symposium: Hamburg 2001*. Springer Verlag Berlin, Heidelberg; 2001: 61–71
6. Tonn T, Herder C, Becker S, Seifried E, Grez M. Generation and Characterization of Human Hematopoietic Cell Lines Expressing Factor VIII. J Hematother Stem Cell Res 2002; 11: 695–704
7. Cameron C, Notley C, Hoyle S, McGlynn L, Hough C, Kamisue S, Giles A, Lillicrap D. The canine factor VIII cDNA and 5' flanking sequence. Thromb Haemost 1998; 79: 317–322
8. Naldini L, Blömer U, Gallay P, Ory D, Mulligan R, Gage FH, Verma IM, Trono D. In vivo gene delivery and stable transduction of nondividing cells by a lentiviral vector. Science 1996; 272: 263–267
9. Scherr M, Battmer K, Blömer U, Schiedlmeier B, Ganser A, Grez M, Eder M. Lentiviral gene transfer into peripheral blood-derived CD34$^+$ NOD/SCID-repopulating cells. Blood 2002; 99: 709–712

Von-Willebrand Factor Cleaving Protease (ADAMTS-13) Activity in Various Thrombotic, Hemolytic and Autoimmune Disorders

M. Böhm, W. Miesbach, M. Krause, Th. Vigh, and I. Scharrer

Introduction

Thrombotic Thrombocytopenic Purpura (TTP) is associated with acquired or congenital deficiency of a plasma von-Willebrand Factor (vWF) cleaving protease [1–5]. The vWF cleaving protease shortens the vWF by cleaving the peptide bond Tyr^{1605}-Met^{1606} within domain A2 [1–2]. The enzyme was recently purified and identified as a new member of the ADAMTS (a disintegrin and metalloproteinase with thrombospondin type I motif) family of metalloproteinases and designated ADAMTS-13 [6–7]. Contemporaneous, Levy et al. [8] performed genome-wide linkage analysis in four pedigrees of humans with familial TTP and mapped the responsible genetic locus to ADAMTS-13 on chromosome 9q34. These findings demonstrated, that congenital TTP is caused by mutations in the gene responsible for the production of vWF cleaving protease. Since then, several mutations in ADAMTS-13 have been reported in patients with familial TTP [9–12]. However, the specificity of ADAMTS-13 deficiency for TTP has been challenged by findings of low activity in physiological and pathological conditions other than TTP e.g. acute inflammation, pregnancy, post-surgery, decompensated liver cirrhosis, renal failure [13], systemic lupus erythematosus, idiopathic thrombocytopenia, disseminated intravascular coagulation [14], metastatic tumors [15], hemolytic uremic syndrome [16] and sepsis [17]. In the present study, we investigated vWF cleaving activity of ADAMTS-13 (ADAMTS-13 activity) in 103 pts with various disorders correlated with thrombocytopenia, hemolysis or auto-antibodies to clarify the specificity of ADAMTS-13 deficiency for acute TTP.

Material and Methods

Study Population

We recruited 32 patients with antiphospholipid syndrome, 25 patients with acute thrombocytopenia and/or hemolysis of unidentified cause, 12 patients with idiopathic thrombocytopenia, 3 patients with HIV or HCV associated thrombocytopenia and 11 patients with compensated liver cirrhosis for the study. We investigated furthermore patients in severe acute clinical conditions: hemolytic uremic syndrome (n=6), myocardial infarction (n=5), sepsis (n=5), ischemic stroke (n=3), acute renal insufficiency (n=3), bone marrow transplantation associated TTP (n=2), dissemi-

I. Scharrer/W. Schramm (Ed.)
33rd Hemophilia Symposion Hamburg 2002
© Springer-Verlag Berlin Heidelberg 2004

nated intravascular coagulation (n=1), purpura rheumatica (n=1), HELLP syndrome (n=1), lung fibroid (n=1), mesenterial vein thrombosis (n=1), catastrophic antiphospholipid syndrome (n=1), pulmonary embolism (n=1) and deep vein thrombosis of the leg (n=1). Results were compared to ADAMTS-13 activity in patients with TTP (n=23) and healthy controls (n=80).

Plasma samples

Venous blood was drawn in citrated collection tubes and centrifuged for 40 min at 4°C and 2500g. The platelet-poor plasma was subsequently stored at -20°C until tested.

ADAMTS-13 activity

ADAMTS-13 activity was estimated by measuring the residual Ristocetin Cofactor activity of the degraded vWF substrate as described previously (13). For assay calibration Imidazole buffer was replaced by heat-inactivated normal human plasma pool (30 min at 60°C and centrifuged for 15 min at 13000 rpm).

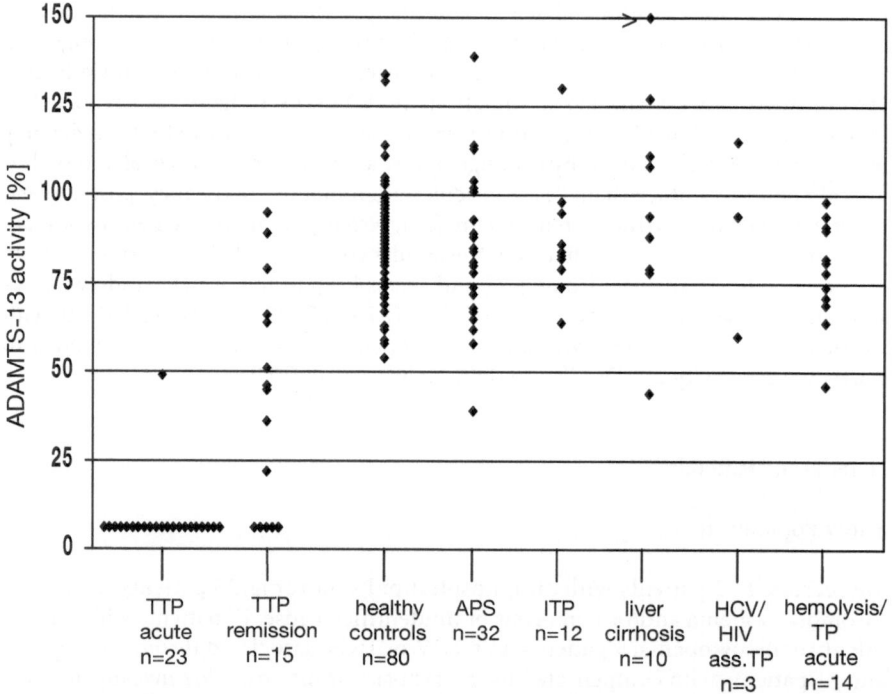

Fig. 1. ADAMTS-13 activity in patients with TTP, normal controls and in patients with APS, ITP, compensated liver cirrhosis, HCV or HIV associated and acute hemolysis and/or thrombocytopenia (TP) of unidentified cause.
> = ADAMTS-13 activity > 150%

Table 1. ADAMTS-13 activity in patients with various thrombotic, hemolytic and autoimmune disorders

Condition	ADAMTS-13 activity [%]		Number
	range	mean+/–SD	
Classic TTP, acute	<6,25 (49)*	<6,25 (49)*	23
TTP in remission	<6,25–108	45 +/– 32	17
Healthy controls	52–134	90 +/– 15	80
Antiphospholipid syndrome (APS)	32–139	84 +/– 21	32
Idiopathic thrombocytopenia	74–130	87 +/– 16	12
Compensated liver cirrhosis	44–188	98 +/– 38	10
HIV or HCV associated thrombocytopenia	60–115	88 +/– 28	3
Hemolysis and/or thrombocytopenia of unidentified cause, acute	64–146	86 +/– 21	14
Hemolytic uremic syndrome (HUS), acute	30–92	67 +/– 24	6
Myocardial infarction, acute	51–98	74 +/– 17	5
Sepsis, acute	21–49	31 +/– 11	5
Ischemic stroke, acute	22–59	37 +/– 16	3
Renal insufficiency, acute	37–48	44 +/– 6	3
Bone marrow transplantation associated TTP, acute	39–62	51 +/– 16	2
Disseminated intravascular coagulation (DIC), acute	33		1
Purpura rheumatica, acute	14		1
HELLP syndrome, acute	25		1
Lung fibroid, acute	37		1
Mesenterial vein thrombosis, acute	42		1
Catastrophic APS, acute	52		1
Pulmonary embolism, acute	75		1
Deep vein thrombosis of the leg, acute	73		1

* 1/23 patients demonstrated measurable ADAMTS-13 activity of 49% during her acute episode

Results and Discussion

Table 1 and Figure 1–2 illustrate the results of ADAMTS-13 activity in the investigated patients. Severe deficiency of vWF cleaving activity of ADAMTS-13 (<6,25%) was restricted to pts with TTP. We found partial deficiency in patients with HUS, sepsis, acute ischemic stroke, renal insufficiency, DIC, Purpura rheumatica, HELLP syndrome, lung fibroid, mesenterial vein thrombosis and in one patient with APS. We confirm therefore data from Bianchi and coworkers [17], who detected partial, but no severe ADAMTS-13 deficiency in 11/68 pts with thrombocytopenic disorders. We contradict data from Remuzzi et al. [16], who found severe ADAMTS-13 deficiency in 5/9 pts with HUS. Our data controvert furthermore the study of Moore et al. [14], who found similar proportions of ADAMTS-13 deficiency in patients with TTP and in patients with other thrombocytopenic disorders like DIC, ITP, and leukemia. In our investigated patient cohort severe ADAMTS-13 deficiency is with 100% specificity and 94% sensitivity strongly correlated to acute TTP. Partial ADAMTS-13 deficiency is there against found in various clinical manifestations associated with multiorgan involvement and acute phase reactions. The reasons for the decreased ADAMTS-13 in this disorders remain obscure. It is noteworthy, that we found in 19/46 patients (41%)

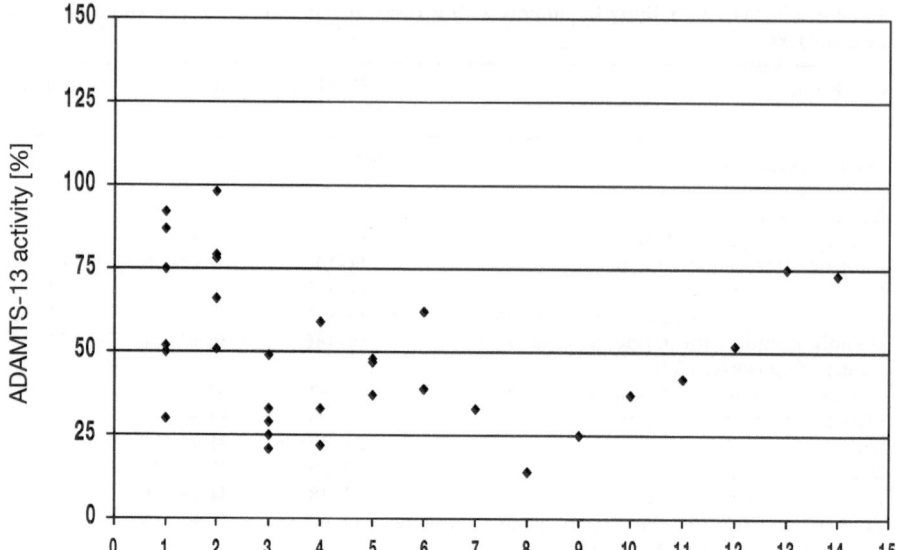

Fig. 2. ADAMTS-13 activity in patients with various, severe clinical conditions: 1 = hemolytic uremic syndrome (n = 6), 2 = myocardial infarction (n = 5), 3 = sepsis (n = 5), 4 = ischemic stroke (n = 3), 5 = acute, renal insufficiency (n = 3), 6 = bone marrow transplantation associated TTP (n = 2), 7 = disseminated intravascular coagulation (n = 1), 8 = purpura rheumatica (n = 1), 9 = HELLP syndrome (n = 1), 10 = lung fibroid (n = 1), 11 = mesenterial vein thrombosis (n = 1), 12 = catastrophic antiphospholipid syndrome, 13 = pulmonary embolism (n = 1), 14 = deep vein thrombosis of the leg (n = 1)

with severe, acute clinical manifestations partial ADAMTS-13 deficiency, whereas only 2/57 patients with compensated disease (APS, compensated liver cirrhosis, ITP, HIV/HCV associated thrombocytopenia) demonstrated impaired ADAMTS-13 activity. We investigated 1 patient with APS and 1 patient with myocardial infarction during acute episode and in remission. Both patients demonstrated a distinct increase of ADAMTS-13 activity in remission from 52 to 107% and from 53% to 78%, respectively (data not shown). Since von-Willebrand Factor is an acute phase reactant, it might be speculated that the loss of ADAMTS-13 activity is due to consumption of the protease. This hypothesis is supported by the recent finding of ADAMTS-13 decrease after infusion of desmopressin [18].

We conclude, that severe ADAMTS-13 deficiency is very specific for acute, classic TTP, thus can be used to characterize the thrombotic microangiopathy. Partial ADAMTS-13 deficiency can on the contrary not yet be linked to a specific disease. Future research is warranted to clarify the pathological relevance of mildly reduced ADAMTS-13 activity in diseases other than TTP.

References

1. Furlan M, Robles R, Galbusera M, Remuzzi G, Kyrle PA, Brenner B, Krause M, Scharrer I, Aumann V, Mittler U, Solenthaler M, Lämmle B. von Willebrand Factor-cleaving protease in thrombotic thrombocytopenic purpura and the hemolytic-uremic syndrome. N Engl J Med 1998, 339: 1578–1584
2. Tsai HM, Lian EC. Antibodies to von Willebrand Factor-cleaving protease in acute thrombotic thrombocytopenic purpura. N Engl J Med 1998, 339: 1585–1594
3. Allford SL, Harrison P, Lawrie AS, Liesner R, Mackie IJ, Machin SJ. von Willebrand Factor-cleaving protease activity in congenital thrombotic thrombocytopenic purpura. Br J Haematol 2000; 111: 1215–1222
4. Veyradier A, Obert B, Houllier A, Meyer D, Girma JP. Specific von Willebrand Factor-cleaving protease in thrombotic microangiopathies: a study of 111 cases. Blood 2001; 98: 1765–1772
5. Böhm M, Vigh T, Scharrer I. Evaluation and clinical application of a new method for measuring activity of von Willebrand Factor-cleaving metalloprotease (ADAMTS13). Ann Hematol 2002; 81: 430–435
6. Fujikawa K, Suzuki H, McMullen B, Chung D. Purification of human von Willebrand Factor-cleaving protease and its identification as a new member of the metalloproteinase family. Blood 2001; 98: 1662–1666
7. Gerritsen HE, Robles R, Lämmle B, Furlan M. Partial amino acid sequence of purified von Willebrand Factor-cleaving protease Blood 2001; 98: 1654–1661
8. Levy GG, Nichols WC, Lian EC, Foroud T, McClintick JN, McGee BM, Yang AY, Siemieniak DR, Stark KR, Gruppo R, Sarode R, Shurin SB, Chandrasekaran V, Stabler SP, Sabio H, Bouhassira EE, Upshaw JD, Ginsburg D, Tsai HM. Mutations in a member of the ADAMTS gene family cause thrombotic thrombocytopenic purpura. Nature 2001; 413: 488–494
9. Kokame K, Matsumoto M, Soejima K, Yagi H, Ishizashi H, Funato M, Tamai H, Konno M, Kamide K, Kawano Y, Miyata T, Fujimura Y. Mutations and common polymorphisms in ADAMTS-13 gene responsible for von Willebrand Factor-cleaving protease activity. PNAS 2002; 99: 11902–11907
10. Schneppenheim R, Budde U, Oyen F, Angerhaus D, Aumann V, Drewke E, Hasenpflug W, Häberle J, Kentouche K, Kohne E, Kurnik K, Mueller-Wiefel D, Obser T, Santer R, Sykora KW. von Willebrand Factor cleaving protease and ADAMTS13 mutations in childhood TTP. Blood 2003; 101: 1845–1850
11. Antoine G, Zimmermann K, Plaimauer B, Grillowitzer M, Studt JD, Lämmle B, Scheiflinger F. ADAMTS-13 gene defects in two brothers with constitutional thrombotic thrombocytopenic purpura and normalization of von Willebrand Factor-cleaving protease activity by recombinant human ADAMTS-13
12. Savasan S, Lee SK, Ginsburg D, Tsai HM. ADAMTS-13 gene mutation in congenital thrombotic thrombocytopenic purpura with previously reported normal vWF cleaving protease activity. Blood, prepublished online February 6, 2003
13. Mannucci PM, Canciani MT, Forza I, Lussana F, Lattuada A, Rossi E. Changes in health and disease of the metalloprotease that cleaves von Willebrand Factor. Blood 2001; 98: 2730–2735
14. Moore JC, Hayward CPM, Warkentin TE, Kelton JG (2001) Decreased von Willebrand Factor protease activity associated with thrombocytopenic disorders. Blood 98: 1842–1846
15. Oleksowicz L, Bhagwati N, DeLeon-Fernandez M. Deficient activity of von-Willebrand's-factor cleaving protease in patients with disseminated malignancies. Cancer Res 1999; 59: 2244–2250
16. Remuzzi G, Galbusera M, Noris M, Canciani MT, Daina E, Bresin E, Contaretti S, Caprioli J, Gamba S, Ruggenenti P, Perico N Mannucci PM for the Italian Registry of Recurrent and Familial HUS/TTP. von Willebrand Factor cleaving protease (ADAMTS-13) is deficient in recurrent and familial thrombotic thrombocytopenic purpura and hemolytic uremic syndrome. Blood 2002, 100: 778–785

17. Bianchi V, Robles R, Alberio L, Furlan M, Lämmle B. von Willebrand Factor-cleaving protease (ADAMTS13) in thrombocytopenic disorders: a severely deficient activity is specific for thrombotic thrombocytopenic purpura. Blood 2002; 100: 710–713
18. Reiter RA, Knöbl P, Varadi K, Turecek PL. Changes in von Willebrand Factor-cleaving protease (ADAMTS-13) activity after infusion of desmopressin. Blood, prepublished online September 19, 2002

VII.   Poster

VIIa. Clinic and Casuistic

Treatment with Interferon Alpha-2a in Patients with Hepatitis C and Hemophilia

R. Zimmermann, A. Huth-Kühne, P. Lages, and B. Kallinowski

Introduction

Already in 1943, Beeson observed a connection between the transfusion of blood products and the emergence of hepatitis [1]. Jaundice developed in 7 patients 1–4 months after the administration of whole blood or plasma. Further reports on the development of hepatitis in hemophilic patients were published in the mid-70s [2, 3, 4]. Today it is generally accepted that the hepatitis C virus causes the majority of cases of post-transfusion hepatitis in the western world. It is responsible for most of the chronic liver disorders observed in hemophilic patients treated with clotting factor concentrates. The hepatitis C infection can be associated with replacement therapy involving clotting factor concentrates applied in the early 1970s [2, 5, 6].

Hepatitis often follows an asymptomatic course, but at least 50% of patients infected with the virus develop chronic hepatitis and up to 30% develop cirrhosis of the liver within 10–20 years following diagnosis. 10% of all those infected develop a liver cell carcinoma within a further 10 years [7, 8]. Of the variants known, 6 more frequently occurring genotypes (types 1–6) are described, although each type can be differentiated further [9]. The 6 most common genotypes have varying nucleotide sequences in the 5-non coding region (NCR).

Alpha-interferon (IFNα-2a) is an effective treatment for chronic hepatitis C, but only 15–30% of patients show a sustained response after treatment. HCV positive hemophiliacs in Europe present mostly with genotype 1a/1b and thus may have an even more poor response rate to IFNα-2a. It has been shown that higher dosage regimens (cumulative dose) are more effective.

The combination of interferon and ribavirin resulted in a higher sustained response rate [12, 13]. Recently the additional use of the antiviral agent amantadine was investigated in pilot studies with improvement of biochemical and virological markers [14].

Patients and Methods

In a first study we treated 14 patients, n = 12 with hemophilia A and n = 2 with von-Willebrand disease with the following dosage regimen: 6 MU s.c. daily for 4 weeks, followed by 6 MU three times per week for 22 weeks; then the dose was reduced to 3 MU three times per week for the next 6 months.

I. Scharrer/W. Schramm (Ed.)
33rd Hemophilia Symposium Hamburg 2002
© Springer-Verlag Berlin Heidelberg 2004

Inclusion criteria were the presence of anti-HCV antibodies, HCV-RNA (detected by nested PCR) and elevated transaminases (ALT). The clinical course, transaminases, quantitative HCV-RNA, HCV-genotype and immunological parameters were evaluated before, 2, 4, 8, 12, 38, 52 weeks after start of treatment and 6 months after discontinuation of therapy.

Because of the disappointing results of the first study, in a second study the combination of interferon alfa-2a, ribavirin and amantadine was investigated in 21 patients with chronic hepatitis C and hemophilia. Patients received 6 MU of interferon alpha-2a s.c. daily for 6 weeks, followed by 6 MU three times/week for 20 weeks; than the dose was reduced to 3 MU three times/week for the next 6 months. Ribavirin was given at a dose of 10 mg/kg bw/d and amantadine 200 mg/d for 52 weeks. Clinical course, transaminases, quantitative HCV-RNA, HCV-genotype and immunological parameters were tested prior and 2, 4, 6, 8, 12, 38 and 52 weeks after start of treatment and 6 months after discontinuation of therapy.

Results

Our first study showed in 10 of the 14 patients a normalization of the ALT-levels. At the end of the study, only 2 of the patients demonstrated a normal behaviour of ALT. After 12 weeks of treatment, ALT could be reduced by 40%.

HCV-RNA could be normalized in 6 of 14 patients (42%) after 12 weeks of treatment. However, at the end of the treatment after 52 weeks only 14% showed further normalization. A sustained response could be demonstrated only in 2 (14%) of the patients 26 weeks after discontinuation of the treatment with interferon (Table 1).

An 80% reduction of the HCV-RNA-values could be measured in our patients after 12 weeks of therapy.

Influenza-like symptoms initially observed in most of the patients disappeared in most of them within a few weeks. In 2 of the patients the interferon dose had to be reduced because of a depression of platelets or leukocytes. 2 patients reported mental depression, and 2 stomatitis and leukoplakia.

The data of our second study are shown in the Tables 2 and 3 and the Figures 1–3. In one of the 21 patients therapy had to be discontinued because of side reactions (one depression). In one patient appendectomy had to be performed with stopping therapy. In 7 of 19 patients a sustained response could be achieved.

Table 1. Response rate in study 1

| Weeks | Response | | |
	CR (%)	PR (%)	NR (%)
2–4	4	39	57
8–26	29	29	42
38–52	14	11	75
58–78	14	7	79

CR = complete response; PR = partial response; NR = non response

Table 2. HCV-Genotypes of the patients in study 2

n = 21	n	%
Type 1a	8	38
Type 1b	11	52
Type 2a	1	5
Type 2b	1	5

Table 3. Response rate in study 2

Weeks	Response		
	CR (%)	PR (%)	NR (%)
2–6	16	47	37
8–26	42	29	29
38–52	41	33	26
Follow up	44	7	49
Study end	37	5	58

A temporary virus elimination could be seen in 56% of our patients. Flue-like symptoms were observed in most of the patients and 35% suffered on psychiatric symptoms.

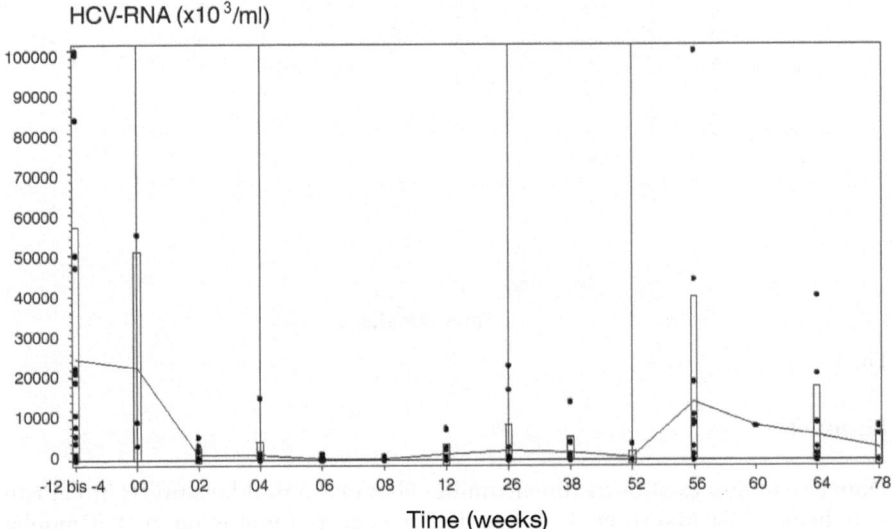

Fig. 1

Δ HCV-RNA (%)

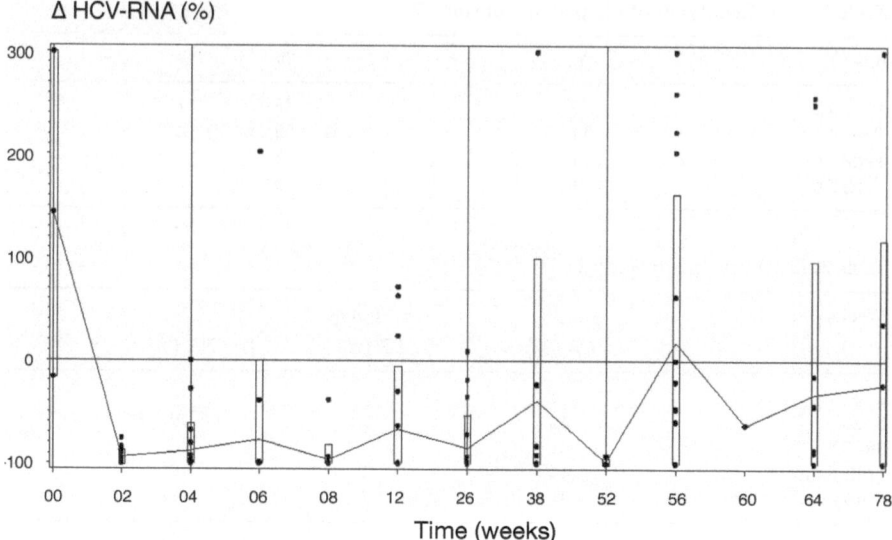

Fig. 2

platelets (x10⁹/L)

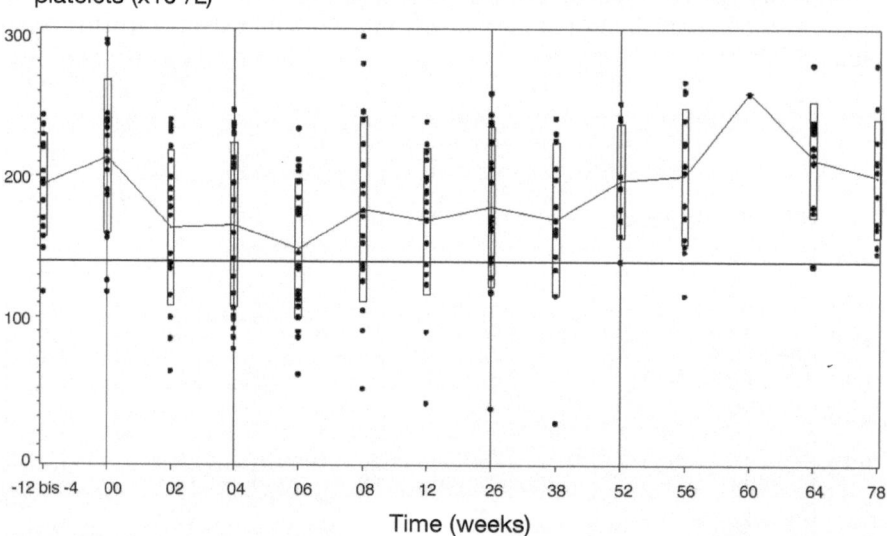

Fig. 3

Discussion

Only few studies exist of treatment studies about chronical hepatitis C in patients with hemophilia. Makris et al. [10] studied the effect of interferon in 18 hemophiliacs and found a sustained biochemical response in only 3 patients. Similar results were reported by Laursen and Coworkers [11]. In the Danish study 47 patients were enrolled and received 3 MU-interferon thrice weekly for 3 months. In 26 non responders the dose was increased to 6 MU TEW for additional 3 months. Only 16% of the patients could be treated successfully with a sustained response documented 26 weeks after discontinuation of therapy.

Also our high dose interferon regimen with an initial treatment of 6 MU daily within the first 4 weeks was not able to induce a higher rate of response. However, we have to consider the high rate of the HCV-genotype 1. 11 of the 14 patients suffered from the type 1a or 1b (79%). The types 2a, 2b and 3a were found in 1 patient respectively. The high incidence of type 1 may explain the poor response rate in spite of the high dosage rate of interferon as well.

In our **second study** 8/21 patients were HCV-RNA negative after 38–52 weeks of treatment. These results appear to be promising with regard to the high prevalence of the genotype 1. Perhaps the prolonged high initial dosage and the combination therapy may have a more pronounced effect and better long time results. At the present time pegylated interferon will be used in our patients as described previously [15,16,17].

Summary

Our data of the here used high dosage treatment with interferon (first study) show that the virus load of HCV-RNA could be reduced in all patients by 80%. HCV-RNA disappeared transiently in 6/14 patients during 12 weeks, but a high reoccurrence has to be considered in most of the patients. A sustained response could be observed only in 2 (14%) of our patients. Influenza-like symptoms could be observed in nearly all patients but disappeared in most of them within a few weeks. Depression of platelets or leukocytes necessitated a dose reduction of interferon in 2 patients. One reason for the lower response rate may be the predominant genotype 1a and 1b in our patient group. The results of the **second study** demonstrated a higher sustained response in 7 of 19 patients.

References

1. Beeson PB. Jaundice occuring one to four months after transfusion of blood or plasma: report of seven cases. J Am Med Assoc 1943; 121: 1332–4
2. Kasper CK, Kipnis SA. Hepatitis and clotting-factor concentrates. JAMA 1972; 221: 510
3. Mannucci PM, Capitanio A, del Nino E, Colombo M, Pareti F, Ruggeri ZM. A symptomatic liver disease in haemophiliacs. J Clin Path 1975; 28: 620–4
4. Schimpf K, Zimmermann K. Hepatitishäufigkeit, serologische Befunde und Leberhistologie nach Therapie schwerer hämorrhagischer Diathesen mit Gerinnungsfaktorenkonzentraten. In: Fibrinogen, Fibrin, and Fibrin Glue. Side effects of the therapy with clottimg factor concentrates. Schimpf K Ed, Schattauer Verlag 1980; 299–308
5. Hasiba UW, Spero JA, Lewis JH. Chronic liver dysfunction in multitransfused haemophiliacs. Transfusion 1977; 17: 490
6. Preston FE, Jarvis LM, Makris M, Philp L, Underwood JCE, Ludlam CA, Simmonds P. Heterogeneity of hepatitis C virus genotypes in haemophilia: relationship with chronic liver disease. Blood 1995; 85: 1259–62

7. Makris M, Preston FE, Triger DR, Underwood JC. The natural history of chronic liver disease in haemophilia: more rapid progression relates to age and mild disease (abstract). Br. J Haematol 1992; 81 (Suppl. 1): 72

8. Zeuzem S, Roth WK, Herrmann G. Virushepatitis C. Z Gastroenterol 1995; 33: 117–32

9. Simonds P, Holmes EC, Cha TA, Chan SW, McOmish F, Irvine B, Beall E, Yap Pl, Kolberg J, Urdea MS. Classification of hepatitis C virus into six major genotypes and a serie of subtypes by phylogenetic analysis of the NS-5 region. J Gén Virol 1993; 74: 2391

10. Makris M, Preston M, Triger DR, Underwood JCE, Westlake L, Adelman MI. A randomized controlled trial of recombinant interferon-α in chronic hepatitis C in hemophiliacs. Blood 1991; 78: 1672–7

11. Laursen AL, Scheibel E, Ingerslev J, Clausen NC, Wantzin P, Oestergaard L, Schou G, Black FT, Krosgaard K. Alpha interferon therapy in Danish hemophilic patients with chronic hepatitis C: results of a randomized controlled open label study comparing two different maintenance regimens following standard interferon-alpha-2b treatment. Haemophilia 1998; 4: 25–32

12. Davis GL, Esteban-Mur R, Rustgi V, Hoefs J, Gordon SC, Trepo C, Shifmann ML, Zeuzem S, Craxi A, Ling MH, Albrecht J. Interferon alpha-2b alone or in combination with ribavirin for the treatment of relapse of chronic hepatitis C. N Engl J Med 1998; 339: 1493–1499

13. McHutchison JG, Gordon SC, Schiff ER, Shiffman ML, Lee WM, Rustgi VK, Goodman ZD, Ling MH, Cort S, Albrecht JK. Interferon alpha-2b alone or in combination with ribavirin as initial treatment for chronic hepatitis C. N Engl J Med 1998, 339: 1485–1492

14. Palmer Smith J. Treatment of chronic hepatitis C with amantadine Dig Dis and Sciences 1997; 42: 1681–1687

15. Zeuzem S, Feinman SV, Rasenack J, Heathcote E, Lai MY, Gane E, et al. Peginterferon alpha-2a in patients with chronic hepatitis C. N Engl J Med 2000; 343: 1666–1672. Abstract

16. Lindsay KL, Trepo C, Heintges T, Shiffman ML, Gordon SC, Hoefs JC, et al. A randomized, double-blind trial comparing pegylated interferon alpha-2b to interferon alpha-2b as initial treatment for chronic hepatitis C. Hepatology. 2001 Aug; 34(2): 395–403. Abstract

17. Manns MP, McHutchison JG, Gordon SC, Rustgi VK, Shiffman M, Reindollar R, et al. Peginterferon alpha-2b plus ribavirin compared with interferon alpha-2b plus ribavirin for initial treatment of chronic hepatitis C: a randomised trial. Lancet 2001; 358: 958–965. Abstract.

Practical Experiences with Therapies for Chronic Hepatitis C in Hemophilia Patients

S. Gottstein, and R. Klamroth

Patients with hemophilia are at risk to be infected with hepatitis C through contaminated blood products. More than 50% of the infections with hepatitis C virus cause in chronic hepatitis. Late complications of chronic hepatitis C are liver cirrhosis and liver cell cancer which can be expected in up to 30% and 10% respectively.

Since 1996 treatment for chronic hepatitis C with interferon alpha has been performed in our hemophilia treatment center. The first patients received a monotherapy with interferon alpha, given three times per week subcutaneously or daily during the first month and three times weekly thereafter. Then Ribavirin was added as peroral antiviral agent. A triple therapy contained also peroral amantadin ("Heidelberger Protokoll"). The development of pegylated interferon alpha lead to the weekly administration of the interferon in combination with Ribavirin.

We report about the treatment of 16 patients in our center. The age was between 18 and 54 years at initiation of the therapy.

They are 13 patients with severe hemophilia A (i.e. FVIII-activity <1%), one patient with mild hemophilia A (FVIII-activity 5%), one patient with subhemophilia A (FVIII-activity 20%) and one patient with severe hemophilia B (FIX-activity <1%).

All patients were infected with hepatitis C through blood products for more than 10 years ago. The diagnosis of chronic hepatitis C was first suspected in the mid '90s by testing for antibodies against hepatitis C. Confirmation by repeated measuring of HCV-RNA was done since 1998. Antiviral therapy was offered to every hemophilia patient with chronic hepatitis below the age of 50 years. It was strongly recommended to those who had constantly elevated liver enzymes or clinical symptoms of chronic infection, f.e. chronic fatigue.

Liver biopsy was not performed. Ultrasound scanning of the upper abdomen was performed before start for antiviral therapy. None of the patients treated had laboratory or imaging criteria for liver cirrhosis. All patients were infected with hepatitis C virus type 1. Accordingly, if virus elimination after 3 months of treatment was achieved, the overall treatment period was 12 months. All patients treated were HIV-negative. The possible consequences of chronic hepatitis C were carefully discussed with the patients as well as common and rare side effects of the antiviral therapy. They were informed about the treatment regimen, the necessity of control examinations and the necessity of contraception during therapy.

The first injection of interferon was performed by the patient in the hemophilia treatment center.

8 patients received the monotherapy (interferon alpha 2a). Only one patient showed a sustained response. The combination with Ribavirin (interferon alpha 2a and Ribavirin) was given in 6 cases. Of these, three patients were Non-Responder and one patient showed a relapse after completed therapy. 2 patients showed virus elimination under therapy and stayed HCV-RNA-negative after the treatment. 3 patients were treated with interferon alpha 2a, Ribavirin and amantadin. In these cases, no virus elimination was seen.

A treatment regimen with pegylated interferon alpha 2b and Ribavirin has lead to virus elimination and has been completed in 4 patients. So far, no relapse has occurred.

There was a broad variability in side effects reported by the patients. Most of them had influenza like symptoms after the injection of interferon alpha. Those patients who received interferon alpha and, in a second attempt, pegylated interferon alpha reported no clear difference concerning headache, muscle pain, malaise and fever. Parallel administration of Paracetamol was effective to reduce these symptoms.

One patient complained about a change of mood in terms of feeling and acting more aggressively than he used to and about sleeplessness. Another patient had nausea and abdominal pains. Local skin irritation with redness and pruritus after the injection of interferon was observed in one case, another patient showed local hair loss. One patient developed a rosacea, another an oral candida-infection. Both required intermittent medical treatment. In one patient a hypothyreosis was found and treated by hormone substitution.

Weight loss at a tolerable grade was observed in all patients (5–10 kg). One patient complained about intermittent coldness of his distal fingers and toes. Duplexsonography of the arteries and capillarmicroscopy showed no abnormalities and a neuropathy is suspected.

Laboratory controls were performed weekly during the first two months, followed by monthly controls. All patients showed a decrease of hemoglobin concentration and leucocyte and thrombocyte count, which indicated a dosis reduction of both drugs in two cases. There was a increase of liver transaminase (ALAT) in one patient after 7 month of therapy (more than 3 times of normal). The therapy was discontinued and the ALAT fell rapidly. Another patient showed an increase in liver parameters after cessation of the antiviral treatment, which resolved spontaneously. Hepatitis C RNA remained negative.

Over all, a reduction of interferon and Ribavirin was necessary in 5 patients because of side effects. No hospitalization was required due to side effects of the antiviral therapy. There was no increase of spontaneous bleedings under the treatment.

The self-application of the interferon by the patients was performed without problems. Except for one patient, the patient compliance was excellent.

The antiviral treatment with interferon alpha in patients with hemophilia and posttransfusional chronic hepatitis C appears safe and easy to perform on an outpatient basis. The additional administration of amantadin showed no benefit in a small group of patients.

Careful information of the patient is necessary to obtain optimal compliance and documentation of side effects.

References

1. Alscher, Bode: Therapie der chronischen Hepatitis C, Sonderdruck Med. Klein. 92 (1997), 147–161 (Nr.3)
2. Zimmermann, Huth-Kühne: Therapieoptimierungsversuch: Behandlung der chronischen Hepatitis C mit Interferon alpha 2a in Kombination mit Amantadinsulfat bei Patienten mit Hämophilie
3. Manns et al.: Peginterferon alfa 2b plus Ribavirin compared with interferon alfa 2b plus Ribavirin. The Lancet 2001, Vol. 358, No. 9286, 958–965

Deep Venous Thrombosis of the Lower Extremity in a 16-Year-Old Girl with Homozygous MTHFR- and Heterozygous Factor V Leiden-Mutation

B. Roschitz, W. Muntean, C. Mannhalter, and M. Koestenberger

Although relatively rare, thromboembolic complications do occur in pediatric patients [1] and cause significant morbidity with occasional mortality. Venous thrombosis is a multicausal disease involving acquired and genetic factors. The pediatric patient with thrombosis has an average of two and some of four or more predisposing and triggering prothrombotic factors [2]. Genetic abnormalities of antithrombin, protein C, protein S, factor V G1691A, prothrombin G20210A and elevated lipoprotein(a) concentration have been reported in children with venous thrombosis [3–5].

In this report we describe the case of a 16-year-old girl with deep venous thrombosis of the left lower extremity homozygous for methylenetetrahydrofolate reductase (MTHFR) T677T- and heterozygous for factor V Leiden-mutation.

Case report

A 16-year-old girl was referred to our department after being diagnosed for deep vein thrombosis of the left lower extremity. The patient was admitted to hospital with sudden pain and numbness in the left leg. Prior to admission no trauma or inflammatory medical condition was found. Her parents were generally healthy and non-consanguineous. Medical history in the family did not reveal any thromboembolic events.

The girl had started computer school and had not got a lot of exercise for two weeks because of mainly sitting activity. Four weeks prior to admission hormonal contraception had been initiated.

Phlebography of the left leg revealed thrombotic occlusion of the veins. Screening for coagulation defects showed normal platelet count, normal aPTT, fibrinogen 627 mg/dl, APCR 1.7. The patient and her mother were found to be heterozygous for factor V Leiden mutation. The girl was also homozygous for a common thermolabile polymorphism in the gene coding for MTHFR. Elevation of homocysteine was found in our patient (fasting homocysteine plasma level: 15.5 µmol/l).

Initially the girl was treated with subcutaneous low-molecular-weight-heparin, meanwhile she is on oral anticoagulation and vitamin supplementation (vitamin B12, folic acid). Good collateralisation of the veins was observed in the last ultrasound control.

Discussion

Because some but not all studies of venous thromboembolism and hyper-homocysteinemia had reported positive associations, it had remained contro-versial whether elevation of homocysteine was an independent risk factor for these events. In contrast the role of hyperhomocysteinemia in arterial disease had been well documented in adults [6] and recent undertaken investigations confirmed that hyperhomocysteinemia was a risk factor in venous thromboembolism [7–11]. Hyperhomocysteinemia in combination with factor V Leiden increases the risk of recurrent thrombosis synergistically in adults [7–11]. Data in MTHFR-muta-tion in children are still sparse and equivocal [12, 13].

Hyperhomocysteinemia may be caused by acquired and/or genetic abnormali-ties of homocysteine metabolism. The most common genetic abnormality of homocysteine metabolism is due to a C to T transition at nucleotide 677 of the gene encoding for MTHFR. As compared with normal individuals, subjects with homozygous MTHFR T677T have decreased MTHFR activity and thermosta-bility, resulting in elevated plasma homocysteine concentrations as well as lower levels of an activated form of folic acid. The role of the MTHFR T-allele in venous thrombosis is still under discussion. Arruda et al., Salamon et al. and others found the homozygous MTHFR T677T-mutation to be a risk factor for venous throm-bosis. Other studies have not shown this association [14–16]. Data of a childhood case-control study suggest that mildly elevated fasting homocysteine concentra-tions are significant risk factors but showed no positive association with MTHFR T677T genotype which was overall rare in the study population and never com-bined with other genetic defects [12].

Our case report is in line with a recent report of Keijzer et al. [8] which has yielded an odds ratio of 18.7 for combined risk of MTHFR T677T and factor V Leiden in adults. So thromboembolic events in childhood might also show positive association with homozygous MTHFR T677T- mutation combined with other thrombophilic traits. Our patient is heterozygous for factor V Leiden and homo-zygous for MTHFR mutation, she had started with oral contraception using a third generation product four weeks prior to the event, and had changed her lifestyle to a more sedentary one.

In any case our report is in line with the recommendation of the SSC-commu-nication of the International Society on Thrombosis and Haemostasis on laboratory testing for thrombophilia in pediatric patients which suggests to test for a full panel of genetic and acquired prothrombotic risk factors, because detection of one throm-bophilic factor does not exclude the existence of a second or third [17].

References

1. Andrew M, David M, Adams M. Venous thromboembolic complications (VTE) in children: first analyses of the Canadian registry of VTE. Blood 1994; 83: 1251–7
2. Nowak-Göttl U, Kosch A, Schlegel N. Thromboembolism in neonates, infants, and children. Thromb Haemost 2001; 86: 464–7

3. Ehrenforth S, Junker R, Koch HG, Kreuz W, Münchow N, Scharrer I, Nowak-Göttl U. Multi-centre evaluation of combined prothrombotic defects with thrombophilia in childhood. Eur J Pediatr 1999; 158: S97–104
4. Nuss R, Hays T, Manco-Johnson M. Childhood thrombosis. Pediatrics 1995; 96: 291–4
5. Bonduel M, Hepner M, Sciuccati G, Torres AF, Pieroni G, Frontroth JP. Prothrombotic abnormalities in children with venous thromboembolism. J Pediatr Hematol Oncol 2000; 22: 66–72
6. Arruda VR, von Zuben PM, Chiaparini LC, Annichino-Bizzacchi JM, Costa FF. The mutation Ala677 Val in the methylene tetrahydrofolate reductase gene: a risk factor arterial disease and venous thrombosis . Thromb Haemost 1997; 77: 818–21
7. Hainaut P, Jaumotte C, Verhelst D, Wallemacq P, Gala JL, Lavenne E et al. Hyperhomocysteinemia and venous thromboembolism: a risk factor more prevalent in the elderly and in idiopathic cases. Thromb Res 2002; 106: 121–5
8. Keijzer MB, Den Heijer M, Blom HJ, Bos GM, Willems HP, Gerrits WB, Rosendaal FR. Interaction between hyperhomocysteinemia, mutated methylentetrahydrofolatereductase (MTHFR) and inherited thrombophilic factors in recurrent venous thrombosis. Thromb Haemost 2002; 88: 723–8
9. Salomon O, Steinberg DM, Zivelin A, Gitel S, Dardik R, Rosenberg N, Berliner S, Inbal A. Single and combined prothrombotic factors in patients with idiopathic venous thromboembolism – prevalence and risk assessment. Arteriol Thromb Vasc Biol 1999; 19: 511–8
10. Falcon CR, Cattaneo M, Panzeri D, Martinelli I, Mannucci PM. High prevalence of hyperhomocyst(e)inemia in patients with juvenile venous thrombosis. Arterioscler Thromb 1994; 14: 1080–3
11. Den Heijer M, Blom HJ, Gerrits WBJ, Rosendaal FR, Haak HL, Wijermans PW, Bos GMJ. Is hyperhomocysteinemia a risk factor for recurrent venous thrombosis? Lancet 1995; 345: 882–5
12. Koch HG, Nabel P, Junker R, Auberger K, Schobess R, Homberger A, Linnebank M, Nowak-Göttl U. The 677T genotype of the common MTHFR thermolabile variant and fasting homocysteine in childhood venous thrombosis. Eur J Pediatr 1999; 158 : S113–6
13. Grow JL, Fliman PJ, Pipe SW. Neonatal sinovenous thrombosis associated with homozygous thermolabile methylene tetrahydrofolate reductase in both mother and infant. J Perinat 2002; 22: 175–8
14. Alhenc-Gelas M, Arnoud E, Nicaud V, Aubry ML, Fiessinger JN, Aich M, Emmerich J. Venous thromboembolic disease and the prothrombin, methylene tetrahydrofolate reductase and factor V genes. Thromb Haemost 1999; 81: 506–10
15. Kluijtmans LA, Den Heijer M, Reitsma PH, Heil SG, Blom HJ, Rosendaal FR. Thermolabile methylenetetrahydrofolate reductase and factor V Leiden in the risk of deep vein thrombosis. Thromb Haemost 79: 254–8
16. Rintelen C, Mannhalter C, Lechner K, Eichinger S, Kyrle PA, Papagiannopolos M, Schneider B, Pabinger I. No evidence for an increased risk of venous thrombosis in patients with factor V Leiden by the 677C to T mutation in the methylene tetrahydrofolate-reductase gene. Blood Coagul + Fibrinol 1999; 10: 101–5
17. Manco-Johnson MJ, Grabowski EF, Hellgreen M, Kemahli AS, Massicotte MP, Muntean W, Peters M, Nowak-Göttl U. Laboratory testing for thrombophilia in pediatric patients. Thromb Haemost 2002; 88: 155–6

Clinical Manifestations of Patients with Highly Elevated Anticardiolipin Antibodies

W. Miesbach, G. Asmelash, and I. Scharrer

The antiphospholipid syndrome (APS) is one of the most common acquired throm-bophilic disorder characterized by arterial and/or venous thrombosis, recurrent preg-nancy losses and the laboratory evidence for antibodies against phospholipids or phospholipid-binding protein cofactors [1]. APS is considered as a disease of the auto-immune system with unpredictably occurring thromboembolism in combina-tion with evidence of antiphospholipid antibodies [2, 3]. This syndrome may be pri-mary or may be associated with other diseases, mainly systemic lupus erythematosus (SLE).

Further clinical manifestations include thrombocytopenia, valvular heart disease and various neurological and gynecological disorders.

A variety of cardiac, neurologic and gynecologic manifestations are associated with the presence of antiphospholipid antibodies (aPL). Thrombocytopenia due to APS does not protect against thrombosis. A particularly serious and often fatal clinical form with a high mortality rate of approximately 50% has been termed catastrophic antiphospholipid syndrome (CAPS), and these patients present with fulminant arterial and venous thrombosis and embolism in mainly the small vessels of the body [6]. This may lead to myocardial infarction, acute respiratory distress syndrome (ARDS), and subsequent death. The extent of APS ranges from asymp-tomatic serologic evidence of antiphospholipid antibodies to life-threatening disease. The deep vein thrombosis is the most common manifestation, whereas stroke and transient ischemic attack are the most common form of arterial throm-bosis in patients with APS [5].

The thromboembolic manifestations can be very heterogenous, may be reflecting the heterogenity of the antiphospholipid antibodies. Common laboratory tests are functional coagulation tests for lupus anticoagulants (LAC) and immunological assays for antibodies against cardiolipin (aCL) and β_2-glycoprotein I (β_2GPI).

In the early 1990 it was reported that antiphospholipid antibodies do not bind to phospholipids (e.g. Cardiolipin) alone but to complexes of phospholipids and protein cofactors, e.g. β_2-glycoprotein I (β_2-GPI) and/or prothrombin [6]. Now it is reported that subgroups of antiphospholipid antibodies bind to the protein cofac-tor without any phospholipids [7]. The finding of cross-reactivity of antiphospholi-pid antibodies with oxidized LDL and antiphospholipid antibodies in 1993 could be a link between coagulation system and lipoproteins [8].

Antiphospholipid antibodies are found in young healthy subjects with a preva-lence of 1–5% [4]. Current studies suggest, that aPL may increase with age and are

I. Scharrer/W. Schramm (Ed.)
33rd Hemophilia Symposion Hamburg 2002
© Springer-Verlag Berlin Heidelberg 2004

often associated with multiple vascular risk factors [10]. Although the presence of aPL in the absence of clinical manifestations does not indicate APS, it is suggested that asymptomatic aPL-positive individuals have a higher risk of developing thrombotic complications and the high titer of aCL may be a significant predictor of thrombosis [11, 12].

The mechanism of thrombosis by antiphospholipid antibodies is unknown, but it is considered as a vasoocclusive thrombotic disease without vessel inflammation [13]. Proposed mechanism include direct endothelial damage, antibody mediated platelet activation and inhibition of endogenous anticoagulants such as thrombomodulin, protein C, protein S, antithrombin or annexin V [14].

Within the pathophysiology of APS, there are apparently infectious, inflammatory and autoimmune factors that contribute to thrombotic manifestation, especially to the progression of atherosclerosis [15].

Leading to the autoimmune origin an infectious cause has been postulated, including the induction by passive transfer of anti-β2-glycoprotein I antibodies induced by common bacteria [16].

Despite the increasing understanding of the mechanism and clinical manifestations of the antiphospholipid syndrome, thrombotic complications are unpredictable and triggering factors are unknown. One important risk factor of thromboembolic complications of APS appears to be a history of thrombosis [11]. Retrospective studies suggest that patients with APS have an increased risk of recurrent thromboembolism [5, 9, 17]. Especially patients with high positive aCL antibodies may have more frequently thrombo-occlusive events after cerebral ischemia [18]. So these patients are recommended to receive oral vitamin K antagonists, like Warfarin to achieve an international normalized ratio (INR) range within the therapeutical level.

Anticardiolipin (aCL) antibodies are considered as specific markers of the antiphospholipid syndrome [1]. The aCL-ELISA is found to be the most frequently performed test in patients with suspected APS.

Up to now it is still unclear, whether IgG-and IgM-isotypes of aCL antibodies are distinct markers of certain clinical manifestations. To study the relationship between clinical presentations of APS and the IgG and IgM isotypes of aCL-antibodies, we included only patients with high elevated titers (more than 8 times elevated than normal), because the higher the anticardiolipin level the greater the likelihood of manifestation of thrombotic disease [19, 20].

Patients

From 1994 until 2002 over 1000 patients were tested positively with elevated titers of IgG- and IgM-aCL in our laboratory by a β_2-glycoprotein I-dependent enzyme-linked immunosorbent assay (Pharmacia ELISA, Freiburg, Germany). Testing for aCL-antibodies was made due to acute or previous thromboembolic disease, in patients with family history of thromboembolic disease or with systemic lupus erythematodes (SLE) or in patients with prolonged PTT.

The group of 48 patients with highly elevated IgG-aCL-titers (IgG-aCL > 100 GPL-U/ml) consisted of 27 female patients and 21 male patients (female:male ratio 1.28 : 1).

The median age at the first examination was 45 years. 18/48 (37%) of the patients were suffering from SLE or SLE-related diseases; 3/48 (6%) of the patients were suffering from malignancies.

The group of 53 patients with highly elevated IgM-aCL-titers (IgM-aCL > 50 MPL-U/ml) consisted of 38 female patients and 15 male patients (female:male ratio 2.53 : 1). The median age at the date of the first examination was 52 years. 22/53 (41%) of these patients were suffering from SLE or SLE-related diseases; 10/53 (19%) of the patients were suffering from malignancies.

Methods

Diagnosis APS was defined by the international consensus criteria (Sapporo criteria) [1].

The aCL-IgG and IgM-antibodies were determined by solid-phase, β_2-glycoprotein-dependent standardized enzyme linked immunosorbent assays (ELISA) [21].

Results

We describe the clinical features of 48 patients with aCL-IgG-titers > 100 GPL (normal range: – 11,7 GPL) and 53 patients with aCL-IgM > 50 MPL (normal range: – 4,8 MPL).

The distribution of the aCL-antibodies of these patients and the frequency of positive lupus anticoagulants is listed in Fig. 1. In 12 patients both, IgG- and IgM-aCL-titers were highly elevated.

The main clinical features of these patients are summarized in Table 1.

The most common clinical manifestations of the patients with high aCL-IgG-titers > 100 GPL were arterial thrombosis (46%), e.g. transient ischemic attacks and strokes (27%), myocardial infarctions (9%) and peripher arterial thromboses (10%).

44% of the patients were presented with venous thromboses, 12% with thrombocytopenia and 12% with fetal loss.

In nearly 23% of the patients no thromboembolic disease could be found.

Cardiolipin-Antibodies (Median)

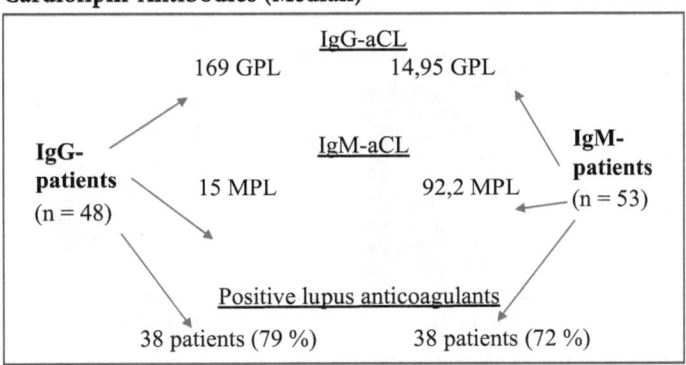

Fig. 1.
Anticardiolipin antibodies and lupus anticoagulants

Table 1. Clinical manifestations of patients with highly elevated aCL-antibodies

%	IgG-aCL > 100 GPL-U/ml	IgM-aCL > 50 MPL-U/ml	
Venous thrombosis	44	26	
Arterial thrombosis	46	40	
Stroke	27	21	
Myocardial infarction	9	8	
Peripheral arterial stenosis	10	11	
Recurrent abortions	12	4	
Thrombocytopenia	12	8	
Without clinical manifestation	23	42	(p < 0,05)

In comparison to that result, in over 42% of the patients with highly elevated aCL-IgM titers no thromboembolic disease could be found (p < 0.05, Fig. 2).

Arterial thrombosis occurred in this group in 40% of the patients. It was the most common clinical manifestation, e.g. transient ischemic attack and stroke (21%). Myocardial infarction (8%) and peripher arterial thrombosis (11%) were less frequent.

26% of the patients were presented with venous thrombosis and 8% with thrombocytopenia.

Recurrent abortions and thrombocytopenia were more frequent in patients with highly elevated IgG-aCL than in patients with highly elevated IgM-aCL (12% vs. 4% and 12% vs. 8%).

Discussion

By including only patients with either highly elevated aCL-IgG or aCL-IgM-titers the prevalence of the clinical features of patients with APS and different aPL antibodies

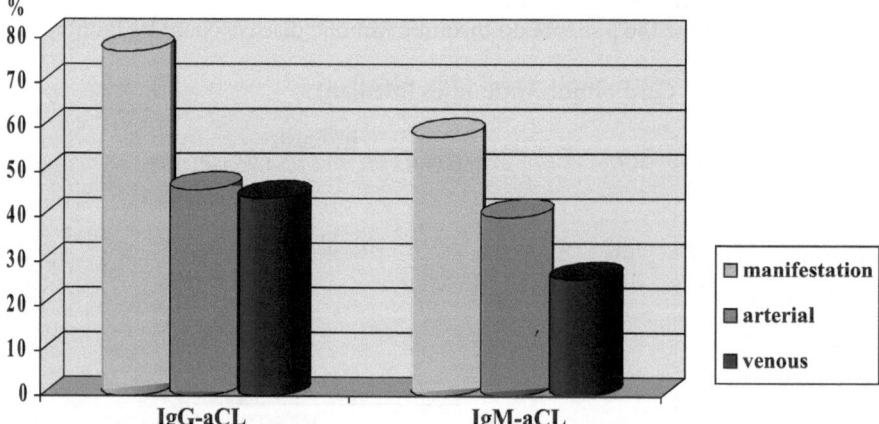

Fig. 2. Rate of clinical manifestations

can be distinguished more clearly. Both groups showed nearly the same median age at the date of the first examination. The female:male ratio was higher in patients with highly elevated IgM-aCL-titers. SLE occurred more often in patients with highly elevated IgM-aCL than in patients with highly elevated IgG-aCL. The rate of malignancies was higher in patients with highly elevated IgM-aCL.

In patients with highly elevated aCL-IgG and aCL-IgM-titers arterial thrombosis occurred more frequently than venous thrombosis. Cerebral ischemic attacks were the most frequent arterial events. IgG-aCL seemed to be the strongest risk factor for thromboembolic disease, especially arterial thrombosis. In contrary, in a recently published study of a large cohort of 1000 patients with definite APS it was reported, that venous thrombosis was the most frequent event in patients with definite APS [5].

The risk of thromboembolic disorders is higher for patients with high aCL-IgG-titer, than high aCL-IgM-titer. In 42% of the patients with high aCL-IgM-titer > 50 MPL a thromboembolic disease could not be found.

Careful identification of aPL antibodies may improve the clinical predictability of the APS. The manifestation of thrombotic disease, especially the risk of arterial thrombosis is higher, the higher the aCL-titer. Further investigations with a large cohort of patients are necessary to demonstrate the characteristics of different groups of patients with APS.

References

1. Wilson WA, Gharavi AE, Koike T, Lockshin MD, Branch DW, Piette JC, Brey R, Derksen R, Harris EN, Hughes GR, Triplett DA, Khamashta MA. International consensus statement on preliminary classification criteria for definite antiphospholipid syndrome: report of an international workshop. *Arthritis Rheum* 1999; 42: 1309–1311
2. Shoenfeld Y. Etiology and pathogenic mechanism of the anti-phospholipid syndrome unraveled. *Trends Immunol.* 2003, 24: 2–4
3. Roubey RAS. Mechanism of autoantibody-mediated thrombosis. *Lupus* 1998; 8: 114–20 (suppl 2)
4. Asherson RA, Cervera R, Piette JC, Font J, Lie JT, Burcoglu A, Lim K, Munoz-Rodriguez FJ, Levy RA, Boue F, Rossert J, Ingelmo M. Catastrophic antiphospholipid syndrome. Clinical and laboratory features of 50 patients. *Medicine (Baltimore)* 1998; 77: 195–207
5. Cervera R, Piette JC, Font J, Khamashta MA, Shoenfeld Y et al. Antiphospholipid syndrome: clinical and immunologic manifestations and patterns of disease expression in a cohort of 1,000 patients. *Arthritis Rheum.* 2002, 46: 1019–27
6. Galli M, Comfurius P, Maassen C, Hemker HC, de Baets MH, van Breda-Vriesman PJ, Barbui T, Zwaal RF, Bevers EM. Anticardiolipin antibodies directed not to cardiolipin but to a plasma protein cofactor. *Lancet* 1990; 335: 1544–7
7. Sheng A, Kandia DA, Krilis SA: Beta2-glycoprotein I: target antigen for »antiphospholipid« antibodies. Immunological and molecular aspects. *Lupus* 1998; 7: 5–9
8. Vaarala O, Alfthan G, Jauhiainen M, Leirisalo-Repo M, Aho K, Palosuo T. Crossreaction between antibodies to oxidized low-density lipoprotein and to cardiolipin in systemic lupus erythematosus. *Lancet* 1993; 341: 923–5
9. Levine JS, Branch DW, Rauch J. The antiphospholipid syndrome. *N Engl J Med* 2002; 346: 752–763
10. Tanne D, D'Olhaberriague L, Schultz LR, Salowich-Palm L, Sawaya KL, Levine SR. Anti-cardiolipin antibodies and their association with cerebrovascular risk factors. *Neurology* 1999; 52 (7): 1368–73

11. Finazzi G, Brancaccio V, Moia M, Ciaverella N, Mazzucconi MG, Schinco PC, Ruggeri M, Pogliani EM, Gamba G, Rossi E, Baudo F, Manotti C, D'Angelo A, Palareti G, De Stefano V, Berrettini M, Barbui T. Natural history and risk factors for thrombosis in 360 patients with antiphospholipid antibodies: a four-year prospective study from the Italian Registry. *Am J Med* 1996;100: 530–6
12. Vaarala O, Mantarri M, Manninen V, Tenkanen L, Puurunen M, Aho K, Palosuo T. Anti-cardiolipin antibodies and risk of myocardial infarction in a prospective cohort of middle-aged men. *Circulation* 1995; 91: 23–7
13. Shoenfeld Y, Sherer Y, Harats D. Atherosclerosis as an infectious, inflammatory and autoimmune disease. *Trends Immunol* 2001; 22: 293–5
14. Cervera R, Asherson RA, Lie JT. Clinicopathological correlations of antiphospholipid syndrome. *Semin Arthritis Rheum* 1995; 24: 262–272
15. DeGroot PG, Oosting JD, Derksen RHWM. Antiphospholipid antibodies: specificity and pathophysiology. *Balliere's Clin Haematol* 1993; 6: 691–709
16. Blank M, Krause I, Fridkin M, Keller N, Kopolovic J, Goldberg I, Tobar A, Shoenfeld Y. Bacterial induction of autoantibodies to β_2-glycoprotein-I accounts for the infectious etiology of antiphospholipid syndrome. *J Clin Invest* 2002; 109: 797–804
17. Petri M. Epidemiology of the antiphospholipid antibody syndrome. *J Autoimmun* 2000; 15: 145–151
18. Levine SR, Salowich-Palm L, Sawaya KL, Perry M, Spencer HJ, Winkler HJ, Alam Z, Carey JL. IgG anticardiolipin antibody titer > 40 GPL and the risk of subsequent thrombo-occlusive events and death. A prospective cohort study. *Stroke* 1997; 28 (9): 1660–5
19. Tanne D, D'Olhaberriague L, Trivedi AM, Salowich-Palm L, Schultz LR, Levine SR. Anticardiolipin antibodies and mortality in patients with ischemic stroke: a prospective follow-up study. Neuroepidemiology 2002 Mar – Apr; 21 (2): 93–9
20. Andreassi C, Zoli A, Riccio A, Scuderi F, Lombardi L, Altomonte L, Eboli ML. Anticardiolipin antibodies in patients with primary antiphospholipid syndrome: a correlation between IgG titre and antibody-induced cell dysfunction in neuronal cell cultures. Clin Rheumatol 2001; 20 (5): 314–8
21. Harris EN, Gharavi AE, Boey ML, Patel BM, Mackworth-Young CG, Loizou S, Hughes GRV. Anticardiolipin antibodies: detection by radioimmunoassay and association with thrombosis in systemic lupus erythematosus. Lancet 1983; 2 (8361): 1211–14.

Progression of an Extensive Deep Vein Thrombosis under High Dose Therapy with low Molecular Weight Heparin of a 13-Year-Old Girl Suffering from Colitis Ulcerosa

M. Deml, C. Bidlingmaier, H. Erhardt, Th. Lang, U. Nowak-Göttl, and K. Kurnik

Introduction

Patients suffering from inflammatory bowel disease (IBD) are known to have a threefold higher risk for thrombotic events compared to standard population. Recent studies show no higher prevalence for genetic thrombophilic risk factors in this group. Compared to patients without IBD manifestation of thrombosis appears earlier in life. Changed coagulation situation during inflammation is suspected to be the major cause. However it is clear that there must be multifactorial genesis.

Case Report

A 13-year-old girl suffering from acute colitis ulcerosa developed severe deep vein thrombosis after two weeks of bed rest under cortisone therapy. Therefore she was transferred to our hospital. Heterocygote prothrombin-mutation was the only genetic risk factor diagnosed for this patient. Lysis was impossible because of massive intestinal bleeding. In spite of high dose subcutaneous therapy with Dalteparin (Anti Xa levels 0,6–0,99 IU/ml) thrombosis grew up to the vena cava. By changing treatment to Enoxaparin and increasing dose up to 220 anti-Xa units/kg body weight subcutaneous given twice a day (anti-Xa levels 0,64–1,42 IU/ml) progression of thrombosis could be stopped. After recovery from colitis ulcerosa gradually dose reduction was possible resulting in comparable anti-Xa levels.

Discussion

Like in standard population genetic risk factors (factor V Leiden, prothrombin mutation, protein C deficiency) are important in genesis of thrombosis of patients with IBD. Well-known risk factors are immobilization, pregnancy, lupus anticoagulant, etc. Our patient was diagnosed of a heterocygote prothrombin mutation G20210A as genetic risk factor. In addition she was bedfast in consequence of the acute colitis ulcerosa. Treatment at time of thrombosis consisted of sulfasalzin and 1,2 mg of prednisolone per kg body weight. Patients with increased cortisone levels are supposed to have a stimulated factor VIII production. In addition factor VIII is increased in inflammation. Our patient had a factor VIII activity of 180% which can

I. Scharrer/W. Schramm (Ed.)
33rd Hemophilia Symposion Hamburg 2002
© Springer-Verlag Berlin Heidelberg 2004

be rated as thrombogenic risk factor. Not sufficiently explained remains the thrombotic progression under high therapeutic anti-Xa levels. After control of the inflammatory reaction by Infliximab anti-Xa values increased over therapeutic levels. In consequence the Enoxaparin dose could be gradually reduced.

Conclusion

This case report shows the extraordinary thrombogenic effect of the changed coagulation system resulting from IBD. Potential other risk factors such as genetic predisposition, cortisone therapy, etc. increase this thrombophilia. To prevent such severe thrombotic events by undertaking an early and sufficient prophylaxis we suggest a standard investigation for thrombophilia at the time of diagnosing IBD.

References

1. Charles N. Bernstein et al.: The incidence of deep venous thrombosis and pulmonary embolism among patients with inflammatory bowel disease: A population-based cohort study. Thromb Haemost 2001; 85: 430–4
2. M. Vecchi et al.: Inflammatory bowel diseases are not associated with major hereditary conditions predisposing to thrombosis. Dig Dis Sci 2000 Jul; 45 (7): 1465–9
3. O. Grip et al.: Inflammatory bowel disease promotes venous thrombosis earlier in life. Scand J Gastroenterol 2000 Jun; 35 (6): 619–23

Hyperfibrinolysis in Hemophagocytic Lymphohistiocytosis

A. Tiede, M. von Depka Prondzinski, H.H. Kreipe, A. Wagner,
A. Ganser, and G. Heil

Introduction

Hemophagocytic lymphohistiocytosis (HLH) is a rare disease of the lymphatic and
reticuloendothelial system that can be inherited (primary or familial HLH) or
acquired (secondary HLH) [1]. Both inherited and acquired HLH are often triggered by infections. The clinical picture is reminiscent of sepsis including fever, splenomegaly, and tricytopenia. Further characteristics are elevated concentration of
serum liver enzymes, triglycerides, ferritin, and cytokines (especially tumor necrosis factor alpha) as well as decreased fibrinogen levels [2]. Biopsy of the bone marrow and other organs typically shows erythrophagocytosis by hyperactive macrophages (histiocytes). Recent studies in familial HLH suggest that abnormal macro-
phage activation results from impaired lymphocyte-mediated cytotoxicity and
defective triggering of apoptosis [3].

Hypofibrinogenemia has been recognized as a typical feature of HLH, although
the underlying coagulopathy is not yet understood. Here, we report a patient with
acquired HLH who developed severe hypofibrinogenemia and hyperfibrinolysis.

Case Report

A 20-year-old German female was admitted with a history of fatigue, fever and swelling of the lower extremities for three months. She reported an episode of diarrhea
due to salmonellosis from that she fully recovered after treatment with ciprofloxa-
cin four months ago. On admission, she presented with continuous fever (about 39
°C), subcutaneous livid nodules of the lower extremities, and hepatomegaly. Under
the suspicion of Löfgren's syndrome (acute sarcoidosis), prednisolone was administered at 30 mg/day without effect. She developed severe tricytopenia and abnormal
coagulation tests (Fig. 1). In addition, elevated transaminases (GOT 109 U/L, GPT
115 U/L), LDH (2584 U/L) and ferritin (35840 µg/L) were observed. Biopsies taken
from the skin, liver and bone marrow demonstrated massive erythrophagocytosis
consistent with HLH. There was no indication of Non-Hodgkin's lymphoma or a
malignant disorder of histiocytes. Blood cultures were repeatedly negative.

Coagulation tests demonstrated moderately prolonged prothrombin time (PT)
and activated partial thromboplastin time (aPTT; Table 1). Fibrinogen was markedly decreased and D-dimers were detected at high plasma concentrations.

I. Scharrer/W. Schramm (Ed.)
33rd Hemophilia Symposion Hamburg 2002
© Springer-Verlag Berlin Heidelberg 2004

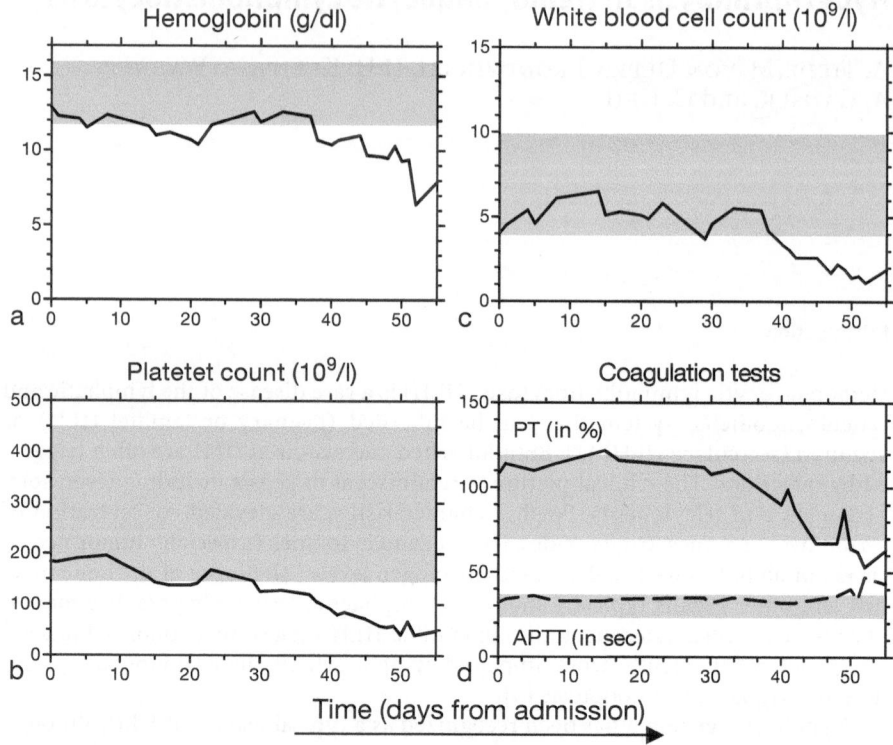

Fig. 1. Development of cytopenia and coagulopathy within the first 50 days of hospitalization. Reference intervals are indicated by gray shading. PT, prothrombin time (Quick) (in %); aPTT activated partial thromboplastin time (in sec.)

Table 1. Coagulation tests

Test	Day 56	Day 58	Day 60	Day 64	Reference
PT (%)	87	64	53	68	70–120
aPTT (sec.)	26	40	47	47	26–35
Fibrinogen (g/l)	0.8	0.7	0.6	1.1	2.0–3.5
Prothrombin (%)	58	40	32	38	70–120
Factor V (%)	>200	116	87	179	65–120
Antithrombin (%)	116		86	103	70–120
D-dimers	>20000	>20000	17978	14406	<500

Prothrombin was also decreased, whereas factor V and antithrombin were normal. There were no clinical signs of bleeding or thrombosis at this time.

Administration of heparin (5000 U/d) and aprotinin (up to 600000 U/h) did not significantly inhibit fibrinolysis as demonstrated by constantly high D-dimers between days 56 and 80. Fibrinogen levels remained low despite of substitution with

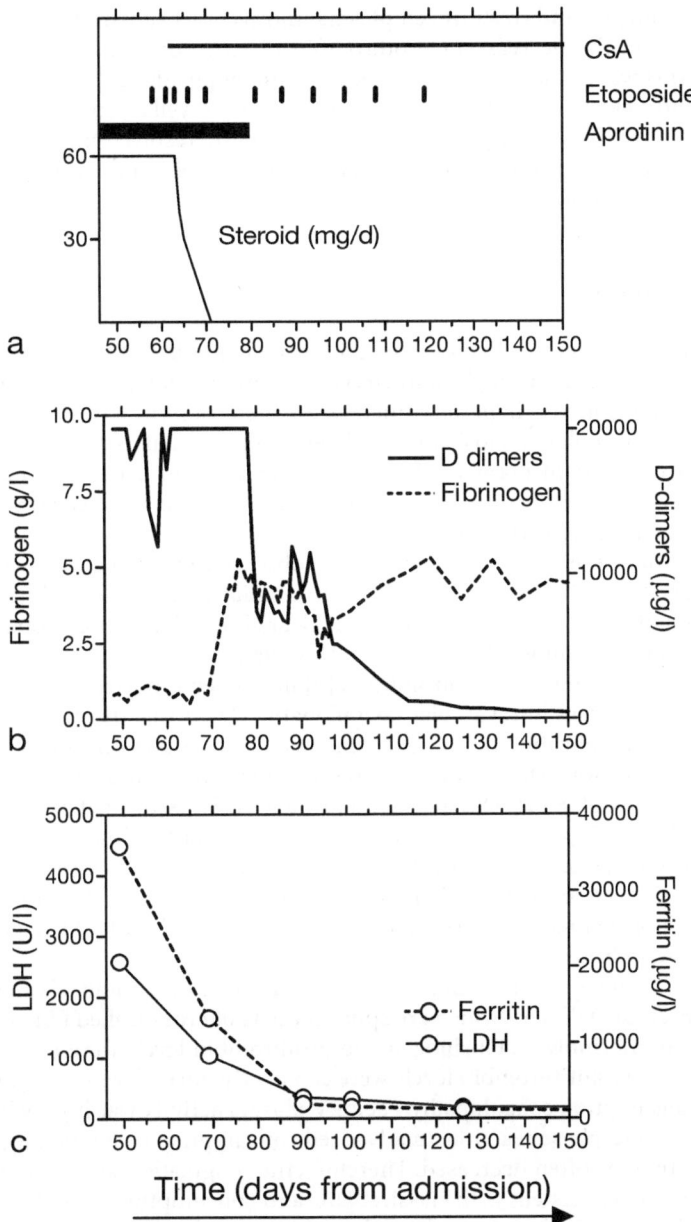

Fig. 2a–c. (a) Therapeutic regimen according to Imashuku et al. [9]. Cyclosporin A (CsA) was administered orally and adjusted to plasma trough levels (150–250 ng/mL). Etoposide was given 150 mg/m² on the indicated days. Aprotinin, which is not included in the HLH-94 protocol, was given at 100 000 to 600 000 U/h. **(b)** Resolution of coagulopathy in response to therapy. **(c)** Resolution of additional laboratory abnormalities (lactate dehydrogenase and ferritin) in response to therapy.

fibrinogen and fresh frozen plasma. Intravenous substitution of vitamin K did not correct the decrease in prothrombin plasma concentration. After a diagnosis of HLH was made, therapy was started with etoposide (150 mg/m^2 body surface area) and ciclosporin A (Fig. 2). Hyperfibrinolysis as well as other pathological laboratory parameters (LDH, ferritin, cytopenia) rapidly resolved under therapy. The patient was discharged from the hospital after four weeks and has been in good health for one year now.

Discussion

In our patient a diagnosis of HLH was made based on the clinical presentation (fever, organomegaly), characteristic laboratory abnormalities (tricytopenia, hypo-fibrinogenemia, hyperferritinemia, elevated transaminases) and the demonstration of erythrophagocytosis in skin, liver and bone marrow. HLH is probably acquired in this patient because of her advanced age and a negative family history. Four weeks before the onset of symptoms salmonellosis had been documented that may have triggered HLH in this case.

Severe hypofibrinogenemia was observed in our patient, which is a common laboratory finding in patients with familial and acquired HLH. The relevance of hypofibrinogenemia in HLH is not clear since clinical coagulopathy is infrequently recognized under this condition. However, cases of HLH complicated by catastrophic bleeding [4] and thrombosis [5] have been reported. In the report by Wu et al. disseminated intravascular coagulopathy (DIC) was diagnosed [4]. DIC is a common complication of sepsis leading to consumption of fibrinogen and other coagulation factors. DIC may also represent a mechanism leading to hypofibrinogenemia in cases of HLH. Others have reported HLH associated with severe thrombotic microangiopathy [6, 7], which may also explain the consumption of fibrinogen in severe cases. In contrast, immunohistochemical studies revealed the presence of fibrinogen antigen in histiocytes in a case of HLH [8]. This indicates that hypofi-brinogenemia may also result from direct uptake of fibrinogen by hyperactive macrophages.

In our patient no clinical signs of bleeding or thrombosis were observed. High levels of D dimers, which are split products of cross-linked fibrin, were indicative of hyperfibrinolysis. Fibrinogen and prothrombin levels were markedly decreased. In contrast, antithrombin levels were constantly normal, which is unusual for DIC and consumption coagulopathy. Factor V plasma activity was high, which may represent an acute-phase reaction. In advanced consumption coagulopathy, however, factor V activity is often decreased. Therefore, the coagulation abnormalities in this patient are not consistent with classical DIC and consumption coagulopathy. It seems possible that fibrinogen and prothrombin are selectively consumed or degraded by proteolytic factors released from activated macrophages. These cells can also bind factor X through Mac-1 receptors [8] suggesting the direct activation of the common coagulation pathway on these cells.

Administration of high doses of the serine protease inhibitor aprotinin were unable to abrogate hyperfibrinolysis in this patient. Therefore fibrin (and fibrinogen) degradation may not result from the action of plasmin in this case, since plasmin is efficiently inactivated by aprotinin. A number of proteolytic enzymes including matrix metalloproteinase are released by or presented on the membrane of activated macrophages.

Importantly, the coagulation abnormalities in this patient rapidly resolved after initiation of an etoposide-containing therapeutic regimen according to the HLH-94 protocol [9, 10]. The topoisomerase-targeting drug etoposide is a potent inhibitor of activated macrophages. The addition of cyclosporin A may correct with the underlying disturbance of lymphocyte regulation in HLH. The role of adjunct therapies including heparin, aprotinin, plasma transfusion and factor replacement remains uncertain.

References

1. Jaffe R. The histiocytoses. Clin Lab Med 1999; 19: 135–155
2. Henter JI, Elinder G, Ost A. Diagnostic guidelines for hemophagocytic lymphohistiocytosis. The FHL Study Group of the Histiocyte Society. Semin Oncol 1991; 18: 29–33
3. Henter JI. Biology and treatment of familial hemophagocytic lymphohistiocytosis: importance of perforin in lymphocyte-mediated cytotoxicity and triggering of apoptosis. Med Pediatr Oncol 2002; 38: 305–309
4. Wu CS, Chang KY, Dunn P, Lo TH. Acute hepatitis A with coexistent hepatitis C virus infection presenting as a virus-associated hemophagocytic syndrome: a case report. Am J Gastroenterol 1995; 90: 1002–1005
5. Inoue Y, Kato M, Ohsuka T, Morikawa A. Successful treatment of a child with inferior vena cava thrombosis using a temporary inferior vena cava filter. Pediatr Cardiol 2002; 23: 74–76
6. Chiang WC, Wu MS, Tsai CC, Lin SL, Tsai TJ, Hsieh BS. Thrombotic microangiopathy in hemophagocytic syndrome: a case report. J Formos Med Assoc 2002; 101: 362–367
7. Kfoury Baz EM, Mikati AR, Kanj NA. Reactive hemophagocytic syndrome associated with thrombotic thrombocytopenic purpura during therapeutic plasma exchange. Ther Apher 2002; 6: 159–162
8. Ooe K. Pathogenesis of hypofibrinogenemia in familial hemophagocytic lymphohistiocytosis. Pediatr Pathol 1991; 11: 657–661
9. Imashuku S, Kuriyama K, Teramura T, Ishii E, Kinugawa N, Kato M, Sako M, Hibi S. Requirement for etoposide in the treatment of Epstein-Barr virus-associated hemophagocytic lymphohistiocytosis. J Clin Oncol 2001; 19: 2665–2673
10. Henter JI, Samuelsson-Horne A, Arico M, Egeler RM, Elinder G, Filipovich AH, Gadner H, Imashuku S, Komp D, Ladisch S, Webb D, Janka G. Treatment of hemophagocytic lymphohistiocytosis with HLH-94 immunochemotherapy and bone marrow transplantation. Blood 2002; 100: 2367–2373

Prolonged Lysis-Therapy of an Arteria Iliaca Externa Thrombosis in a very Low Birth Weight Infant with a Variant in the Factor-XIII-Gene

C. BIDLINGMAIER, A.W. FLEMMER, B. KAMMER, M. DEML,
U. NOWAK-GÖTTL, and K. KURNIK

Background

Very-low-birth-weight infants (VLBW) have – compared to children of other age-groups – an increased risk for thromboembolic diseases [1]. The importance of diagnosis and management of these high risk patients is growing due to higher survival rates of previously untreatable diseases and complications. But diagnosis and management differs greatly from other age groups. Arterial angiography is rarely used since the risk of inducing another thromboembolic events and embolectomy has a high failure rate.

Patient

A male newborn (birth weight 910 g, gestational age 27 weeks) underwent operation due to a necrotizing enterocolitis. After placement of a peripheral arterial catheter for monitoring, he developed a right arteria iliaca externa thrombosis in the first postoperative night. Only hours after the operation foot swelling quickly occurred although pulses were still detectable. In the following days the perfusion of the leg decreased rapidly (Fig. 1) and the malperfusion finally extended up to the hip.

Laboratory Findings

Thrombocytosis (up to 930 000/μl) and hyperfibrinogenemia (up to 550 mg/dl) were found after the operation (Fig. 2).

Examination for inherited or acquired thrombophilia of the parents and the patient did not reveal pathological findings for: Quick, PTT, antithrombin, protein C/S, plasminogen, prothrombin mutation (G20210A), factor V Leiden (G1691A), lipoprotein (a), MTHFR (C677T heterozygous), lupus inhibitors, CDG-syndrome, GPIa- and HPA-polymorphisms.

Only a PAI-polymorphism (4G4G) and a variant of the factor XIII-gene (Val-34-Leu) were found.

I. Scharrer/W. Schramm (Ed.)
33rd Hemophilia Symposion Hamburg 2002
© Springer-Verlag Berlin Heidelberg 2004

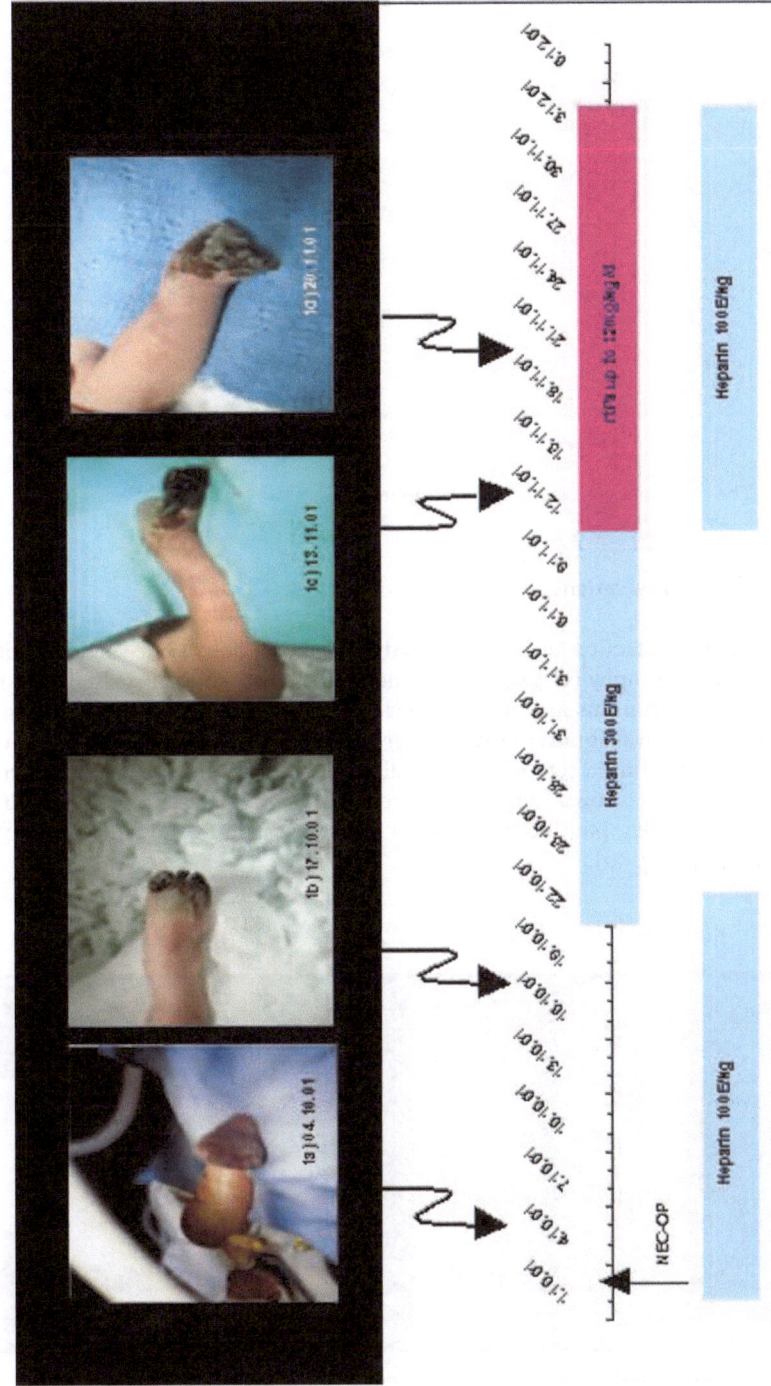

Fig. 1. and 3. (lower graph). The clinical course and the timepoints of intervention

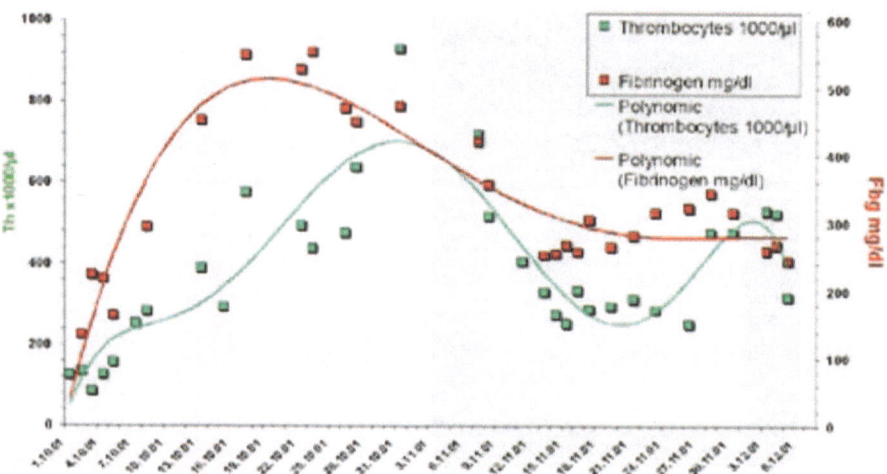

Fig. 2. The thrombocyte-counts and fibrinogen levels

Radiological Observations

Sonographic detection of the suspected thrombosis failed, but venous digital subtraction angiography (vDSA) – performed for the first time in such a small infant – showed the thrombus and the vascular status of the entire extremity (Fig. 4a–c). The thrombus was found in the right arteria iliaca externa [4a] and reperfusion of the arteria profunda femoralis via collaterals descending from the arteria iliaca interna could be shown [4b]. vDSA revealed the vascular status of the entire – unaffected – left leg [4c]. Retrospectively it was possible to show the thrombus with sonography (Fig. 4d).

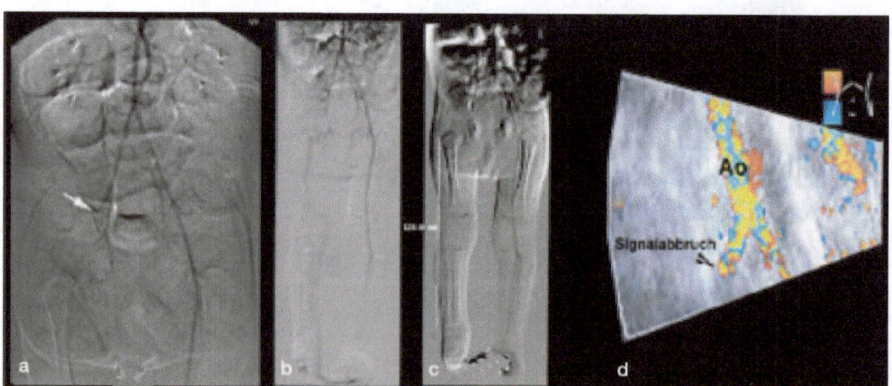

Fig. 4. Radiological diagnostics

Therapy

Neither standard heparin (100–300 U/kg/d) nor low molecular weight heparin (LMWH, Dalteparin, up to 250 anti-Xa U/kg/d) could stop the process. Finally rtPA-lysis (up to 12 mg/kg/d) was performed and the leg beside the foot could be saved (Fig. 3). At 1-year-follow-up under LMWH-prophylaxis the leg shows only light growth retardation. The function of the leg is only mildly affected. The patient is still treated with LMWH for prophylaxis.

Discussion

We showed – for the first time in such a small child – that it is possible to evaluate the vascular status of the lower extremity in VLBW infants via vDSA. Therefore vDSA forms a save and effective alternative to the more invasive arterial DSA [2]. Thrombocytosis and hyperfibrinogenemia formed the risk factors for thrombosis in our patient, along with the activated hemostasis after the operation. Whether the peripheral arterial catheter added to the risk can only be speculated but seems plausible. As inherited risk factors a PAI-polymorphism which is widely accepted to increase the risk for thrombosis was found. The Val-34-Leu variant of the factor XIII gene is currently controversially discussed for being either protective or a potential risk factor [3]. There are some single-case reports describing a prolonged lysis in patients with myocardial infarctions [4]. In our case the progression of the ascending thrombosis was only mitigated and finally stopped by rtPA lysis therapy. This regimen is highly invasive in VLBW infants due to the high risk of intracerebral bleeding and should in our opinion only used as ultima ratio. This case stresses the need for limited use of arterial catheters in these high risk patients, especially since information about possible inherited thrombophilia is usually not available at the beginning of treatment.

References

1. Nowak-Göttl et al.: Thrombolysis in newborns and infants. Thromb Haemost 1999; 82 Suppl 1: 112–6
2. Parker et al.: Intravenous digital subtraction angiography: its use in evaluating vascular injuries in children. J Pediatr Surg 1989; 24 (5): 423–7
3. Ariëns et al.: Role of factor XIII in fibrin clot formation and effects of genetic polymorphisms. Blood 2002; 100 (3): 743–754
4. Roldán et al.: Effect of factor XIII Val34Leu polymorphism on thrombolytic therapy in premature myocardial infarction. Thromb Haemost 2002; 88: 354–355

Modified Immunsuppression in a Case of Acquired Hemophilia – Case Report

H. Krebs, C. Domsch, W. Schramm, and M. Spannagl

Patient

A 62-year-old female patient with suspicion on ovarial carcinoma was introduced. An unclear bleeding disorder persisted for about six months. In addition a mama carcinoma (pT1b, pN0, pM0) without indications of a relapse or metastases is known since 1988. Furthermore a compensated heart insufficiency as well as a compensated renal insufficiency was diagnosed. Bodily findings showed a female patient in good health condition; size: 154 cm; weight: 60 kg; vital parameters: RR 110/80 mmHg, HF 99/min, RF 19/min; Cor 2/6 systolicum p.m AK. A big tumor in the right underbelly was palpable and large hematomas at extremities and body were visible. Laboratory diagnostics adduced several pathological parameters: Hb 6,6 g/dl; ESR 88/150 mm; CRP 7,25 mg/dl; Cr 1,8 mg/dl; aPTT 75,4 sec; BT 350 sec; FVIII below 1%; inhibitor against FVIII 90 BU. CT-diagnostics showed a irregular bordered and septed structure in the area of the fossa ovarica right strengthening the suspicion of a peritoneal carcinosis, infiltration of the small and large intestine and ascites. The sonography showed thickens jejunum loops for a length of about 22 cm and a thickness of about 8 to 12 cm, conformable to a bleeding into the intestinal wall. An ovarial tumor (7 x 6 x 6 cm³) of unknown dignity and ascites showed up in the gynecological sonography. An explorative laparatomy and removal of the tumor was carried out.

Diagnosis

- Acquired inhibitor against factor VIII
- Ovarial cystadenofibrome and intestinal bleeding
- Compensated renal insufficiency
- Compensated heart insufficiency

Pre-, PPeri- and Postoperative Hemotherapy

Preoperative management of bleeding and therapy of the inhibitor:
- Six red cell concentrates
- Initial infusion of NovoSeven 100 µg/kg all six hours

I. Scharrer/W. Schramm (Ed.)
33rd Hemophilia Symposion Hamburg 2002
© Springer-Verlag Berlin Heidelberg 2004

- Immunoglobulin 25 g/day
- Decortin H 60 mg/day

Peri- and Postoperative Hemotherapy (Explorative Laparatomy)

- Continuous infusion of NovoSeven 50 µg/kg/h perioperative
- Infusion of NovoSeven 240 µg/kg every six hours as bolus → hemoglobin drop and bleeding
- Aprotinin 1.000.000 I.U. and 200.000 I.U. all four hours as bolus
- Eleven red cell concentrates and eleven fresh frozen plasma concentrates
- Fibrogammin (FXIII) 1250 I.U.

Peri- postoperative hemotherapy due to postoperative complications (intraabdominal bleeding/4l blood loss) and relaparatomy:

- Continuous infusion of NovoSeven 150 µg/kg/h perioperative up to the third postoperative day
- Two red cell concentrates and 3 fresh frozen plasma concentrates
- Infusion of NovoSeven 300 µg/kg every two hours as bolus up to the fifth postoperative day.

Recommended Medicinal Therapy

Recommendations for the immunosuppressive therapy of acquired hemophilia suggest the following drug combinations [1]:

Primary Therapy:

- Prednisolone 1 mg/kg +- Cyclophosphamide 50–100 mg/d oral or Cyclophosphamide i.v.
- Prednisolone mg/kg +- Azathioprin 100 mg/day oral

Secondary Therapy:

- Immunoglobulin 2 mg/kg for 2–5 days
- Cyclosporin A 10–15 mg/kg/d +- Prednisolon 1 mg/kg

Conducted Medicinal Therapy

Week	Cyclophosphamide [mg]	Prednisolone [mg]	Azathioprine [mg]	Cyclosporin A [mg]
initial	50 i.v.	60	–	–
1.–4.	100 oral	60	–	–
5.–24.	–	60/40/30/20	–	–
24.–30.	–	10	100	–
30.–38.	–	10	–	50–0–50
39.–42.	–	10	–	75–0–75

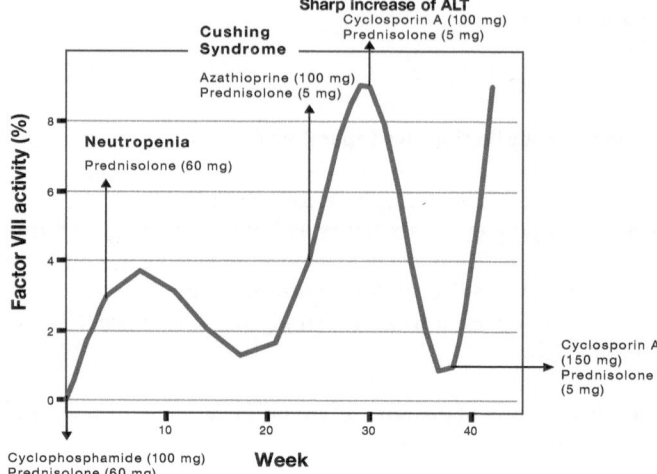

Fig. 1. Change of Faktor VIII activity during therapy

Discussion

The attempt of reducing the inhibitor by drugs induced serious adverse reactions forcing a repeated change of therapy regimes. Cyclophosphamide led to a neutropenia with leucocyte numbers below 1000/µl. The subsequent monotherapy with Prednisolone induced a Cushing Syndrome and diabetes after a few weeks, requiring a significant reduction of Prednisolone dosage. Simultaneously the therapy was expanded by Azathioprin, which involved a sharp increase of ALT. The application of Cyclosporin A in a reduced dosage (50 ng/dl) due to the compensated renal insufficiency showed no positive effect. Factor VIII again dropped below an activity of 1% resulting in a relevant risk of bleeding. Thereupon systemic Cyclosporin A levels were lifted to 75 ng/dl leading to 9% factor VIII activity at last. Relevant adverse effect of this therapy could not be observed up to now (Fig. 1).

Conclusion

An immunosuppressive therapy in acquired inhibitor patients requires due to the possible adverse reactions a strict guidance of patients. The adoption of Cyclosporin A as an alternative in this case was efficient in a reduced dosage. By monitoring the drug level the optimal dosage finding is much more easier and helps to minimize possible adverse reactions. Nevertheless these adverse reactions often require a reduction of recommended dosages.

References

1. Guideline (2000), the Diagnosis and Management of Factor VIII Inhibitors: A Guideline from the UK Hemophilia Center Doctors' Organization (UKHCDO). British Journal of Haematology, 111, 78–90

Life-Threatening Bleeding after Vaccination as a First Manifestation of Hemophilia A

C. WERMES, M. VON DEPKA-PRONDZINSKI, K. WELTE, A. GANSER, and K.-W. SYKORA

Background

Vaccinations can lead to local reactions. In about 15% of all cases, pain or swellings, as well as fever up to 38.0° C are observed during the first 72 hours. Normally they are caused by allergic reactions or inflammations.

We report about two boys with initially unknown diagnosis of hemophilia A, who developed severe bleeding complications after a vaccination.

Patient I

The boy was three months old, when he received his first vaccination in his left thigh. During the following 12 days he developed a local swelling and show a reduced movement of the leg. Finally he developed fever for 3 days and was sent to a hospital, for a suspected abscess. After surgical removal of a big hematoma, the patient developed a severe bleeding anemia (hemoglobin 5.6 g/dl). Therefore, he received a red cell blood concentrate. On the following day the boy had a secondary hemorrhage accompanied by a further decrease of the hemoglobin. In total, two weeks after the onset of the swelling, which was caused by a hemorrhage, for the first time a hemostaseological investigation was performed and the diagnosis of hemophilia A (factor VIII < 1%) was made. After transfusion of factor VIII concentrates and an additional red cell blood concentrate the bleeding stopped.

The boy is the first child of healthy parents without consanguinity. They are from Kasachstan. In the family, coagulation disorders are unknown. Therefore, this case represents a case of sporadic hemophilia (de novo factor VIII gene mutation).

Patient II

At an age of 5 months the boy got an intramuscular injection (vaccination) in his left thigh. Three days later the parents recognized a swelling of the thigh and reduced movement of the left leg. Six days after the vaccination the parents went to the doctor. The diagnosis of a local vaccination reaction was made. Because of additional fever up to 38.8 °C and a common cold, the boy received antibiotic treatment with amoxicilline. Two days later, the boy's condition did not improve, again the physician was contacted. He sent the patient to a special surgeon for ultrasound exami-

I. Scharrer/W. Schramm (Ed.)
33rd Hemophilia Symposion Hamburg 2002
© Springer-Verlag Berlin Heidelberg 2004

nation. The swelling was punctured under ultrasound guidance and 10 ml blood could be aspired. Then the boy was sent to a hospital for exclusion of a bone fracture by x-ray examination. Finally, an evaluation of the clotting system including several clotting assays led to the diagnosis of severe hemophilia A (F VIII activity < 1%). In total, 8 days after the beginning of the swelling, which was caused by a bleeding, the boy received treatment with factor VIII concentrates resulting in rapid recovery. In addition, a transfusion with a red cell blood concentrate was necessary.

The history of his own and of his family concerning bleeding disorders was inconspicuous. Nevertheless there have been only female descendants on his mother's side. Obviously, this is another case of sporadic hemophilia.

Discussion

In both children life-threatening bleedings occurred after vaccinations in early infancy. Swellings and a reduced movement of the limb were the main symptoms. Classical blue colored hematoma were not seen because of the deep localization of the bleedings, so that experienced pediatricians themselves did not diagnose the complication immediately. Although it is described in the literature that hemophiliacs can develop bleedings after intramuscular injections as e.g. vaccinations [1, 2], this is not the first bleeding complication in most cases leading to the diagnosis of hemophilia. In those children with inconspicuous family history diagnosis of hemophilia is usually made in the second half of the first year of life [3], and the vaccinations of the first months of life have been made apparently without any bleeding complications. Prothrombotic risk factors could be protective against bleedings especially in young babies [3]. In addition, possibly part of the bleedings are not recognized by parents and physicians and are diagnosed as harmless vaccination reactions because of the atypical symptoms.

Conclusion

Swellings after vaccinations or other intramuscular injections expecially when the ultrasound shows a fluid accumulation should be suspected to be local bleedings. Because of the deep intramuscular localization of the bleeding, clinical presentation may be atypical.

References

1. Goyal R. Intramuscular vaccination in hemophilia. Indian Pediatr 2000; 37 (5): 569
2. Klinge J.M. et al. Hämophilie – Symptomatik, Diagnostik, Therapie. Päd. Praxis 2001; 59 (2): 223–240
3. Ettingshausen CE et al. Symptomatic onset of hemophilia A in childhood is dependent on the presence of prothrombotic risk factors. Thromb Haemost 2001; 85: 218–220

Administration of Protein C Concentrate (Ceprotin, Baxter) in Purpura Fulminans as the First Clinical Manifestation of Galactosemia

A. Zyschka, C. Escuriola-Ettingshausen, D. Klarmann, D. Heller, S. Becker, W. Müller, C. Königs, S. Figura, A. Zubcov, T. Klingebiel, and W. Kreuz

Introduction

The classic galactosemia is a severe inherited metabolic disease with an early onset of symptoms. The incidence of galactosemia is 1: 60 000 in newborn.

Inactivity of the enzyme galactose-1-phosphat-uridyltransferase (gal.-1-PUT) causes an increase of galaktose-1-phosphat in the liver, brain, kidney and the eye lens.

Affected newborns as well as older infants are usually affected by one or more of the following symptoms: Jaundice, hepatomegaly, vomiting, hypoglycemia, convulsion, lethargy, irritability, feeding difficulties, poor weight gain, amonoaciduria, cataracts, vitreous hemorrhage, hepatic cirrhosis, ascites, splenomegaly, or mental retardation. Patients with galactosemia are at increased risk for neonatal sepsis caused by E. coli; the onset of sepsis and/or coagulopathy often precedes the diagnosis of galactosemia [1].

Case Report

We report about a 5-day-old female newborn, who developed purpura at the entire right foot.

The baby was the first child of a Caucasian, non-consanguineous relation, born in the 38th week of gestation after normal pregnancy. Delivery was without complications. Postpartal adaptation of the baby was very good. After birth Konakion 2 mg was administered per os twice. Immediately the baby was breast fed. At the age of 3 days the baby was admitted home in a good physical state.

Second day at home her mother noticed a dark blue discoloration of the entire right foot. The child was brought to the next local hospital immediately. At admittance the baby was still in good physical state, and drank well.

There was no evidence of trauma or infection (no leucocytosis or leukopenia, and no thrombopenia, CRP and differential white blood count was in range). Bilirubin, liver enzymes (GOT, GPT) were within the upper normal ranges or slightly elevated. Blood glucose was 47 mg/dl. The coagulation parameters at admittance to the periphere hospital were strongly disturbed (TPZ: 22%; aPTT: 96 s.; TZ: 32 sec.; fibrinogen 167 mg/dl; D-dimer: 6,4 μg/ml; protein C activity : 25%; AT 48%).

I. Scharrer/W. Schramm (Ed.)
33rd Hemophilia Symposion Hamburg 2002
© Springer-Verlag Berlin Heidelberg 2004

Initial therapy included the administration of fresh frozen plasma (FFP), AT-concentrate, vitamin K (intravenously) and low-dose heparin (100 IU/kg bw) as well as antibiotic therapy. Further more blood was taken for the newborn screening (e. g. Galactosemia).

Under the therapeutic strategy mentioned above the clinical course as well as the coagulation parameters did not improve: Protein C activity dropped to 5% during the following 3 days. It was decided to transfer the patient to our hospital (University Hospital Frankfurt/Main, Department of Pediatrics).

At arrival at our department the patient was listless and floppy and started vomiting after breastfeeding. The entire right foot showed a dark-blue discoloration. The coagulation parameters and clinical chemistry at admittance to our hospital were: TPZ: 37%; aPTT: 54 s.; TZ: 26 s.; fibrinogen: 250 mg/dl; protein C activity: 4,06%; AT 48%; Bilirubin total: 14,5 mg/dl; GOT: 72 U/l; GPT 40 U/l; Gamma – GT: 28 U/l; AP: 1500 U/l; ammonica: 107 μmol/l; normal ranges: glucose; electrolyte; creatinin, CRP. A metabolic disease, particularly galactosemia was suspected and breastfeeding was stopped immediately. Specific diagnostic tests were performed.

The severely enhanced microcirculation of the right foot caused by severe acquired protein C deficiency had been deteriorated continuously.

Therefore we decided to give a plasma derived protein C concentrate (Ceprotin, Baxter). The PC administration was started with an intravenous bolus injection (60 IU/kg body weight), followed by continuous infusion of 9 IU/kg bw/hour.

Our aim was to keep protein C activity >80% during the initial phase of treatment.

Antibiotic therapy as well as FFP, AT concentrate and heparin were discontinued.

Under the single use of PC concentrate the activity of protein C increased immediately towards the aimed ranges. The global hemostatic parameters normalized as well and the enhanced microcirculation improved continuously. PC dosage was reduced subsequently and was stopped after 6 days (Table 1). The foot recovered completely without any following complications and consequences.

Table 1. Coagulation parameters before and under treatment with protein C concentrate

Days of treatment	day 0	day 1	day 2	day 3	day 4	day 5	day 6
Protein C (IU)		Bol. 150 4x140	4x140	4x110	4x110	4x60	4x60
TPZ (%)	22	37	30	40	92	72	93
aPTT (sec.)	103	54	78	71	38	53	39
Fibrinog. (mg/dl)	98	250	237	219	119	200	202
Thromb. (x10/μl)	normal	173	213	211	209	249	273
Protein C activity (%)	4,06	3,43	90	119	104		104

The ophthalmologic examination revealed leucoria of the right eye caused by a bleeding in the vitreous body. Venous and arterial microthrombosis of the retinal circulatory system were found during pars plana vitrectomy of the right eye. The development of the microthrombosis may be attributed to the severe acquired PC deficiency. In spite of PC replacement therapy the patient lost her sight of the right eye.

The diagnostic tests in order to detect a metabolic disease revealed a positive Beutler test. In the Beutler enzyme spot test, GALT enzyme activity is monitored with the aid of phosphoglucomutase and glucose-6-phosphate dehydrogenase (G6PD) and the visualization of the fluorescence of reduced NADP+ under ultraviolet light [2]. Galactose-1-phosphat-uridyltransferase activity was not detectable.

The molecular genetic analysis of the GALT-genes revealed the patient to be homozygous for the mutation Q188R. The parents were heterozygous.

The elevated liver enzymes, hyperbilirubinemia and hyperammoniemia turned towards normal ranges under galactose and lactose free nutrition.

Long-term Outcome

Under dietetic nutrition with Milupa SOM the patient showed a normal development. The parents underwent nutricial advisement.

During follow-ups PC activity was within age-dependent normal ranges. The child got a blind right eye caused by retinal microthrombosis.

Discussion

Coagulopathy, particularly disseminated intravascular coagulopathy (DIC) are often observed in patients with galactosemia. However, purpura fulminans as the first clinical manifestation is rarely reported. The strongly enhanced microcirculation (foot, retina) can be attributed to the severe acquired PC-deficiency. The occurrence of purpura fulminans and retinal thrombosis with consecutive loss of sight is also reported in patients with severe and congenital PC-deficiency.

In this situation the administration of FFP solely is often not sufficient to restore microcirculation. With the administration of PC concentrate the normalization of coagulopathy and restoration of microcirculation was achieved.

However damage of the retina was irreversible. This observation is comparable to the outcome of retinal thrombosis in patients with severe congenital PC deficiency [4]. However, in purpura fulminans efficacy was excellent in all cases.

Protein C (PC) is a natural anticoagulant that, when activated by a thrombomodulin/thrombin complex on vascular endothelium, inactivates coagulation factors Va and VIIIa, limiting coagulation and simultaneously enhancing fibrinolysis by inhibition of PAI 1 (Plasminogen activator inhibitor) and downregulation of TAFi (thrombin activatable fibrinolysis inhibitor) [3].

References

1. Nelson. Textbook of Pediatrics. Fourteenth Edition. Behrmann 1992; 8: 359–362
2. Beutler E, Baluda MC. A simple spot screening test for galactosemia. J Lab. Clin Med 1966; 68: 137–141
3. Esa Rintala et. al: Protein C substitution in sepsis-associated purpura fulminans. Critical Care Medicine 2000; 28: 2373–2378
4. Moritz et al: The efficacy and safty of Protein C concentrate (human) vapor-heated in the treatment of severe congenital Protein C deficiency with or without purpura fulminans. ASH 2000 poster pres
5. Fields PA et al. (1994): Use of Protein C concentrate to treat severe homozygous deficiency. Br J Haematol 87 (suppl.1)
6. Conard J et al. (1993): Normalization of markers of coagulation activation with a purified Protein C concentrate in adults with homozygous Protein C deficiency. Blood 82; 1159–1164

Case Report: Successful Treatment of a Spontaneous Acquired Inhibitor Against Factor VIII in a 73-Year-old Patient

R. Klamroth, F. Seibt, and S. Gottstein

Background

Acquired hemophilia is a spontaneous autoimmune disease in which patients develop antibodies against clotting factors, mostly against factor VIII. Inhibitor formation is rare with an incidence of 0,2–1 per 1 million persons per year. Approximately 50% of cases have no underlying disease.

Bleeding episodes associated with acquired hemophilia could be life-threatening and the mortality rate is approximately 14–22%. There are two main goals in treatment, first to control the acute bleedings and second to achieve immune tolerance (IT). The first goal, therapy of hemorrhage is successful and well established with recombinant factor VIIa (rFVIIa) or activated prothrombin complex concentrates, the second goal, permanent elimination of the inhibitor remains a reason for discussion and modification. First of all immunosuppressive drugs like corticosteroids and cyclophosphamide are given for IT induction. As part of the Malmö treatment protocol and its modifications they are combined with intravenous immunoglobulins (IVIG), immunoadsorptions (IA) and presentation of the causative antigen, in most cases factor VIII. The antigen presentation with high doses of factor VIII remains controversial and does not seem to be mandatory. This case report describes the successful, permanent inhibitor elimination in a patient with an acquired inhibitor against factor VIII according to the modified Malmö treatment protocol.

Treatment Regimen

1. Therapy of acute hemorrhage with rFVIIa (bolus 90 μg/kg BW).
2. Immunosuppressive therapy with 1 mg/kg BW per day prednisolone and 2 mg/kg BW per day cyclophosphamide
3. Extracorporeal IA (Ig Therasorb) on three consecutive days each week to achieve an IgG level below 0,5 g/dl (adsorption of 3 times the plasma volume per day)
4. IVIG 0,2 g/kg BW (Octagam, Octapharma) on three consecutive days starting one day after the last IA

Patient

A 73-year-old patient (90 kg, 176 cm) was admitted to regional hospital with hematoma on both legs without any previous trauma. Laboratory diagnostics revealed

I. Scharrer/W. Schramm (Ed.)
33rd Hemophilia Symposion Hamburg 2002
© Springer-Verlag Berlin Heidelberg 2004

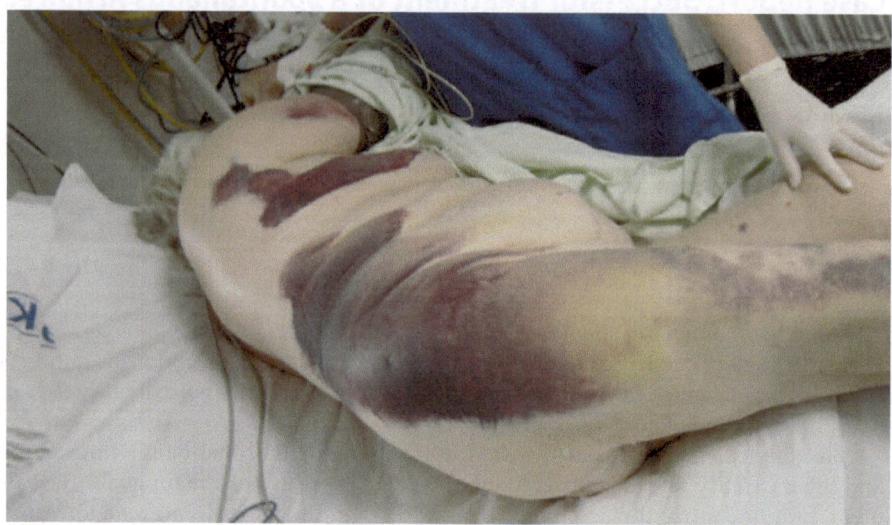

Fig. 1. Patient with a spontaneous acquired inhibitor against factor VIII (1)

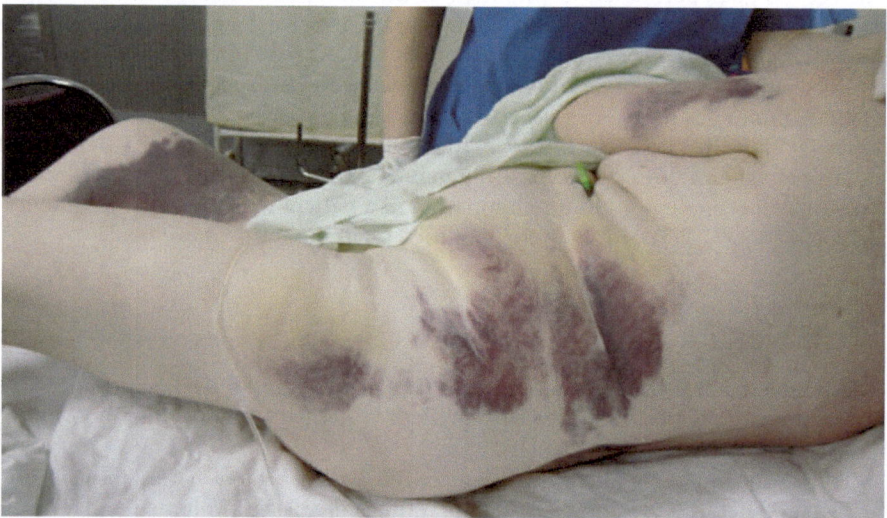

Fig. 1. Patient with a spontaneous acquired inhibitor against factor VIII (2)

prolongation of aPTT and analysis in our laboratory showed a factor VIII level of 5% and an inhibitor against factor VIII of 15,7 B.U. The patient was transferred to our hospital due to excessive bleeding. Six packed red cells were already given before admission in our department .

At admission the patient showed hematomas at both legs, right hip and right shoulder. A CT-scan revealed a hugh hemorrhage in the left iliopsoas muscle.

Treatment

Acute bleeding was treated with several boli of rFVIIa and due to recurrent bleeding the therapy with rFVIIa was continued for seven days. According to the modified Malmö treatment protocol we initiated immunosuppression with cyclophosphamide (2 mg/kg BW) and prednisolone (1 mg/kg BW).

Due to persistent recurrent bleedings after reduction of rFVIIa we decided to start IA at day six. We needed three absorptions to reduce the IgG levels below 0,5 g/dl. In the next three days we replaced IVIG (0,2g/kg BW).

Results

After only two IA (two days) we could stop treatment with rFVIIa because the excessive bleeding disappeared. After five IA (one and a half week) the inhibitor against factor VIII disappeared in the Bethesda test, after 12 IA (four weeks) we achieved an endogenous factor VIII level higher than 70%. Immunosuppressive treatment with prednisolone and cyclophosphamide was finished two months later. Even 12 months after the last IA there was no evidence for recurrence of the inhibitor.

Discussion

This case report shows as an example the opportunity of fast elimination of an inhibitor against factor VIII in combination with IA. This could be useful and cost effective in patients with excessive bleedings and high consumption of rFVIIa to control these bleedings. After only two IA we were able to stop the ongoing treatment with rFVIIa.

High doses of factor VIII (according to the modified Malmö treatment protocol) do not seem to be mandatory to induce immune tolerance in patients with acquired inhibitors against factor VIII.

References

1. Green D, Lechner K: A survey of 215 non hemophilic patients with inhibitors to factor VIII. Thromb Haemost 45 (1981), 200
2. Hay CRM, Negrier A, Ludlam A: The treatment of bleeding in acquired hemophilia with recombinant factor VIIa: A multicenter study. Thromb Haemost 78 (1997), 1463
3. Huth-Kühne A, Lages P, Zimmermann R: A new therapeutic option for inhibitor elimination in patients with acquired hemophilia. In Scharrer I, Schramm W (Eds), 30th Hemophilia Symposium Hamburg 1999, Springer Verlag Berlin Heidelberg 2000
4. Knöbl P, Derfler L, Koninger L, Kapiotis S, Jäger U, Maier-Dobersberger T, Hörl W, Lechner K, Pabinger I: Elimination of acquired factor VIII antibodies by extracorporeal antibody based IA (Ig Therasorb). Thromb Haemost 74 (1995), 1035
5. Nilsson IM, Berntorp E, Freiburghaus C: Treatment of patients with factor VIII and IX inhibitors. Thromb Haemost 72 (1994), 155

VIIb. Hemophilia and Hemorrhagic Disorders

Medical Need and Quality of Life in Patients with Hemophilia A

K. Hespe-Jungesblut, M. von Depka Prondzinski, and A. Dörries

Introduction

Quality of life studies are an important and well accepted aspect in evaluating the health status of population groups. In times of financial constraints in the health care system, quality of life studies may even become one of the factors to influence priority setting in a health care system based on the aspect of solidarity.

Our quality of life study is the first part of a project divided into two parts, financed by the DFG (DFG; Na 184/6–1) about medical need and the option to use medical need as a basis for allocation in the German health care system.

As a clinical example, we have chosen hemophilia A as a model disease because it is a very costly chronic disease with a successful prospect for treatment and thus an excellent example for the question of priority setting.

Method

The first part of the study is a health-related quality of life study of the hemophilia A patients at the outpatients department of hemostasis at the Hanover Medical School (MHH). The second part will be a qualitative interview with patients, doctors, nurses and members of the health insurance system, as well as self-help groups, about medical need.

The first part, the health-related quality of life is determined by demographic, self-developed hemophilia A specific questions and the Short Form 36 (SF-36), a multiple-choice questionnaire, which assesses physical functioning, physical role, bodily pain, general health, vitality, social functioning, and emotional role items. Results from this study collected in September 2002 are shown. The study provides information on the situation of the patients, their quality of life and treatment.

Results

For the quality of life study, 107 adult patients (18–80 years) with hemophilia A were asked to answer hemophilia A specific, demographic and health-related quality of life questions (SF-36). 56% of the patients answered (N=60).

Results of the demographic and hemophilia A specific questions:

The average age of the patient is 43 years (19–76 years).

I. Scharrer/W. Schramm (Ed.)
33rd Hemophilia Symposium Hamburg 2002
© Springer-Verlag Berlin Heidelberg 2004

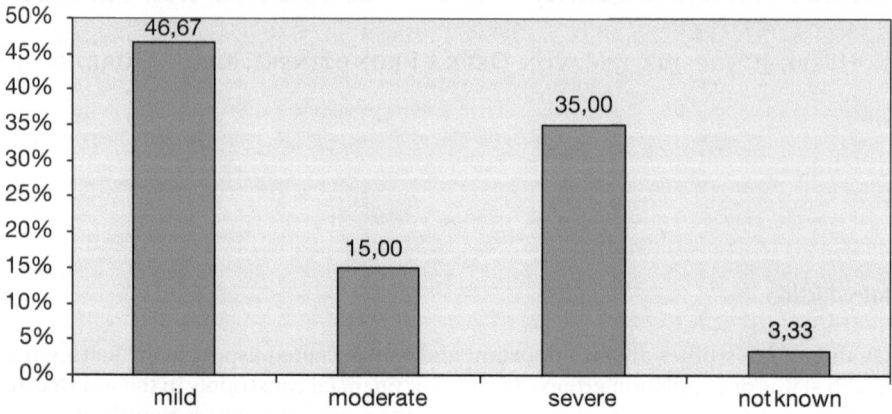

Fig. 1. Severity of hemophilia A (n=60)

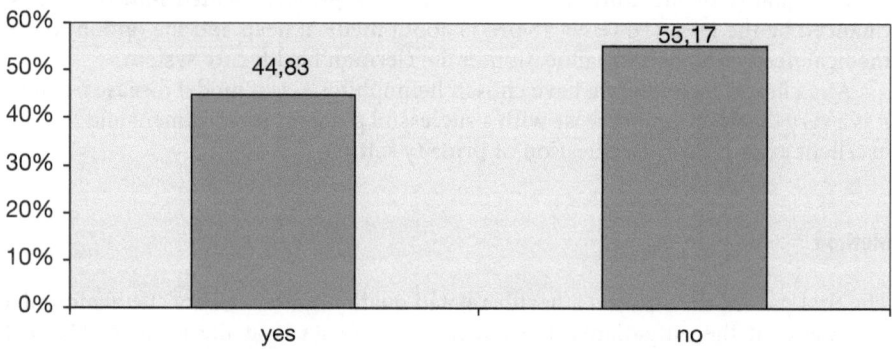

Fig. 2. Self-treatment at home (n=60)

Almost 50% of the patients suffer from a »mild«, 35% from a severe and 15% from a moderate hemophilia A (Fig. 1).

55% of the patients practice factor replacement therapy in home-self-treatment (Fig. 2). The majority of these patients suffer from severe hemophilia A.

70% of the study group receive factor on demand and 20% prophylactic (Fig. 3).

About one third (32%) of the patients suffer from chronic pain (Fig. 4). There is no correlation between chronic pain and the severity of the hemophilia A disease.

Almost half the patients (48%) did not receive out-patient treatment because of their hemophilia A in the last twelve months (Fig. 5).

Most patients (83%) have not been admitted to hospital during the last twelve months. (Fig. 6).

15% of the patients are involved in a hemophilia self-help group. The majority of the patients joining self-help groups suffer from severe hemophilia A.

65% of the patients did not have any days off work due to hemophilia during the last 12 months.

Half the study group (52%) works full-time and 13% receive disability or invalidity pension.

55% of the patients suffer from some further disease caused by the treatment with factor concentrate.

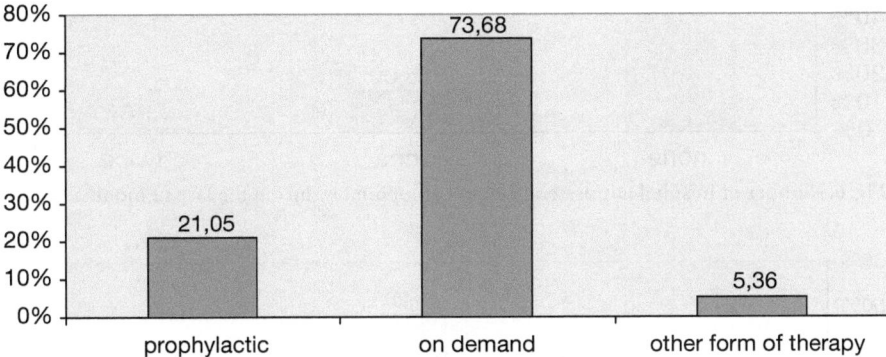

Fig. 3. Form of replacement therapy (n=60)

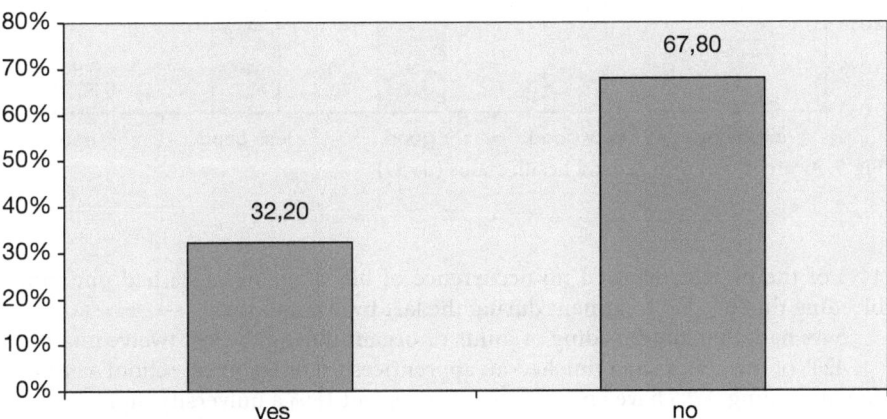

Fig. 4. Chronic pain (n=60)

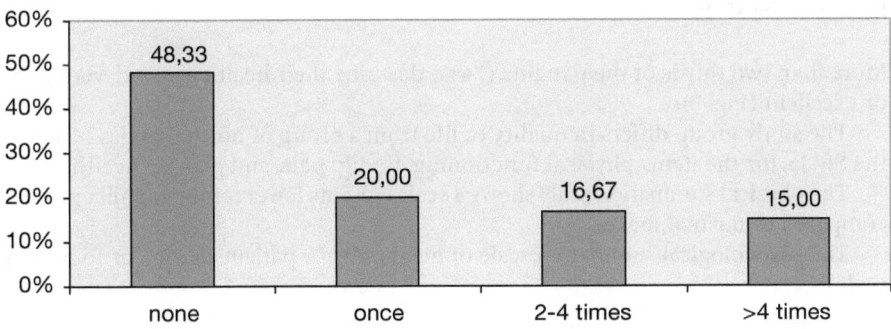

Fig. 5. Number of treatments in outpatient centers in the last 12 months (n=60)

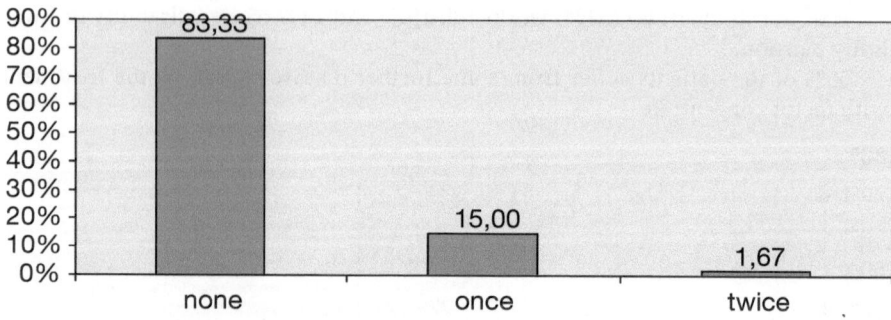

Fig. 6. Number of hospital admissions due to hemophilia A during the last 12 months (n=60)

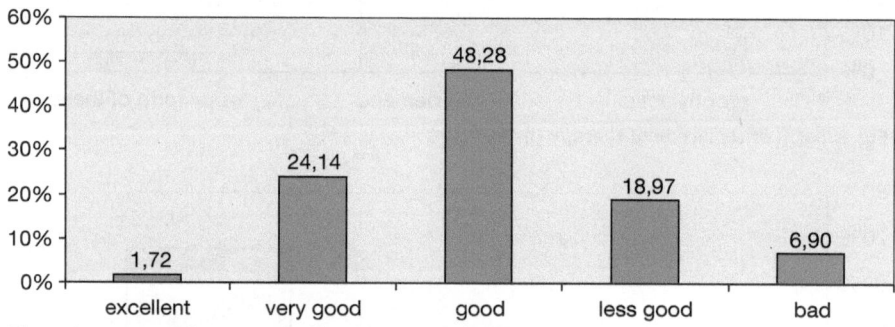

Fig. 7. Awareness of own general health status (n=59)

44% of the patients showed no occurrence of bleeding, and 22% had one minor bleeding that needed treatment during the last twelve months.

59% had no major bleeding of joints or organs during the last twelve months.

42% of the cohort had finished an apprenticeship or technical school as professional training, 17% have an academic degree, and 18% a university diploma.

Results of the SF-36

More than two thirds of the patients (74%) describe their health as good, very good or excellent (Fig. 7).

The study group differs in quality of life from a group of normal males tested by the SF-36, for the items physical functioning, bodily pain and general health.

The physical summation scale shows a scale 6 points lower for hemophilia patients compared to normal males.

The psychological summation scale of hemophilia A patients is similar to normal males.

Discussion

Even though 74% of the patients describe their health status as good, very good or excellent (Fig. 7), the results of the SF-36 show a lower quality of life for a hemophilia A patients than a group of German normal healthy males in all of the eight items tested (physical functioning, physical role, bodily pain, general health, vitality, social functioning, emotional role). While the patients show a significant lower quality of life for the items physical functioning, bodily pain and general health, they only differ marginally from the healthy population in the item of mental health. All the other items mentioned show a bias towards a lower quality of life in the study group.

The physical summation scale evaluated by the SF 36 shows a lower scale for hemophilia A patients than for a healthy males. Comparing the physical and psychological summation scales of hemophilia patients with patients suffering from other diseases tested with the SF-36 (Bullinger M., Kirchberger I., 1998), it can be seen that there are many patient groups showing a similar physical summation scale to hemophilia A patients (e.g. patients with impaired vision, backache, cancer, hypertonia). However the psychological summation scale of hemophilia A patients is higher than all other diseases in the comparison.

Compared to the average male population in Lower Saxony, the study group shows a higher percentage of academic and university degrees. The reason for this is unknown. It could perhaps be explained by the existent or expected limitation of body functioning caused by hemophilia.

The medical treatment of the study group seems to be good. This would explain the small number of hospital admissions and doctor visits during the last twelve months and the relatively large percentage of patients who did not have any bleedings needing treatment during the last year.

Conclusions

The patients of our study group show a lower quality of life than German healthy males. While hemophilia A patients show a significantly lower quality of life in the items physical functioning, bodily pain and general health, there are nearly no differences in the psychological quality of life.

The quality of life study is our basis for the subsequent qualitative interviews with patients, doctors, nurses and members of the health insurance system as well as self-help groups about medical need, which will be done at the beginning of 2003.

References

1. Bullinger M., Kirchberger I. SF-36 Fragebogen zum Gesundheitszustand (Handanweisung), Hogrefe, Verlag für Psychologie, Göttingen-Toronto-Seattle
2. Hege H. (01) Die Politik muss entscheiden. Deutsches Ärzteblatt, Jg 98, Heft 5, 2.2.01, S. 185–188
3. Janischowski A. (1999) Budgetierung und medizinische Notwendigkeit aus der Sicht des Krankenhausmanagements. Aus: Ratajczak, Schwaz-Schilling, Medizinische Notwendigkeit und Ethik, MedR Schriftenreihe Medizinrecht, Springerverlag, S. 91–101r

Quality of Life Autoevaluation of Hemophilia Patients in Romania

D. Mihailov, M. Jernea, V. Serban, S. Arghirescu, M. Serban, W. Schramm, and D. Lighezan

Introduction

The problem of quality of life in chronic patients remains a concern for the health care system, its improvement being an aim as important as the discovery of new therapeutic methods. Furthermore, quality of life is used in health planning, health economics and medical decision-making.

Quality of life can be assessed using both objective criteria (e.g. chronic arthropathy, mobility, work capacity, etc) and subjective ones, by the own modality of integrating these realities by the subject.

A number of studies mention significant differences between the subjective perceptions of individual life quality versus objective assessments. Quality of life has various dimensions with multiple meaning for people, so that these differences derive on the one hand from individual expectations, and on the other hand from personal life experience.

The existence of a correlation between personality and quality of life, life satisfaction and well-being was demonstrated by several studies.

Aim of the Study

Starting from hemophiliac' status in Romania (high rate of chronic arthropathy, high number of transfusion-transmitted diseases and of neuro-sensitive and sensorial sequels) we aim to carry out a quality of life autoevaluation in hemophilia patients.

On the basis of these objective realities we aimed to evaluate their perception on quality of life and to establish the domains and facets where quality of life is affected in hemophilia patients.

Material and Methods

This study reports on the field testing, using the Word Health Organization Quality of Life instrument (WHOQOL-100) on:
- study group (SG): 50 hemophilia patients, registered and treated in the IIIrd Pediatric Clinic Timisoara and in the Clinical Center for Evaluation and Rehabilitation Cristian Serban Buzias.
- blind group (BG): 50 males subjects, without chronic pathology.

I. Scharrer/W. Schramm (Ed.)
33rd Hemophilia Symposion Hamburg 2002
© Springer-Verlag Berlin Heidelberg 2004

Inclusion Criteria

- age: more than 18 years
- IQ >100

The WHOQOL instrument (Table 1) contains different five-point response scales concerned with intensity (not at all - extremely), capacity (not at all - completely), frequency (never - always) and evaluation (very satisfied - very dissatisfied, very good - very poor). The mean age was 25.42 years (SG) and 25.92 years (BG).
The data was assessed using the Australian algorithm.
Statistical analysis employed non-parametric comparison methods, U test.
We considered statistically significant $p<0.05$

The distribution of the patients was: 94% cases hemophilia A and 6% hemophilia B. The coagulopathy was severe in 82% cases, moderate in 12% cases and mild in 6% cases.

Table 1. The structure of the WHOQOL-100

Domain	Facet	
	Overall quality of life and general health	
1. Physical health	F1	Pain and discomfort
	F2	Energy and fatigue
	F3	Sleep and rest
2. Psychological health	F4	Positive feelings
	F5	Thinking, learning, memory and concentration
	F6	Self-esteem
	F7	Body image and appearance
	F8	Negative feelings
3. Level of independence	F9	Mobility
	F10	Activities of daily living
	F11	Dependence on medicinal substances and medical aids
	F12	Work capacity
4. Social relationships	F13	Personal relationships
	F14	Social support
	F15	Sexual activity
5. Environment	F16	Freedom, physical safety and security
	F17	Home environment
	F18	Financial resources
	F19	Health and social care: accessibility and quality
	F20	Opportunities for acquiring new information and skills
	F21	Participation in and opportunities for recreation/leisure activities
	F22	Physical environment (pollution, noise, traffic, climate)
	F23	Transportation
6. Spirituality	F24	Spirituality/religion/personal beliefs (single facet)

The functional joint score of hemophilia patients was: 1.52 right ankle, 2,16 left ankle, 6.77 right knee, 6.05 left knee, 4.44 right elbow and 5.02 left elbow.

Neuro-sensitive-sensorial sequels were found in 10 patients from the SG: sensorial neuropathy (3-), optic nerve atrophy (2-), blindness (1-), epilepsy (1-), pyramidal syndrome (1-), facial nerve paralysis (1-), lateral popliteal nerve paralysis (1 cases).

The transfusion-transmitted diseases in SG revealed that 48% of the patients presented HCV infection, 12% had both HCV and HBV infection, and all patients were HIV-negative.

Results

In life quality domains we noticed statistically significant differences in overall quality of life and general health ($p = 0.01$), physical health ($p < 0.001$), level of independence ($p < 0.001$) and social relationships ($p < 0.001$) domains, while psychological health ($p = 0.69$), environment ($p = 0.47$) and spirituality ($p = 0.31$) domains showed no statistically significant differences.

The results in life quality domains are represented in Fig. 1–5.

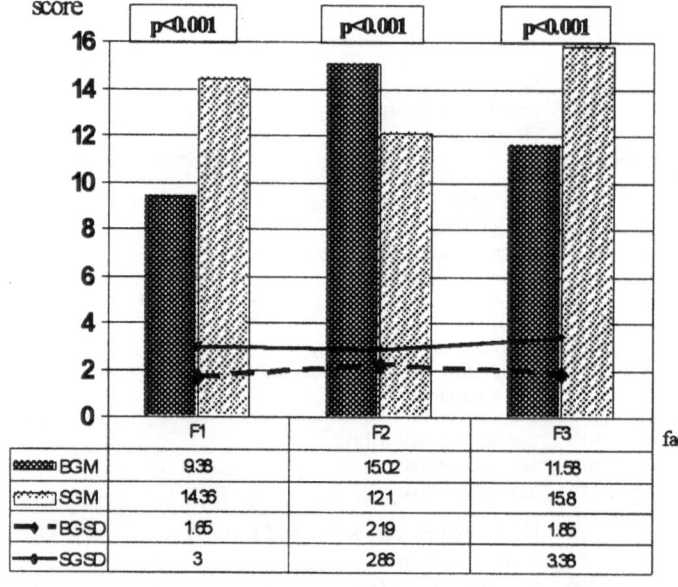

	F1	F2	F3
BGM	9.38	15.02	11.58
SGM	14.36	12.1	15.8
BGSD	1.65	2.19	1.85
SGSD	3	2.86	3.38

Fig. 1. Mean scores and standard deviations in physical health domain

Discussions and Conclusions

As predicted, our data confirm that general life quality level is affected in hemophiliacs, but the differences were not so important as we expected, supporting the data from the literature regarding objective-subjective differences.

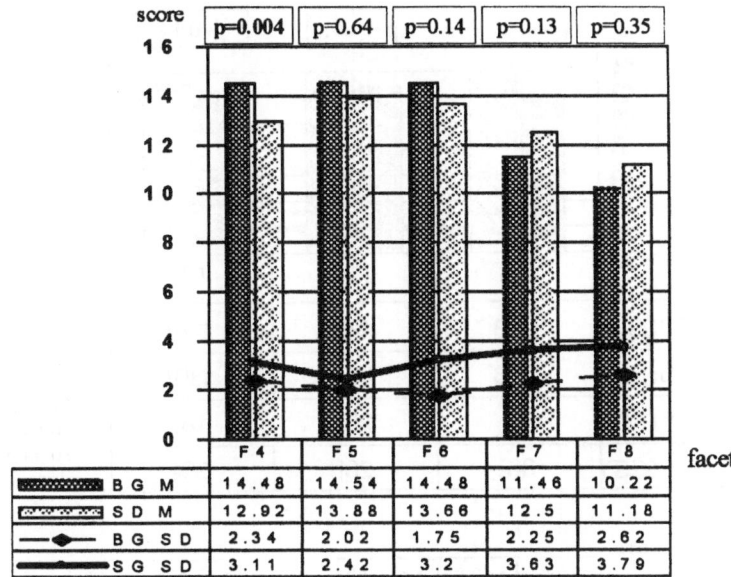

Fig. 2. Mean scores and standard deviations in psychological health domain

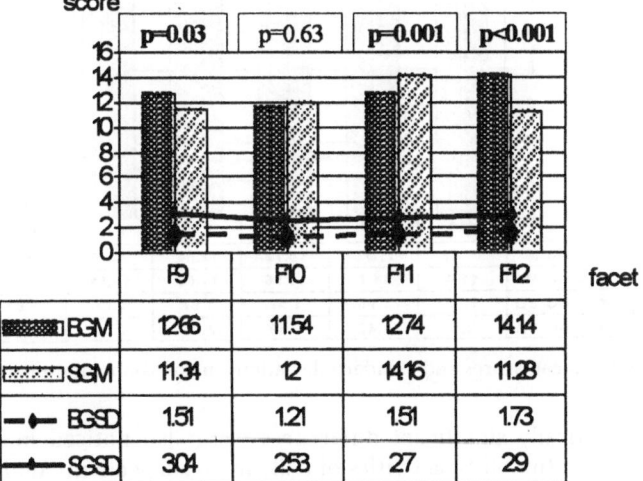

Fig. 3. Mean scores and standard deviations in level of independence domain

It was found that physical health, level of independence and social relations domains made a significant impact on perception of general quality of life related to health.

The results in physical domain accurately reveal the consequences of the deficiencies in hemophilia treatment in our country (absence of prophylactic therapy, inadequate doses and duration of the »on demand« therapy).

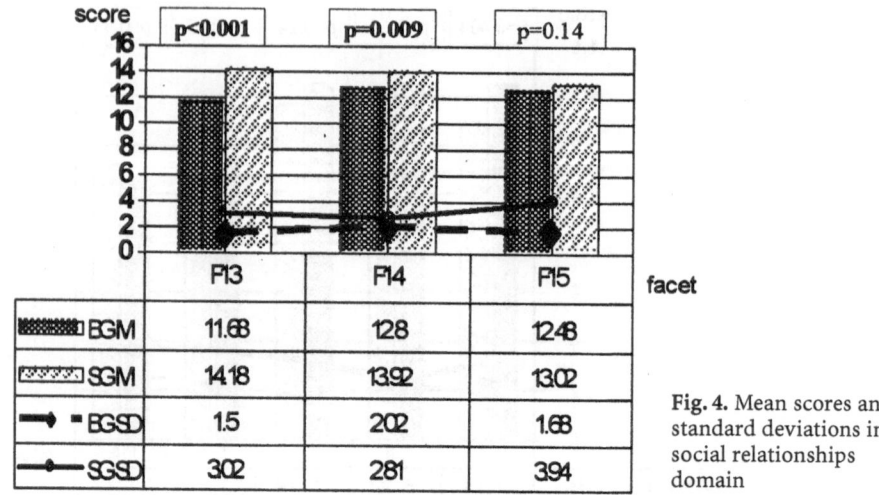

Fig. 4. Mean scores and standard deviations in social relationships domain

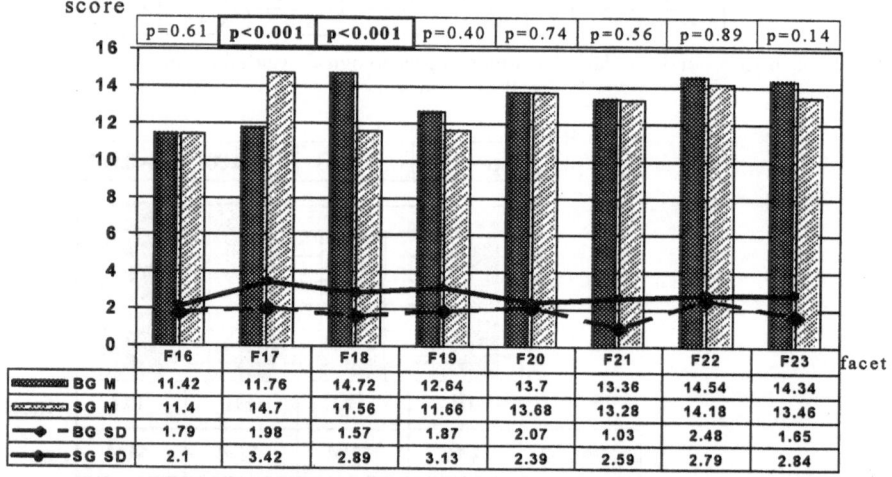

Fig. 5. Mean scores and standard deviations in environment domain

Statistically significant differences were also noticed in level of independence domain (mobility, activities of daily living, dependence on medical substances and medical aids, work capacity), expressing in this regard an actual important limitation of Romanian hemophiliacs (patient with chronic complication of the disease, depending on his parents, in most cases single and presenting social life integration difficulties).

Our patients also declare their unsatisfaction in social relations domain, which examines feelings in family, couple, friendship, relationships and satisfaction; they are also unsatisfied with practical social support. These needs are correlated with other facets which, although they belong to a domain without generally statistical significant differences (environment), are affected: home environment and financial resources.

In the psychological domain we did not notice statistically significant differences. We expected a high anxiety, depression and worries level, coded in negative feelings facet (also unaffected). But statistically significant differences appeared in positive feelings facet, which expresses hope in the future and confidence, and which underlines in fact the same idea.

The spirituality domain did not show statistically significant differences, personal beliefs, religion and spirituality being an important support for our patients, offering them a sense of existence.

Another surprisingly unaffected facet is health and social care. An explanation could be that our study is carried out in a rehabilitation center, where hemophilia patient assistance includes psychological support and alternative therapy.

Our results support the objective data of hemophiliacs life quality in Romania and underline the necessity of developing national long-term programs in order to improve their life quality.

A further development of this study, both in enlarged age groups and by associating it with a needs questionnaire to detect practical needs addressed to the family, health system and society should be fulfilled.

By involving decision making factors, these data could become a real basis of some special programs, in order to improve hemophilia treatment and to reduce complications rate, increasing the patients independence level by a better social life integration.

References

1. Carr AJ; Gibson B; Robinson PG. Measuring quality of life: Is quality of life determined by expectations or experience? BMJ 2001 May 19; 322 (7296): 1240–1243
2. Hagberg M, Hagberg B, Saveman BI. The significance of personality factors for various dimensions of life quality among older people. Aging Ment Health 2002 May; 6 (2): 178–185
3. Royal S, Schramm W, Berntrop E, Giangrande P, Gringeri A, Ludlam C, Kroner B, Szucs T. Quality-of-life differences between prophylactic and on-demand factor replacement therapy in European hemophilia patients, Hemophilia, 2002 Jan; 8 (1): 44–50
4. Schramm W, Berger K. Linking medicine an economics: health economics and quality of life in hemophilia care, Haemophilia, 2002 May; 8 (3): 217–220
5. Skevington SM, Carse MS, Williams AC. Validation of the WHOQOL-100: pain management improves quality of life for chronic pain patients, Clin J Pain, 2001 Sep; 17 (3): 264–275
6. Skevington SM. Investigating the relationship between pin and discomfort and quality of life, using the WHOQOL, Pain 1998 Jun; 76 (3): 395–406
7. Trippoli S, Vaiani M, Linari S, Longo G, Morfini M, Messori A. Multivariate analysis of factor influencing quality of life and utility in patients with hemophilia, Haematologica, 2001 Jul; 86 (7): 722–728

Valproate-Induced Type I von-Willebrand Disease – a Common Occurrence?

V. AUMANN, G. LUTZE, F. WIEN, and U. MITTLER

Introduction

An increased bleeding tendency and its possible consequences have a considerable impact on the lives of the people concerned. This is shown by restrictions in daily life, e.g. in sports activities, by the increased risk associated with operative procedures or accidents but also by the necessary treatment measures.

If the disturbances of the coagulation system are a consequence of drug therapy, a careful benefit-to-risk assessment is called for. For a responsible decision comprehensive data on the drug concerned are essential.

Valproic acid or valproate sodium or valproate calcium (Convulex, Convulsofin, Ergenyl, Leptilan, Orfiril) are widely used as antiepileptics in neuropediatrics. The indications are

- treatment of generalized seizures in the form of absences, myoclonic and tonic-clonic seizures,
- treatment of focal and secondary generalized seizures,
- combination treatment of other forms of seizures, if these do not respond to conventional antiepileptic treatment.

Side-effects on the coagulation system have been described [3, 7]. Effects on components of the FVIII/von-Willebrand-factor complex such as those found in type I von-Willebrand disease were observed by Kreuz et al. [8, 9] in 67 % of the children on valproate therapy. However, an as yet unpublished study by Eberl et al. [6] was not able to confirm these results.

The aim of our investigations was to determine the incidence of von-Willebrand disease type changes in our own neuropediatric patient population.

Methods

Patients

45 patients from the neuropediatric outpatient clinic of the Center for Pediatric Medicine at the University of Magdeburg were included in the investigations. The median age at the time of beginning valproate therapy was 9 years and 7 months.

I. Scharrer/W. Schramm (Ed.)
33rd Hemophilia Symposion Hamburg 2002
© Springer-Verlag Berlin Heidelberg 2004

Coagulation Studies

In all patients a full coagulation status including the components of the FVIII/von-Willebrand-factor complex was obtained. In 43 patients baseline findings were obtained before beginning treatment. In 36 patients follow-up data were obtained after intervals of at least three months.

Statistical Analysis

In line with the objective of our study, factor VIII activity (VIII:C), von-Willebrand-factor antigen (vWF:Ag) and ristocetin cofactor (vWF:RCo) were statistically analyzed. For this purpose patient groups were formed, values less than 50% of normal being regarded as pathological [6]. The patient groups were compared with each other before and after beginning valproate therapy. This was performed by frequency tables and cross tables with regard to the group behaviour and by comparisons of means at the different time points.

Results

The changes in the parameters VIII:C, vWF:Ag and vWF:RCo are shown graphically in Figures 1–3. Values above 50% of normal were found at baseline in 88% of the cases. In the course of the valproate therapy considerable deviations from baseline, both increases and decreases, were observed in individual cases. Thus, »migration« of individual patients between the pre-determined groups was observed. In one

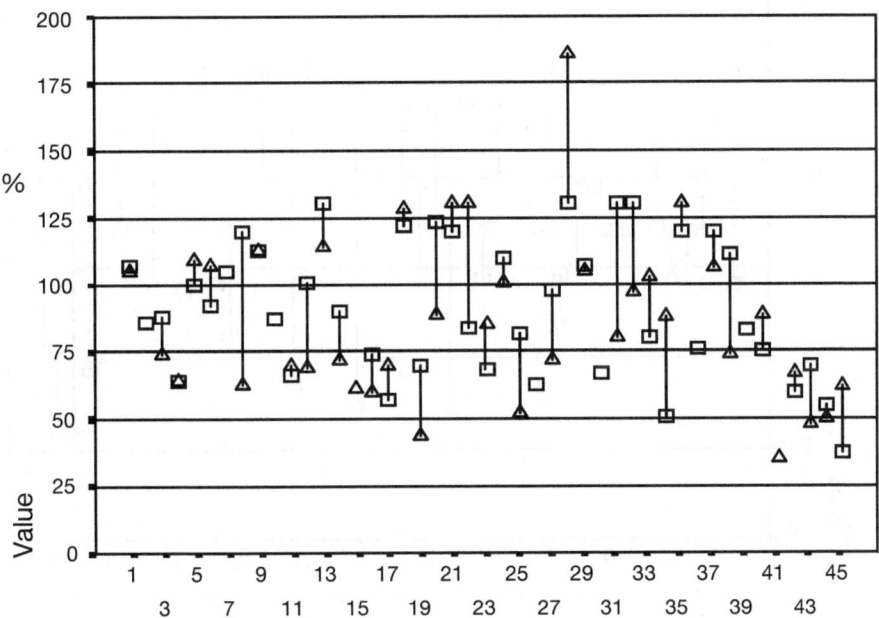

Fig. 1. VIII:C in patients before (□) and during (△) valproate therapy

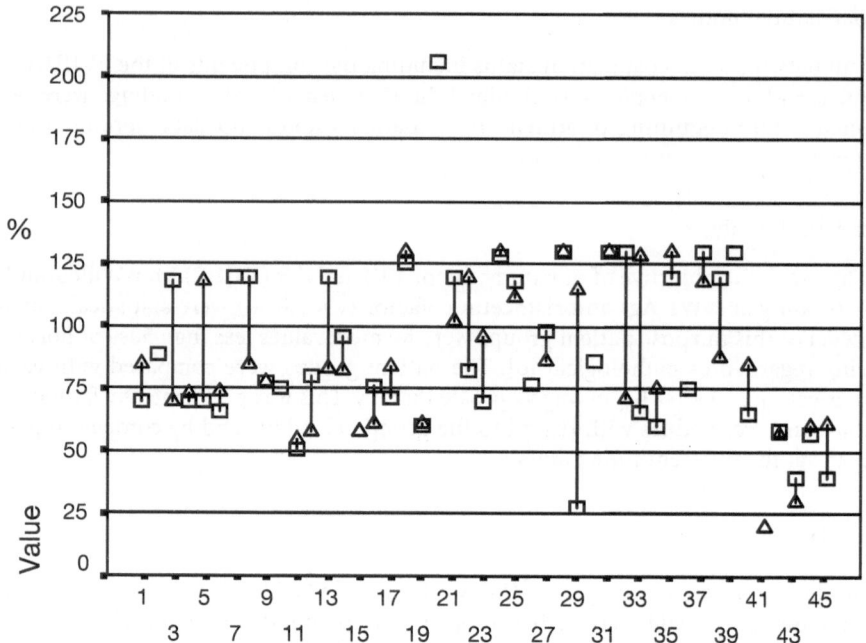

Fig. 2. vWF:Ag in patients before (□) and during (△) valproate therapy

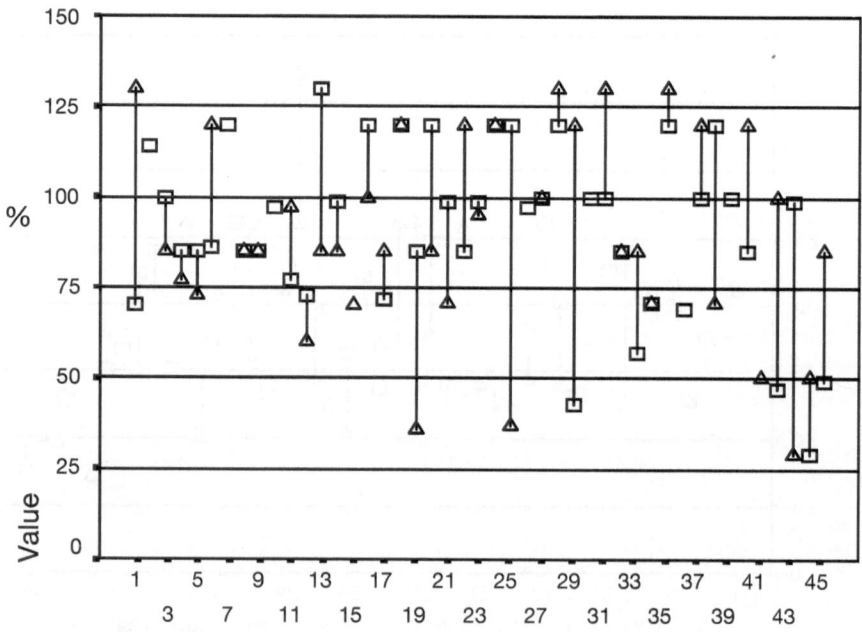

Fig. 3. vWF:RCo in patients before (□) and during (△) valproate therapy

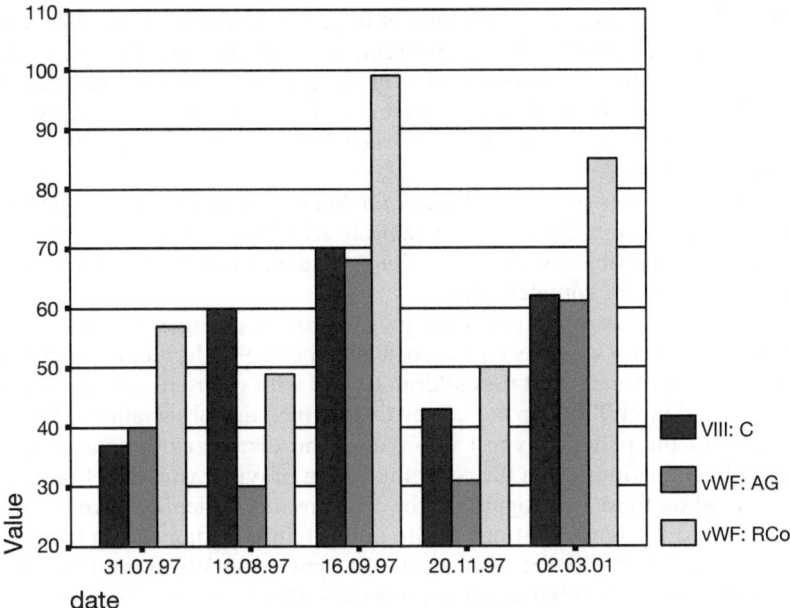

Fig. 4. VIII:C, vWF:Ag and vWF:RCo in the same patient at different times during valproate therapy

patient the initially reduced factor VIII activity became normal, in three patients with normal VIII:C findings at baseline the values fell to below the 50% mark. Ristocetin cofactor (vWF:RCo) became normal in three of four patients with originally depressed values, while in three patients who had had normal findings before starting valproate therapy the values became pathological. Only one patient showed a possibly valproate-related reduction in vWF:Ag. The changes were significant in the individual patients. However, this was not the case when the patients were regarded as a whole as decreases and increases in the parameters were approximately balanced. Therefore, the latter form of consideration fails to do justice to the individual as clinically relevant findings can be concealed behind apparent normality. This is the case, for example, in the three patients in whom vWF:RCo fell to below 35% during the treatment.

Fig. 4 shows the parameters VIII:C, vWF:Ag and vWF:RCo in the same patient at different times of treatment with valproate. The substantial differences in the findings at the different time points stand out. In this respect the patient is not an exception.

Discussion and Conclusions

Reports on studies investigating the effects of valproate on the coagulation system go back about 30 years. Monographs on valproic acid [3, 7] described global coagulation disturbances as a consequence of impaired synthesis in toxic liver failure, qualitative and quantitative platelet disorders and reductions in fibrinogen. Monitoring of the coagulation by determination of the prothrombin time, fibrinogen and the platelet count has been proposed, together with the consequence of discontinuation of the valproate therapy in the case of marked disturbances of these values or the occurrence of bleeding.

The guidelines of the *Gesellschaft für Neuropädiatrie* (Neuropediatrics Society) [1] do not mention side-effects of valproic acid. The American RxList Monographs [10] do not describe any effects of valproic acid on factor VIII or the factor VIII/von-Willebrand-factor complex either.

Kreuz et al. were the first to draw attention to changes in the factor VIII/von-Willebrand-factor complex on valproate therapy [8, 9]. They found reductions in factor VIII activity in 33% of the children treated with valproate, reductions in vWF:Ag in 83% and in vWF:RCo in 66%. They then termed this observation, which was made in 67% of the patients, type I von-Willebrand disease as these acquired findings resembled the findings in the congenital form of type I von-Willebrand disease.

Based on these investigations, the *Vademecum Antiepilepticum* [11], following the revised recommendations of the Königstein Working Group for Epileptology of 1995 and 2000 [5], drew attention to a type I von-Willebrand disease induced by valproate. Its incidence was given as 20–30%. Performance of the appropriate coagulation tests was recommended. Platelets, aPTT, prothrombin time and fibrinogen were to be determined 3 and 6 months after beginning therapy. It was suggested that a full coagulation status, including bleeding time and special tests for von-Willebrand disease, should be performed before operations. If necessary, prophylaxis or treatment with clotting factors (factor VIII concentrate) or desmopressin should be performed, although the latter can provoke epileptic seizures.

The data sheet for valproate [4] mentions an effect on and the need for examination of coagulation by determining the platelet count, prothrombin time, aPTT, fibrinogen, factor VIII and factor VIII-associated factors.

However, Banerjea et al. [2] found relatively little effect of valproate therapy on von-Willebrand-factor. Likewise, Eberl et al. [6], who performed a multicenter study in children treated with valproate, found no changes justifying a diagnosis of von-Willebrand's disease. These studies thus contradict the results and classifications of previous authors [8, 9].

We can thus conclude that effects of valproate on blood coagulation do exist and that, with regard to hepatotoxic actions not presented here and to the occurrence of hypofibrinogenemia and thrombocytic disorders, these effects require hemostaseological attention. However, as regards the development of type I von-Willebrand disease as a result of valproate therapy, we were not able to confirm the reported incidence. On the other hand, nor were we able to establish the complete absence of any effect on FVIII/von-Willebrand-factor. In our own investigations we found that significant changes typical of type I von-Willebrand disease were not present on overall analysis of the patients but were present in individual patients. Changes in the components of von-Willebrand-factor are thus possible. However, the decision criteria for evaluation must be uniformly defined. The results obtained suggest that clinical consequences are possible. However, in the few patients with reduced VIII:C and vWF:RCo in our study no increased bleeding tendency was found. The diagnostic and therapeutic recommendations were additionally complicated by the individually varying, sometimes considerable fluctuations in the coagulation findings in one and the same patient at different times of treatment.

With regard to an influence of valproate therapy on the components of the FVIII/von-Willebrand-factor complex the following recommendations are made:

- Before beginning treatment with valproate a full coagulation work-up should be performed to detect high-risk patients. The presence of type I von-Willebrand disease is not a contraindication to clinically indicated use of valproate.
- Routine determination of coagulation parameters during treatment with valproate to test for von-Willebrand disease is not recommended, but only if disturbances were existing before beginning treatment.
- The necessary coagulation parameters should be determined before operations or other situations associated with an increased bleeding risk.
- If clinically necessary, replacement therapy with FVIII concentrates containing von-Willebrand-factor should be carried out.
- The term »valproate induced von-Willebrand disease« should not be used.

References

1. Arbeitsgemeinschaft der Wissenschaftlichen Medizinischen Fachgesellschaften (AWMF). Leitlinien der Gesellschaft für Neuropädiatrie: Diagnostische und therapeutische Prinzipien bei Epilepsien im Kindesalter. AWMF online 1996. www.uni-duesseldorf.de
2. Banerjea MC, Diener W, Kutschke G, Schneble HJ, Korinthenberg R, Sutor AH. Pro- and anticoagulatory factors under sodium valproate-therapy in children. Neuropediatrics 2002; 33: 215–220
3. von Czettritz G, Weinmann HM. Gerinnungsstörungen unter Valproinsäure. In: Krämer G, Laub M (eds). Valproinsäure. Springer Heidelberg New York 1992; 210–216
4. Desitin Arzneimittel GmbH. Gebrauchsinformation Orfiril®long 150 mg; 08/99
5. Doose H et al. Früherkennung von Komplikationen einer Valproattherapie im Kindesalter. Empfehlungen des Königsteiner Arbeitskreises für Epileptologie. Päd Prax 1986; 33: 581–582
6. Eberl W, Budde U, Bentele K, Bergmann F, Christen H, Fehr V, Hassenpflug W, Knapp R, Kurzeia A, Schneppenheim R. Valproat-induziertes von Willebrand Syndrom (in Vorbereitung)
7. König SA, König I. Nebenwirkungen von Valproinsäure an Leber, Pankreas und am blutbildenden System. In: Krämer G, Walden J (eds). Valproinsäure. Springer Berlin Heidelberg New York 2002; 367–380
8. Kreuz W, Linde R, Funk M, Meyer-Schrod R, Föll E, Nowak-Göttl U, Jacobi G, Scharrer I. Induction of von Willebrand disease type I by valproic acid. Lancet II 1990: 1350–1351
9. Kreuz W, Linde R, Funk M, Meyer-Schrod R, Föll E, Nowak-Göttl U, Jacobi G, Vigh Z, Scharrer I. Valproate therapy induces von Willebrand disease type I. Epilepsia 1992; 33: 178–184
10. RxList Monographs: Valproic Acid: Warnings. Adverse Reactions. www.rxlist.com 2002
11. Schneble H, Ernst JP. Pharmakotherapie der Epilepsien. Vademecum Antiepilepticum 2001/2002. Deutsche Sektion der Internationalen Liga gegen Epilepsie

Bleeding Symptoms in Carriers of Hemophilia A – Association to the Factor VIII Gene Mutation?

W. Miesbach, Th. Vigh, I. Stier-Brück, J. Oldenburg, and I. Scharrer

Hemophilia A is an X-linked recessive bleeding disorder of variable severity that is caused by a deficiency of coagulation factor VIII (FVIII). The disease results from mutations in the FVIII gene which are heterogenous both in type and position within the gene.

The disease occurs almost exclusively in males who have only one X chromosome; females with one abnormal FVIII gene mostly are asymptomatic carriers. The frequency of hemophilia A is 1–2 in 10 000 male births in all ethnic groups.

The daughters of men with hemophilia are obligate carriers. Carriers have a 50:50 chance of passing on the condition to a son and a 50:50 chance that a daughter will be a carrier.

Since the mutation occurs very rarely in female germ cells, nearly all mothers of patients with hemophilia A are carriers of FVIII deficiency. Members of the same family usually have the same factor level and the severity of hemophilia within a family remains mostly constant.

Over the last 20 years the advances in molecular biology and prenatal diagnostic techniques have faciliated the diagnosis of hemophilia.

The gene for factor VIII was cloned in 1984 [1–3]. The FVIII gene is 186 kb in size and contains 26 exons.

Factor VIII is expressed in the liver, spleen, lymph nodes and a variety of human tissues [4].

Presumably the genetic diversity accounts for the heterogenity in clinical severity of hemophilia A. Severity of the disease is determined by the amount of FVIII coagulant activity present in plasma leading to the classification of mild, moderate or severe hemophilia A with corresponding activity levels.

In hemophilia A subjects many mutations in the FVIII gene have been identified including deletions, point mutations or mutations resulting in stop codons [5]. FVIII gene inversion mutations were identified in 45% of severe hemophiliacs [6].

In about 5% of the patients with hemophilia A there are large (more than 100 nucleotides) deletions in the FVIII gene [7]. Deletions almost always produce severe hemophilia A. Small deletions or insertions in the coding region of the factor VIII gene that result in frameshifts may cause severe hemophilia A, too.

Carrier detection in hemophilia A can give definite answers in 80–90% of cases after DNA analysis. The tests sometimes require blood samples from other members of the family, particularly the person with hemophilia and an unaffected male. It is not always possible to exclude carrier status by measuring a woman's FVIII level.

I. Scharrer/W. Schramm (Ed.)
33rd Hemophilia Symposion Hamburg 2002
© Springer-Verlag Berlin Heidelberg 2004

These levels fluctuate in normal people under stress, during pregnancy and for those under oral contraceptives. Therefore, for these tests calculations are made after taking blood samples on several separate occasions.

Levels of FVIII and vWF:Ag in normal women are approximately equal. The level of vWF:Ag in carriers is normal (for it is controlled by genes on autosomes) and, because FVIII production may be subnormal, vWF is often higher than FVIII. If a potential carrier's FVIII level is definitely below the normal range, she may be designated a carrier. If her FVIII level is within the normal range, but her vWF:Ag level is higher, and the discrepancy is greater than is ever found in normal women, she may be designated a carrier, too. Moreover vWF-Ag is helpful for detecting carriers of hemophilia A, who have the ratio of FVIII/vWF:Ag around 0.5 while in normal women it is around 1. A ratio less than 0.7 is indicative of carrier status.

Although carriers have only one affected chromosome, a wide range of values have been reported [8] as a result of random inactivation of one of the two X chromosomes, i.e. lyonization [9].

Most carriers of hemophilia A have levels of FVIII within the normal range but symptomatic carriers of hemophilia A with low levels of factor VIII can have bleeding symptoms like a male patient with mild hemophilia A. A small number of carriers may have very low levels of FVIII [10] due to co-inheritance of a variant von-Willebrand-factor allele (i.e. von-Willebrand disease Normandy), homozygosity for hemophilia gene [11] or extreme lyonization.

The aim of this study was to investigate the incidence of bleeding symptoms of hemophilia A carriers and their correlation to the activity of FVIII and the FVIII gene mutation.

Patients

We studied bleeding symptoms of 29 carriers of hemophilia A. FVIII gene analysis was done by Dr. Oldenburg, Würzburg/Frankfurt: 9 carriers with an inversion mutation in intron 22, 19 carriers with a single point mutation (17 carriers with a missense mutation and 2 carriers with a nonsense mutation) and 1 carrier with a small deletion. The median age of the carriers with an inversion mutation in intron 22 was 40 years (33–74 years), the median weight was 67 kg (50–89 kg). The median age of the carriers with a single point mutation was 38 years (15–63 years), the median weight was 69 kg (50–95 kg). The single carrier with the small deletion was 50 years old and the weight was 72 kg.

The following bleeding events were reported: bleeding after trauma and surgery, bleeding when giving birth, bleeding associated with teeth coming in and dental extraction, nose and gums bleeding, recurrent hematoma, heavy and long menstrual bleeding.

Methods

Factor VIII was tested by an one stage method (Instrument ACL 300, normal range:

64%–167%). The FVIII binding test was made by an ELISA (normal range: > 65 %). von-Willebrand factor antigen (vWF-Ag) was tested by a homemade ELISA (normal range: 82%–138%).

Results

6/9 (67%) of carriers with an inversion mutation of intron 22 were suffering from bleeding symptoms. The median activity of FVIII was 39% (17%–80%), median antigen of von-Willebrand-factor was 86% (40–234%). The ratio vWF/FVIII-activity was 2.2 (Table 1).

9/19 (47%) of carriers with a single point mutation were suffering from bleeding symptoms. The median activity of FVIII was 53% (20%–91%), median antigen of von-Willebrand-factor was 92% (66–233%). The ratio vWF/FVIII was 1.7.

Table 1. Association of FVIII and vWF-Ag with bleeding events

Median	Intron 22 Inversion	Single point mutation	Deletion
Factor VIII-Activity	39% (33–74)	53% (20–91)	30%
Factor VIII-binding test*	89% (80–94)	116% (83–127)	
vWF-Ag	86% (40–234)	92% (66–233)	50%
Ratio vWF-Ag/factor VIII	2,20	1,7	1,7
Bleeding events	6/9 (67%)	9/19 (47%)	yes

* factor VIII-binding test was made of 4 carriers with an inverse mutation in intron 22 and of 9 carriers with single point mutation.

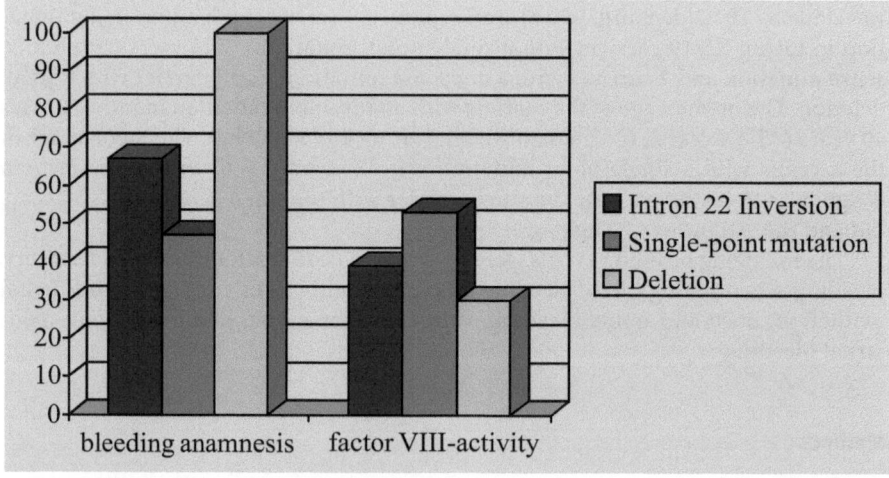

Fig. 1. Bleeding anamnesis and FVIII-activity

The single carrier with the small deletion was suffering from bleeding symptoms. Activity of FVIII was 30% and vWF-Ag was 50%. The ratio vWF/FVIII was 1.7.

The frequency of bleeding symptoms differed significantly among carriers with an inversion mutation in intron 22 and carriers with a single point mutation dependent on the factor VIII activity ($p < 0.05$). The risk of bleeding is higher in carriers with an inversion of intron 22 than in carriers with a single-point mutation (OR 2.28, 95% CI 1.3–4.0, Fig. 1).

Discussion

Most carriers of hemophilia A have levels of FVIII within the normal range but symptomatic carriers of hemophilia A with low levels of factor VIII can have bleeding symptoms like a male patient with mild hemophilia A. Our study showed that the incidence of bleeding symptoms of hemophilia A carriers is correlated to the activity of FVIII and the underlying FVIII gene mutation. Carriers with low levels of FVIII are at risk of excessive bleeding from surgery or other invasive procedures, such as dental extractions, biopsies, etc. Genotypic analysis to determine the underlying genetic defect should be taken to identify the carriers. The precise determination of the carrier status by direct gene analysis allows a better understanding of the possible bleeding risk of carriers of hemophilia A.

References

1. Gitschier J, Wood WI, Goralka TM, et al. Characterization of the human factor VIII gene. Nature 1984;312: 326–30
2. Wood WI, Capon DJ, Simonsen CC, et al. Expression of active human factor VIII from recombinant DNA clones. Nature 1984; 312: 330–7
3. Toole JJ, Knopf JL, Wozney JM, et al. Molecular cloning of a cDNA encoding human anti-hemophilic factor. Nature 1984; 312: 342–7
4. Wion KL, Kelly D, Summerfield JA, Tuddenham EGD, Lawn RM. Distribution of factor VIII mRNA and antigen in human liver and other tissues. Nature 1985; 317: 726–9
5. Higuchi M, Kochhan L, Schwaab R, Egli H, Brackmann HH, Horst J, Olek K. Molecular defects in hemophilia A: identification and characterization of mutations in the factor VIII Gene and family analysis. Blood 1989; 74: 1045–51
6. Lakich D, Kazazian HH, Antoarakis SE, Gitschier J. Inversions disrupting the factor VIII gene are a common cause of severe hemophilia A. Nature Genetics 1993; 5: 236–41
7. Antonarakis SF, Kazazian HH Jr. The molecular basis of hemophilia A in man. Trends Genet 1988; 4: 233–7
8. Rapaport SI, Patch MJ, Moore FJ. Anti-hemophilic globulin levels in carriers of hemophilia A. J Clin Invest 1961; 39: 1619–25
9. Lyon MF. Sex chromatin and gene action in the mammalian x-chromosome. Am J Hum Genet 1962; 14: 135–48
10. Lusher JM, McMillan CW. Severe factor VIII and factor IX deficiency in females. Am J Med 1978; 65: 637–48
11. Graham JB, Barrow ES, Roberts HR, et al. Dominant inheritance of hemophilia A in three generations of women. Blood 1975; 46: 175–88

Recombinant Human Interferon α-2b Therapy, for Refractory Immune Thrombocytopenic Purpura in Children

M. Serban, V. Borla. C. Petrescu, S. Arghirescu, I. Cuca, and W. Schramm

Summary

The study was designed to evaluate the effect of a-IFN, in patients with chronic immune thrombocytopenic purpura (ITP) who did not respond to conventional therapy; there were included 10 patients; 5 of them associated a chronic B or C hepatitis. The patients received IFN α-2b (3×10^6 U/m²/dose, sc., 3 times per week) for 6–18 months. We observed a good immediate response (increase of platelet count after 1 month of therapy) in 8 patients, followed by relapse after discontinuing IFN in 4 out of 7 responsive patients; 3 cases presented long-term remission; 2 out of 4 cases with chronic B hepatitis achieved seroconversion after 6–12 months of IFN.

In conclusion, α-IFN may be an alternative therapy in patients who did not respond to standard therapy. It may be beneficial especially in patients who associate a chronic hepatitis, attempting to achieve a long-term remission and the seroconversion at the same time.

Keywords: refractory immune thrombocytopenic purpura (ITP), treatment with IFN, child.

Introduction

Immune thrombocytopenic purpura (ITP) represents the most frequent hemorrhagic diathesis in childhood; up to 30% of patients are regarded as refractory to standard therapy and have a chronic evolution [1, 2]; 1% of them can present life-threatening hemorrhage mostly with intracranial origin [1].

Although its mechanism has not been well documented [4], α-interferon (IFN) was presented as a treatment with promising results for these patients [2, 3]; due to its immunomodulatory properties, α-IFN increases Th1 activity, modifies the citokines production (IL_2, IL_4, IL_{10}) and decreases the antiplatelet antibody production [4].

The objective of the study was to evaluate the effect of α-IFN in patients who did not respond to conventional therapy (corticosteroids) or to other treatments (iv immunoglobulins, danazol, cyclosporine).

I. Scharrer/W. Schramm (Ed.)
33rd Hemophilia Symposion Hamburg 2002
© Springer-Verlag Berlin Heidelberg 2004

Patients and Methods

This retrospective evaluation included 10 patients (13.69%) selected from the total cases (73 patients) with chronic ITP, treated in our clinic between 1990–2002: 9 cases with chronic ITP and 1 case with subacute ITP; 1 case was in stage I, 6 cases in stage II and 3 cases in stage III; there were 7 boys and 3 girls, aged between 5–13 years.

The *inclusion criteria* were: refractory ITP lasting more than 6–12 months (excepting 1 case, which had a history of 3 months), platelet (PLT) count ≤ 50 x 10^9/l in spite of conventional therapy: corticosteroids, immunoglobulins, danazol, cyclosporine (Table 1).

The *treatment schedule* was: IFN α-2b (3×10^6 U/m^2 per dose), subcutaneously, 3 times per week for a period of 6–18 months (excepting 1 new case, who underwent 2 months of therapy). *We assessed* the patients according to the clinical criteria and the PLT counts on the 28th day of therapy and then reevaluated them after 3, 6, 12 and 18 months (Table 2).

Table 1. Therapeutic modalities used before IFN

Therapeutic modalities	No. of patients
corticosteroids	10
iv immunoglobulins	7
danazol	7
cyclosporine	2

Table 2. Types of treatment response

Treatment response	Complete Remission /CR	Partial Remission /PR	Satisfactory response	Failure
Clinical criteria				
– petechiaes	–	–	±	+
– tourniquet test	–	±	+	+
– evident bleedings	–	–	±	+
Biological criteria	≥ 150	$\geq 100 < 150$	$\geq 50 < 100$	< 50
– PLT counts x 10^9/l				

Results

Considering the best response achieved by each patient, we registered different results:
1. 2 cases with complete response (PLT ≥ 150 x 10^9/l) and 1 case with partial response (PLT ≥ 100 x 10^9/l) throughout the treatment period (6–18 months), also followed by long-term remission (12–18 months); 1 case with complete response during IFN (2 months) and is continuing the treatment (Fig. 1);
2. 1 case with transient partial response (PLT ≥ 100 x 10^9/l) followed by relapse after discontinuing IFN;

PLT x 10^9/l

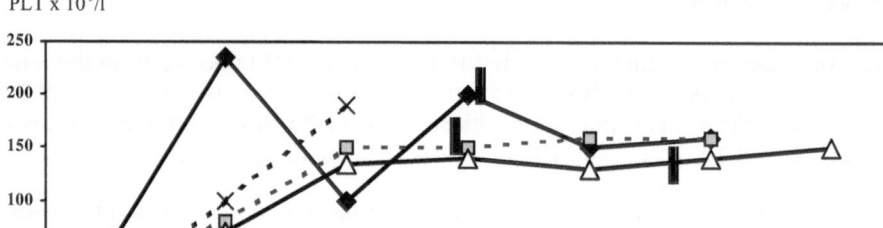

Fig. 1. 3 cases – CR/PR during IFN, followed by long-term remission (12–18 months) 1 case – CR for 2 months and is continuing the treatment

PLT x 10^9/l

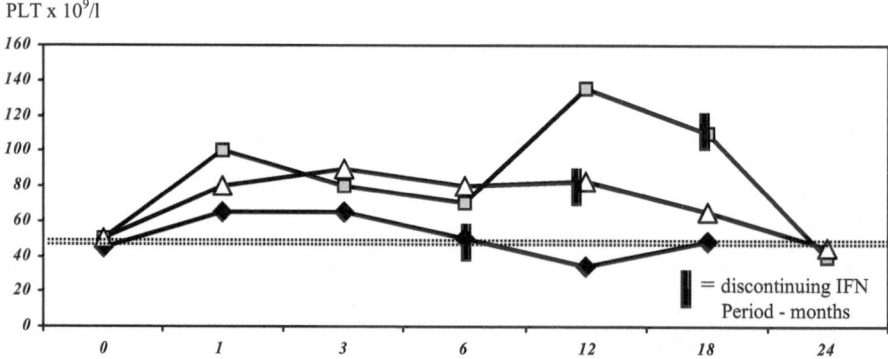

Fig. 2. 3 cases – satisfactory response during treatment, followed by relapse after discontinuing IFN

PLT x 10^9/l

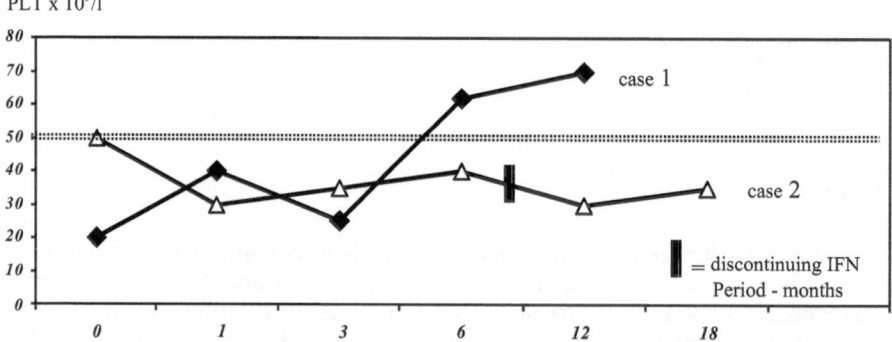

Fig. 3. case 1- belated satisfactory response (after 3 months) – is continuing the treatment; case 2- worsening thrombocytopenia

3. 3 cases with satisfactory response (PLT $\geq$ 50 x 10^9/l) during therapy, then subsequent decrease of PLT values (Fig. 2); 1 case with satisfactory response obtained later (after 6 months) and maintained due to the ongoing treatment (Fig. 3);
4. 1 case with worsening thrombocytopenia (Fig. 3). The median PLT count rose significantly after 1 month of IFN (p = 0,002), from 42 ± 12 x 10^9/l to 106 ± 53 x 10^9/l, in 8 patients. In these 8 responders, during the whole treatment period, the maximum PLT values achieved was 158 ± 47 x 10^9/l. In contrast with the good immediate results, relapse was noticed in 4 out of 7 patients after discontinuing IFN; 2 cases are continuing the treatment.

Four cases were associated with chronic B hepatitis and 1 case with chronic C hepatitis; 2 of those with B hepatitis achieved seroconversion after 6–12 months of IFN. The therapy was well tolerated; a mild to moderate flu-like syndrome was the only side-effect observed.

Discussions

IFN is generally not accepted as a common therapeutic indication for autoimmune diseases, because itself can induce thrombocytopenia as adverse effect [5]. Paradoxically, due to an insufficient elucidated mechanism [4] it may prove beneficial in refractory ITP, especially in children. The clinical trials mention that independent of the treatment schedule: 1 [6] or 3 administrations per week [2, 7], in a low -1.5 MIU [6], medium -3 MIU [2, 7] or high dose -5 MIU [1], there can be reached good results especially on a short and medium term; a significant rise of PLT count is achieved promptly after maximum 7–14 days of treatment [1].

Our experience was initiated by observing the favorable consequences of IFN in thrombocytopenia, in a patient who associated a hepatitis infection; the results obtained were similar with those presented in literature.

Conclusions

α-IFN may be an alternative therapy in patients who did not respond to conventional therapy; it can be used when immunosuppressive treatment or splenectomy are disconsidered or contraindicated.

IFN treatment may be beneficial especially in patients who associate a chronic hepatitis, attempting to achieve long-term remission and seroconversion at the same time.

The treatment is better tolerated in children than in adults; there were only minor side effects observed.

In spite of these good results obtained on our small cohort, especially on a short period of time, the role of IFN in the treatment of refractory ITP remains to be established and requires further studies.

References

1. Dikici B, Bosnak M, Kara IH et al.- Interferon-alpha therapy in idiopathic thrombocyto-penic purpura. *Pediatr Int*, 2001 Dec; 43 (6): 577–80
2. Dubbeld P, Hillen HF, Schouten HC- Interferon treatment of refractory idiopathic throm-bocytopenic purpura. *Eur J Haematol* 1994 Apr ; 52 (4): 233–5
3. Yesilipek MA, Yegin O- Interferon-alpha therapy for refractory idiopathic thrombocytope-nic purpura in children. *Turk J Pediatr*, 1997 Apr-Jun; 39 (2): 173–6
4. Crossley AR, Dickinson AM, Proctor SJ et al.- Effects of interferon-alpha therapy on immune parameters in immune thrombocytopenic purpura. *Autoimmunity* 1996; 24 (2): 81–100
5. Dourakis SP, Deutsch M, Hadziyannis SJ- Immune thrombocytopenia and alpha-inter-feron therapy. *J Hepatol* 1996 Dec; 25 (6): 972–5
6. Fujimura K, Takafuta T, Kuriya S, et al.- Recombinant human interferon α–2b therapy for steroid resistant idiopathic thrombocytopenic purpura. *Am. J. of Hematology*, 1998; 51: 37–44
7. Donato H, Kohan R, Picon A, et al.- Alpha-interferon therapy induces improvement of platelet counts in children with chronic idiopathic thrombocytopenic purpura. *J Pediatr Hematol Oncol*, 2001 Dec ; 23 (9): 598–603

Review on Bleeding Episodes in Hemophiliacs Receiving no Primary Prophylactic Replacement Therapy

C. A. Petrescu, M. Serban, C. Jinca, and P. Tepeneu

Introduction

Primary prophylactic replacement therapy, recommended by the WFH and EHC for hemophilia patients with severe disease, is not yet applied in our country. Furthermore, on demand therapy is frequently inadequate, both from the qualitative and quantitative point of view. Under these circumstances, bleeding episodes are very frequent and diverse, with a high risk of immediate and late complications and sequelae.

Objectives

The objective of the present study consists on the evaluation of the frequency, clinical aspects and associated risks and complications of different type of bleeding episodes, correlated with the severity of the disease and patient's age, in hemophiliacs receiving almost exclusively on demand treatment, with no primary prophylactic replacement therapy.

Material and Methods

The study was conducted on a cohort of 212 hemophilia patients from all over the country, treated in Hemophilia Center Timisoara between 1990–2000. The median follow-up period was 7.44 years. Almost half of the patients (43.87%) were diagnosed in the period of study. Hemophilia A was 5.6 times more frequent than hemophilia B. Severe forms represented about half of the cases (51.89%). The familial and sporadic forms were almost equally represented; this aspect is very important for the clinical practice. The age at admission varied between 1 month and 24 years.

Replacement therapy was administered almost exclusively on demand. »Classic« virally inactivated blood products (fresh frozen plasma – Pl, cryoprecipitate – Cr) were exclusively used before 1992. Factor concentrates (FC) were used beginning with 1992 (FVIII), respectively 1993 (FIX), and were almost exclusively administered for four years (1993–1996). After that period (1997–2000), Pl and/or Cr were mainly used in hemophilia A patients. More than half of the bleeding episodes (63.79%) were treated exclusively with Pl/Cr. The medium FVIII/ FIX consumption/patient/

I. Scharrer/W. Schramm (Ed.)
33rd Hemophilia Symposion Hamburg 2002
© Springer-Verlag Berlin Heidelberg 2004

year was 2.54 to 6.38 times smaller, in case of Pl/Cr administration, compared to FC; in those cases, the medium doses/administration were constantly lower than 20 IU/kg. Only a quarter (24.79%) of the registered bleeding episodes were treated exclusively with FC, the medium doses/patient/year being significantly lower, compared to those used in developed countries. FC were used mostly in case of dangerous bleedings (intracranial-IC, gastrointestinal – GI, intraperitoneal – IP, massive hematomas – HM, especially those of iliopsoas and retroperitoneal, internal organs HM, cervical, tongue, pharyngeal HM, etc.).

Results and Discussions

In the studied period, 1,964 bleeding episodes were registered, the majority in patients with severe hemophilia. The number of registered bleeding episodes was smaller than the real number; patients presenting mild, and often moderate bleedings, hemarthrose, epistaxis (HA, EPI) often didn't come for treatment. Especially for those patients coming from far-off zones, the registered number corresponds to that of severe bleedings. HA were the most frequent accidents (61.3% of patients, 50.4% of bleeding episodes), followed by HM and wound bleeding (Fig. 1).

About two thirds of the registered bleeding episodes were encountered in patients aged 3 to 17 years, most frequently in patients aged 10 to 13 years. HM were the

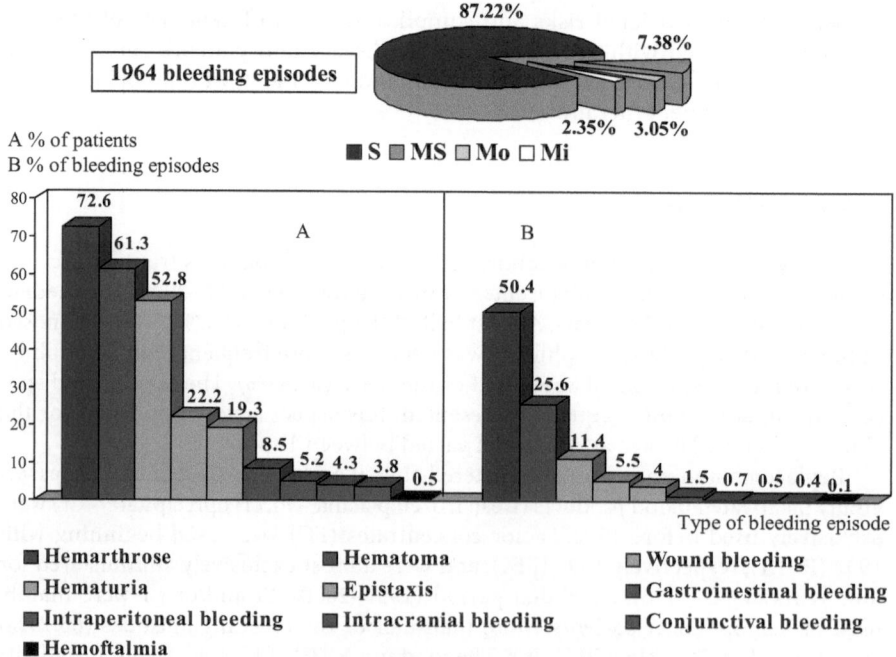

Fig. 1. The frequency and type of bleeding episodes in studied patients

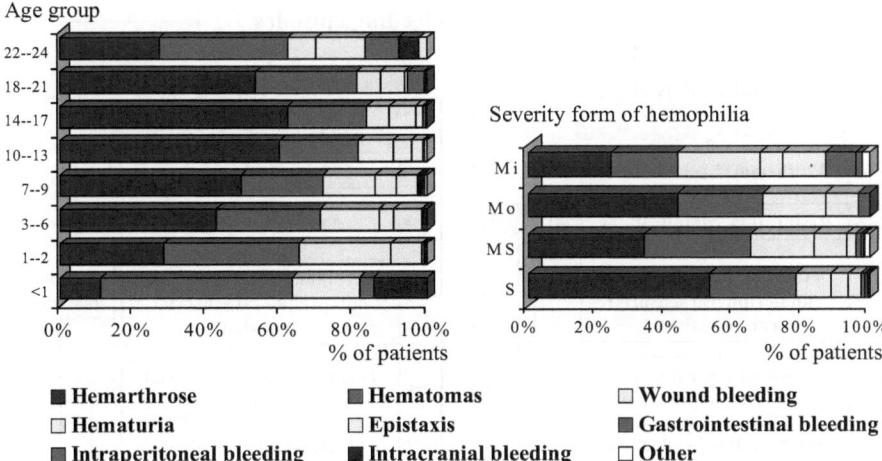

Fig. 2. The distribution of bleeding episodes in different age groups and severity forms of hemophilia

most frequent accidents in infants, usually occurring after intramuscular injection; bleedings from oral cavity (gums, tongue, lips, dental eruption, rupture of tongue or lips frenulum) were also very frequent; IC hemorrhage was the most frequent before the age of 1 year, when it usually appeared secondary to birth trauma. HA were the most characteristic bleeding events in patients aged 3 to 21 years. In older patients, HM occupied again the first place, represented mostly by iliopsoas HM. GI and IP bleedings were characteristic for older patients (Fig. 2). The great majority (87.22%) of the registered bleeding episodes were noted patients with severe hemophilia. HA were the most frequent accidents in all severity forms of hemophilia.

Bleeding episodes are sources of different complications, some of that life-threatening. Death may occur from severe anemia, respiratory distress or IC bleeding. Permanent damages resulting from bleedings create physic or neurosensorial handicaps. Psychological handicap may directly result from intracranial bleeding, or may be the consequence of the stress associated with repeated bleedings, pain, hospitalization, invalidity, social or familial problems (Fig. 3).

The aim of primary prophylaxis is to prevent bleedings, and thus, their immediate and late consequences. Inadequate replacement therapy in case of bleeding episodes (late administration, small doses, and short duration) is a favouring factor for the apparition of complications and sequelae.

Posthemorrhage anemia was the most frequent complication (23.98% of bleeding episodes, 51.88% of patients). Bacterial infections were encountered in more than a quarter of patients. Hematomas were responsible for the majority of immediate complications – more than one third of posthemorrhage anemia cases, 58.62% of hemorrhagic shock cases, including one death (rupture of a spleen hematoma), more than half of bacterial infections, the majority of blood cysts and all the respiratory and peripheral neurovascular complications (Fig. 4).

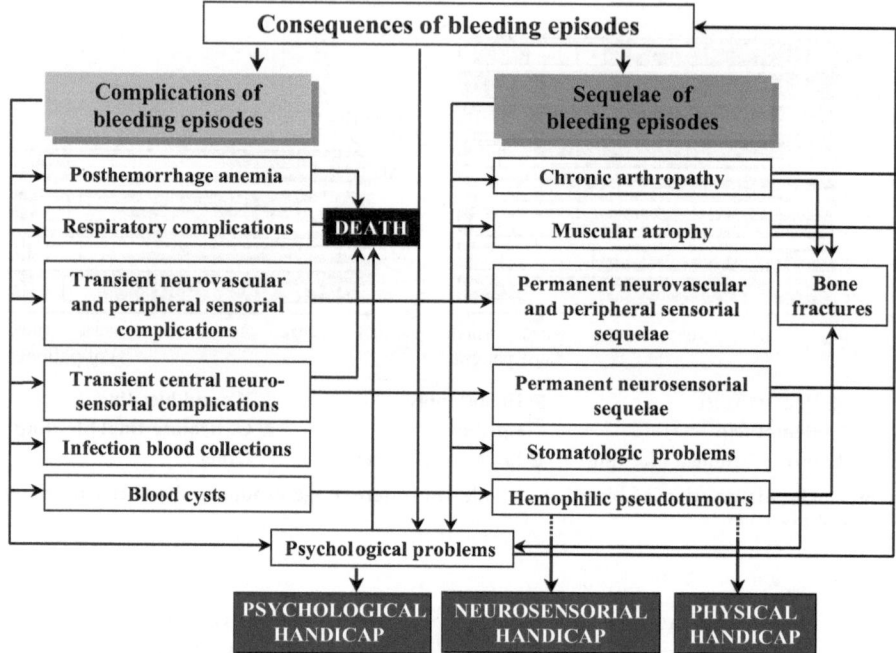

Fig. 3. The consequences of the bleeding episodes

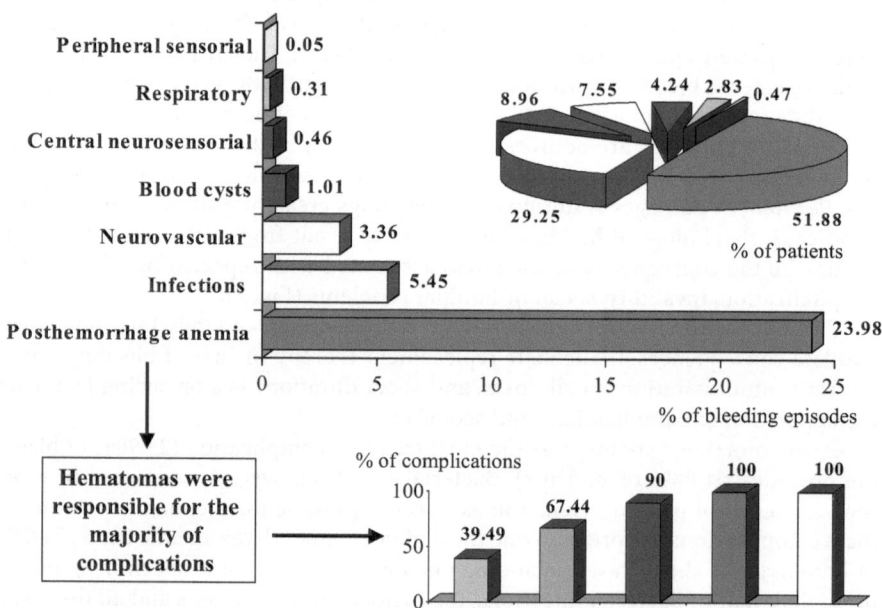

Fig. 4. The complications of bleeding episodes

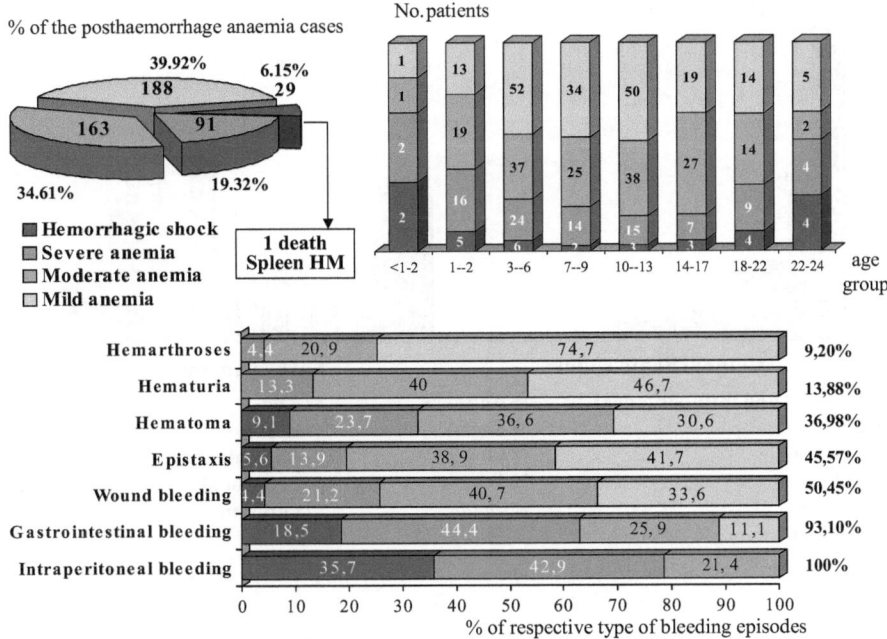

Fig. 5. The severity forms of posthemorrhage anemia, and their distribution in different age groups and type of bleeding episodes

Severe anemia appeared in 19.32% of bleeding episodes, and hemorrhagic shock, in 6.15% of cases. Posthemorrhage anemia complicated 78.34% of the bleedings in patients with severe hemophilia; severe anemia and posthemorrhagic shock were mostly encountered in these patients (86.21%, respectively 72.53% of the corresponding severity forms of anemia) (Fig. 5).

Severe anemia and hemorrhagic shock were more frequent in patients from the extreme age groups, infants (66.67% of the anemia cases), respectively patients older than 22 years (53.33% of the anemia cases). This aspect is explained by the high frequency of bleedings predisposing to the apparition of anemia; in infants, HM represented 51.85% of bleedings, the majority affecting important muscles (57.14% localised at buttocks and thights); in patients older than 22 years of age, HM (61.29% affecting the iliopsoas muscle), together with GI and IP bleedings, represented 49.44% of the bleeding episodes (Fig. 5).

Taking into account the associated risk of severe anemia and hemorrhagic shock, for different types of bleedings (Fig. 5), GI hemorrhages were the most dangerous isolated bleedings – determining severe anemia or hemorrhagic shock in 62.96% of the cases (Fig. 5). Infection with H.pylori was diagnosed in more than half of the patients with this type of bleeding (62.5%). In 29.41% of cases, no suggestive clinical symptoms were noted. The real frequency of H.pylori infection in hemophiliacs seems to be the same as in general populations, but the risk for GI hemorhage is higher [1, 3, 20]. IP bleeding was constantly associated with iliopsoas, retroperito-

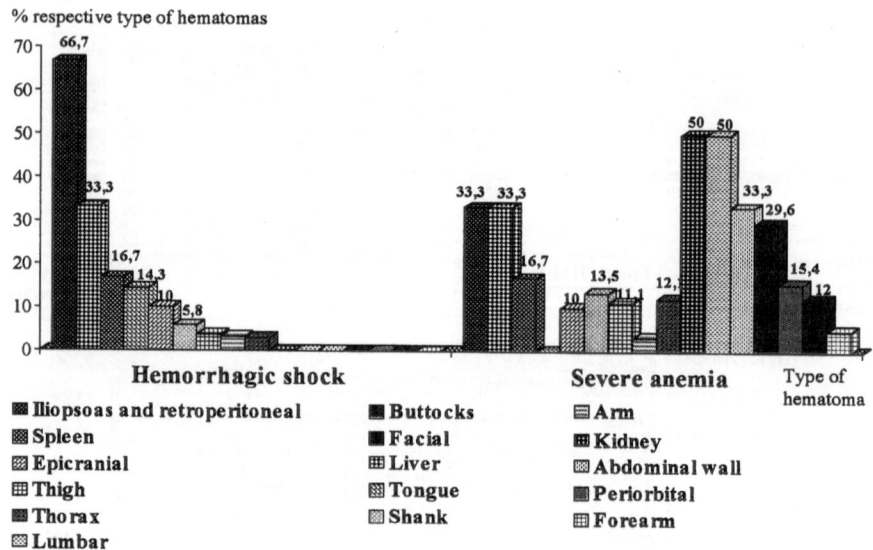

Fig. 6. Hemorrhagic shock and severe anemia in different type of hematomas

neal, or intraperitoneal organs HM. IP bleedings directly resulting from the rupture of liver or spleen HM appeared in young children, and were extremely severe (determining the death of a 5 years old patient); those produced indirectly, by the passing of blood from retroperitoneum, in case of iliopsoas or retroperitoneal HM, were moderate, and seen in older patients.

Internal organs and iliopsoas HM associated or not with IP bleeding were the most severe types of bleedings, from the point of view of severe anemia and hemorrhagic shock; other severe HM were localized in the abdominal wall, buttocks, thigh, and shank muscles (Fig. 6).

HM, the second most frequent bleeding episodes, were strongly characteristic for patients with severe hemophilia (86.28% of patients), having very diverse locations. HM of the extremities represented almost a half (45.92%) of the total. HM of the trunk, head and neck, were also frequent (Fig. 7). In infants, HM after muscular injections (usually vaccination) were characteristic (41.93 of HM). Before the age of 2 years, head and neck HM were the most frequent. The majority of epicranial HM (76.67%), and severe tongue, sublingual, and pharingeal HM (83.33%), appeared before the age of 6 years. In patients aged between 7–17 years, extremities and trunk HM appeared in 69.09% of cases. After 17 years, ilipsoas and retroperitoneal HM were the most frequent (42.59%) (Fig. 7).

Iliopsoas HM (Fig.8) had a high tendency to relapse and to cystic transformation, an otherwise known aspect for this type of bleedings [9, 10, 13].

Almost a half of the registered iliopsoas HM (64.10%) appeared in patients having this type of bleeding before; blood cyst formation was encountered in 30.77% of the patients with this type of HM (Fig. 9). Iliopsoas HM were sometimes misinterpreted as coxofemoral HA. The importance of prolonged secondary pro-

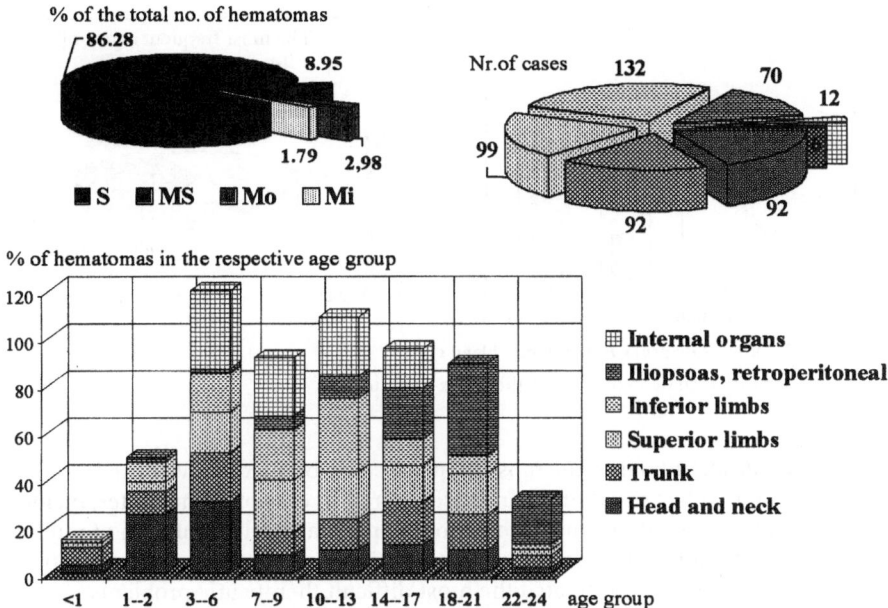

% of the total no. of hematomas

Fig. 7. The distribution of hematomas in different severity forms of hemophilia, and age groups

phylaxis after iliopsoas HM, until the complete resorption was clearly undelined [9, 10, 13]; it was also applied in the last five years in our patients, proving efficient. Cystic transformation was rarely encountered in other type of HM (epicranial, laterocervical, extremities). The formation of blood cysts, potentially severe complications of HM (risk of evolution to pseudotumours), was favoured by the unsufficient replacement therapy.

Bacterial infections of blood collections were the second complications in our patients (25% of patients, 5.94% of bleeding episodes). HM were most frequently infected (68.08% of cases), especially in young patients (53.13% in children aged under 7 years). Reported to the total number of registered HM, less than 10% were

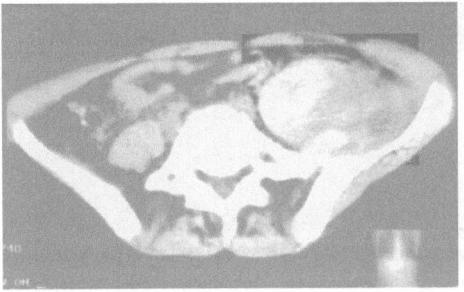
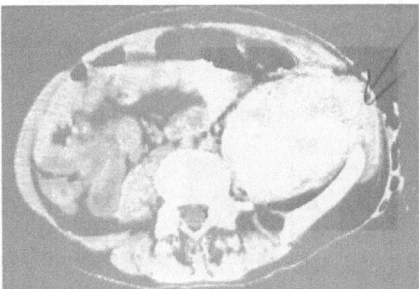

Fig. 8. Iliopsoas hematomas

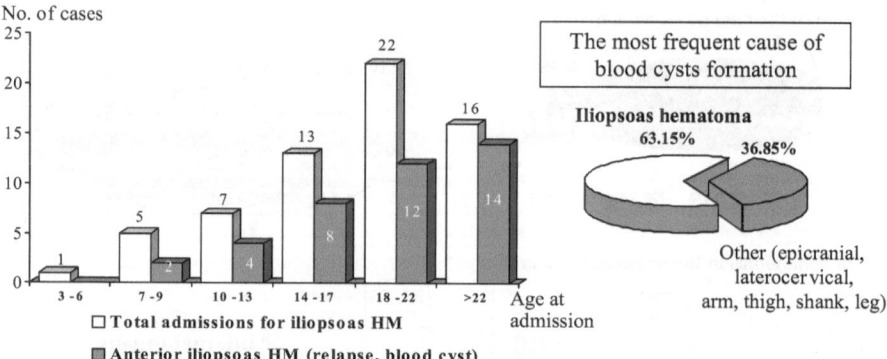

Fig. 9. The characteristic evolution of iliopsoas hematomas

infected (6.36%). In infants, the most frequent cause of infection was the intramuscular injection; other situations were encountered in case of animal bites, incidental or operatory wounds. Bacterial infections complicating the evolution of multiple distal pseudotumours (PT) seen consecutively, in a patient with severe hemophilia A and high inhibitor level, created the most difficult therapeutic problems.

The sequelae of bleeding episodes were very diverse (Fig. 10), resulting in different type of handicaps, sometimes transforming the patients in major invalids. Compared to the high risk for immediate complications, characteristic for HM, HA were responsible for the most frequent sequele – chronic arthropathy (ChA).

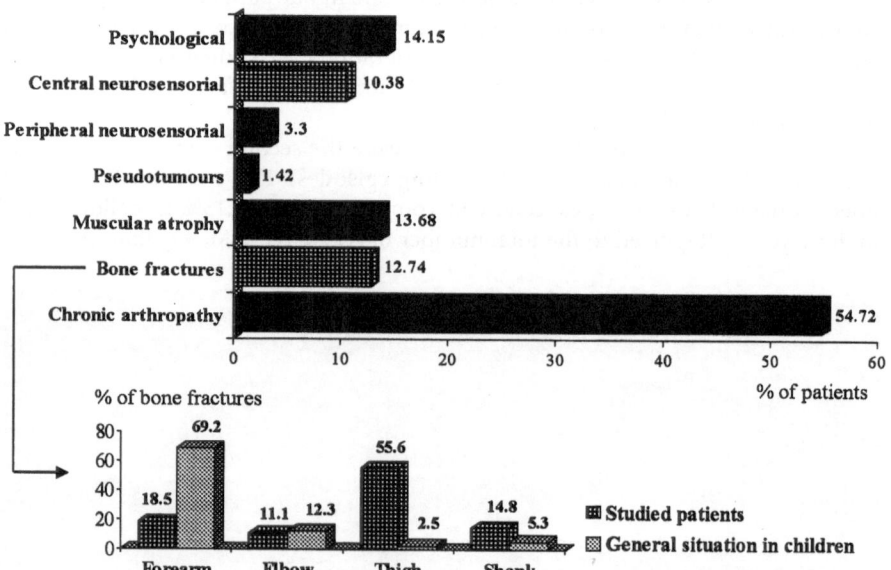

Fig. 10. The sequelae of bleeding episodes

Together with the muscular atrophy, ChA predisposed to bone fractures, having distinct features, compared to those generally seen in children; while forearms and elbows fractures usually represent more than 90% in children [5], in our patients thigh and shank fractures were 20 times, respectively 2.7 times more frequent (Fig. 10). Bone fractures determined more permanent sequelae in 29.62% of cases (angulation, coxa vara, permanent nerve paralysis, muscle retraction, diasthasis), usually because of the inadequate orthopedic treatment.

HA were the most frequent bleeding episodes, appearing in 91.82% of the patients with severe hemophilia, and 81.58% of those with moderate-severe disease; in these patients, HA appeared apparently spontaneous, affecting different joints. In patients with moderate or mild hemopilia, HA appeared in 50% in a single joint, usually after trauma, or associated with bone fractures. The number of registered HA was smaller than the real one, in many patients that didn't present for treatment in case of mild or moderate HA; the difficulties and costs of the travel, the prolonged hospitalization in case of the treatment with Pl and Cr, interfering with the parents' presence at jobs and childrens' presence at school, were some of the reasons for this aspect. HA appeared in patients as young 7 months of age; almost one eight of patients younger than 3 years had HA. Their frequency increased significantly until the age of 13 years. Knee HA were more than twice more frequent, than those of elbows and ankles. The frequency of HA declined with patients age, in contrast to that of ChA (Fig. 11). This aspect is explained by the progressive atrophy of the synovial membrane, in advanced ChA [14–16].

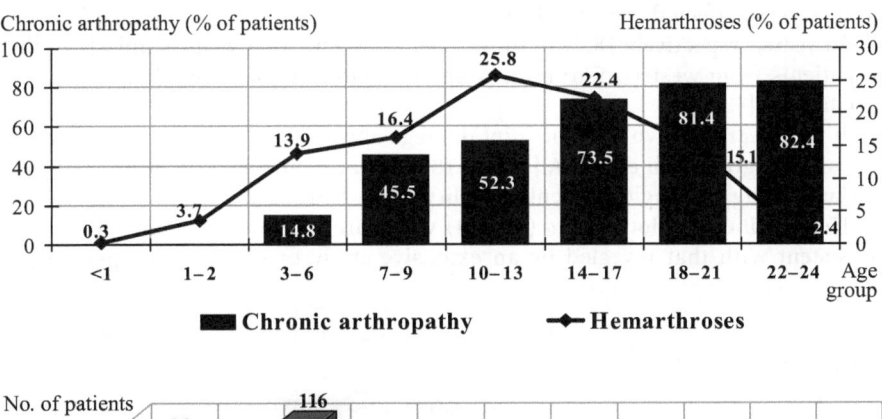

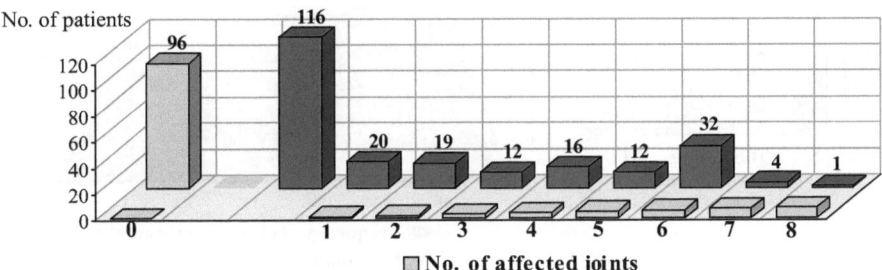

Fig. 11. Hemarthroses and chronic arthropathy

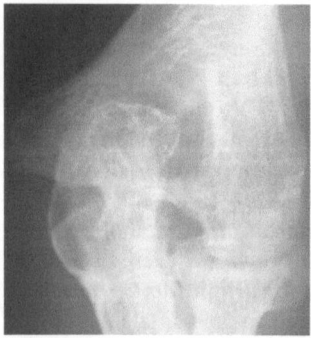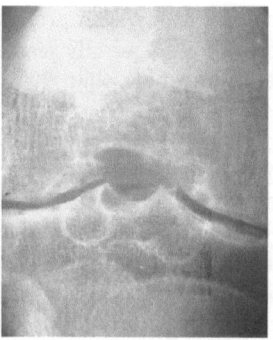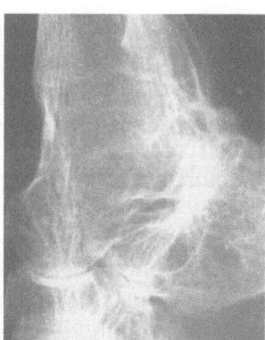

Fig. 12. Chronic arthropathy of elbow, knee, and ankle

The consequence of the impossibility to apply primary prophylaxis in our patients is best reflected by the high frequency of chronic arthropathy (Fig. 11, 13).

ChA (Fig. 12) appeared mostly in patients with severe and moderate-severe disease (Fig. 13). ChA was observed as early as in patients aged 3 to 7 years and progressively increased with age, so that more than half of our patients aged between 10–14 years, respectively more than three quarters of those aged more than 14 years had ChA (73.53–82.35%). The majority of patients (82.76%) had more than one affected joint, and almost half, more than four joints with ChA. Looking at the severity of ChA, appreciated using the WFH scoring system, the knees were again more severly affected. The total joint score was 12.77 for patients aged between 10–15 years, respectively 18.98 in those aged between 16–21 years, similarly to that of patients from western European countries before the introduction of primary prophylaxis [12].

It was clearly shown that the joint damage appear very early, after the first few HA, and progress with each HA [14–16, 18], the early introduction of primary prophylaxis being the single efficient modality to prevent the apparition of ChA.

Hemophilic pseudotumours (Fig. 14) were rare (1.42% of patients), an aspect consistent with that revealed by an extensive study over a 25 years period [9].

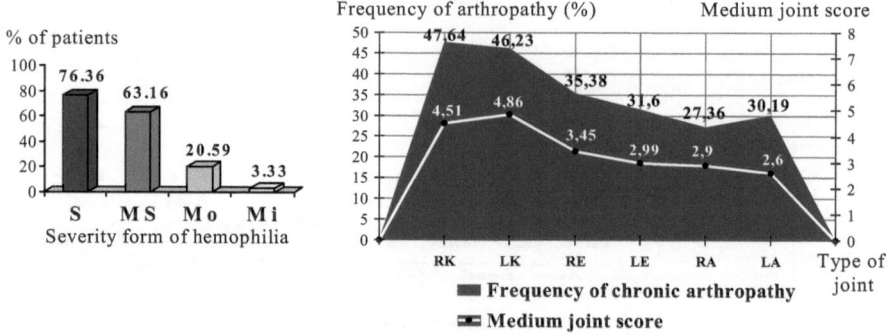

Fig. 13. The frequency and severity of chronic arthropathy

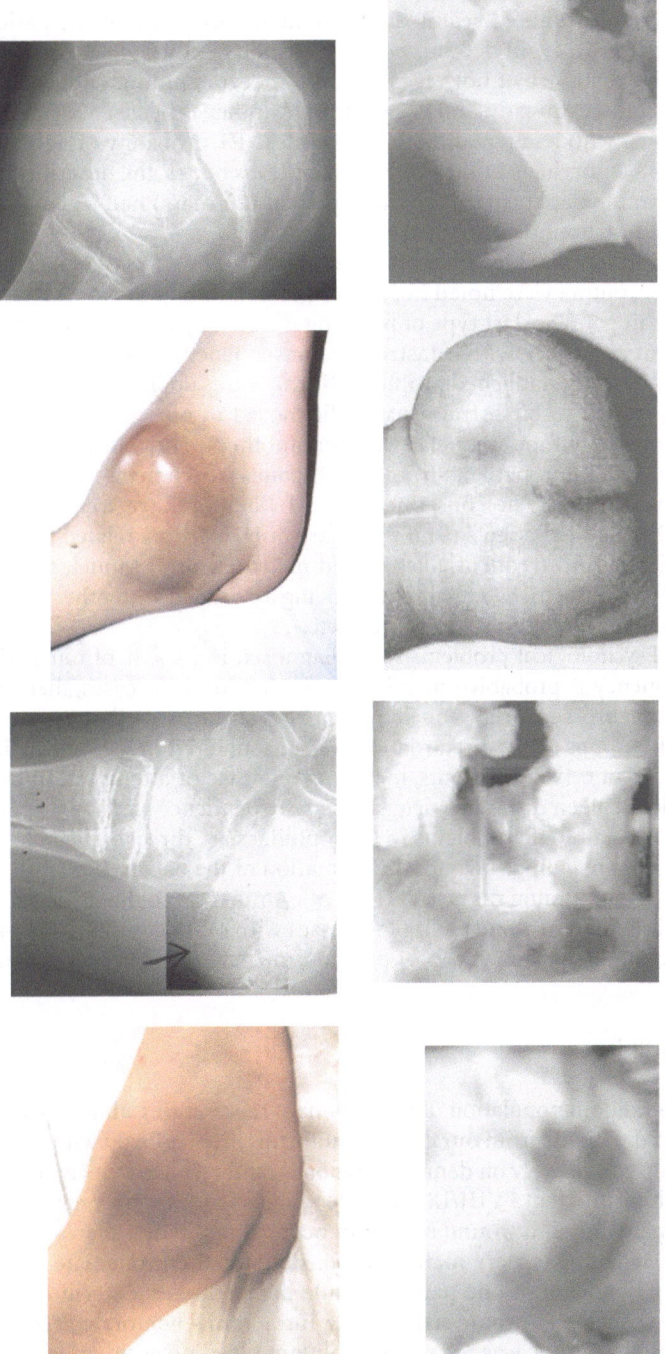

Fig. 14. Hemophilic pseudotumours of legs (A–D), mandible (E, F), and pelvis (G, H)

Nevertheless, we cannot ignore the fact that our study was conducted on children and adolescents; it seems quite probable that some of the patients with relapsed iliopsoas HM will develop pelvic PT in the next years. One patient had four consecutive distal PT of both legs and left knee, beginning with 8 years of age; this is a rare but yet already noted aspect [6]. Another rare case was seen in a five years old patient who had a mandible PT. All these PT probabily orriginated from subperiosteal hemorrhage in the growing spongious bones, the described characteristic type for young patients [13]. An older patient (20 years) had a giant pelvic PT with massive destruction of the iliac bone.

Intracranial bleedings (IC) were rare (8.49% of patients). IC bleeding related to birth trauma were noted in 3.3% of patients, being the most frequent (38.89% of IC bleedings). This last type of bleeding is noted by other authors to appear with a frequency of 1–4%, with catastrophic consequences [2, 4, 7, 8], and there are programmes of well established prophylactic measures applied in many countries. IC bleeding related to birth trauma was diagnosed in our service in a single patient, that recovered without sequelae with prompt therapeutic measures. The rest of the cases appeared all in patients from far-off zones where there is no specific assistance for hemophiliacs. The consequences of IC hemorrhage were extremely severe, with 72.22% of the patients (91.67% in case of IC bleeding related to birth trauma) having different and frequently associated neurosensorial sequelae. Epilepsy appeared in 76.92% of the cases, in half of that being associated with other severe troubles (hydrocephalus, hemiparesis, blindness, etc.).

Psychological problems were diagnosed in 14.15% of our patients but their real frequency is probably much higher; in 50% of these cases, there was an association with neuro-sensorial sequele, and in 20% of the cases, they appeared in patients with IC bleedings. Mental retardation was encountered in 4.2% of patients, emotion disorders in 6.1% of patients, including one case of attempted suicide. Behavioral disorders, spleen disorders, drug abuse or dependence were other noted problems.

Stomatologic problems in hemophiliacs are direcly related to the disease; repeated gum bleedings favour the formation of the bacterial plaque and the apparition of the parodontal disease [11, 17, 19]. Almost three thirds of our patients (70.28%) had cavities, in almost half of the cases with other complications. Dental extractions were necessary in 29.72% of patients, in 64.39% of cases of permanent teeth.

Conclusions

In a random population of hemophiliacs representing almost one quarter of the registered patients from our country, at the moment, mostly with severe disease, treated almost exclusively on demand, preponderantly with plasma and cryoprecipitate, often with insufficient FVIII/IX dose, bleeding episodes were very diverse, hemarthroses, hematomas, and wound bleedings occupying the first places.

Hematomas were mainly responsible for the immediate complications, (including the death of one patient), while hemarthroses determined the most frequent late sequelae – chronic arthropathy. Intracranial hemorrhage, especially that related to birth trauma, was the most invalidant bleeding accident.

The high frequency, extreme diversity, severe immediate and late risks of the bleeding episodes, beginning with the moment of birth and persistent until older age, are evident and strong arguments used in our intensive effort of initiating primary prophylactic replacement therapy in hemophiliacs from our country.

References

1. Arai M: Gastrointestinal bleeding in hemophilic patients. Haemph Forum, Discussion Forum Topic 06.2000
2. Berry E: Intracranial hemorrhage in the hemophilic neonate – the case for prophylaxis. Haemoph Forum, Discussion Forum Topics, 06.1999
3. Braden B, Wenke A, Karich HJ et al: Risk of gastrointestinal bleeding associated with Helicobacter pylori infection in patients with hemophilia or von Willebrand's syndrome. Helicobacter (USA) 3 (3):184, 1998
4. Bray GL, Luban NLC: Hemophilia presenting with intracranial hemorrhage. Am J Dis Child 141: 1215, 1987
5. Cristu-Ionescu L: Fractures of dyaphiseal bones in children. Bucuresti: Ed. Medicala, 1988
6. Heim M, Horoszovski H, Schulman S et al: Multifocal pseudotumor in a single limb. Haemophilia 3:50, 1997
7. Kulkarni R, Lusher J, Henry RC: A review of cranial hemorrhages in neonatal hemophilia. Haemophilia 4:172, 1998
8. Kulkarni R, Lusher JM: Intracranial and extracranial hemorrhages in newborns with hemophilia: A review of the literature. J Pediatr Hem Oncology 21:289, 1999
9. Magallon M, Monteagudo J, Altisent A et al: Hemophilic pseudotumor: multicenter experience over a 25 year period. Am J Hematol 45:103, 1994
10. Martinowitz U: Pseudotumor surgery in hemophilia patients. Haemoph Forum, Discussion Forum Topic, 03.1999
11. Onisei D, Serban M: Control of the bacterial plaque in children with hemophilia. Timisoara Medicala vol.XL, 1–2: 62, 1995
12. Nilsson IM, Hemophilia. Stockholm: Pharmacia, 1994.
13. Rodriguez-Merchan EC: The hemophilic pseudotumour. Haemoph Forum, Discussion Forum Topic, 06.2001
14. Rosendaal G, Vianen ME, van den Berg HM et al: Cartilage damage as a result of hemarthrosis in a human in vitro model. J Rheumatol 24:1350, 1997
15. Rosendaal G, Vianen ME, Marx JJM et al: Blood-induced joint damage: a human in vitro study. Arthritis Rheum 42:1025, 1999
16. Rosendaal G, van den Berg HM, Lafeber FPJG et al: Pathologie der Synovitis und hämophilen Arthropathie. Der Orthopäde 28:323, 1999
17. Socransky SS, Haffajee AD: Effect of therapy on periodontal infections. J Periodontol 64:8, 1993.
18. Tekoppele JM, Vianen ME et al: Articular cartilage is more susceptible to blood-induced damage in young than in old age. In Scharrer I, Schramm W: 30th Hemophilia Symposium Hamburg 1999. Berlin Heidelberg: Springer Verlag, 2000: 182
19. Voigt I, Wendisch J, Weissbach G: Komplexe zahnärztliche Betreuung von Kindern und Jugendlichen mit Blutgerinnungsstörungen. In Scharrer I, Schramm W: 23. Hämophilie-Symposion, Hamburg 1992. Berlin Heidelberg: Springer-Verlag, 1993:119.
20. Von Depka Prondzinski M, Wenke A, Braaden A, Scharrer I: Prävalenz und klinische Relevanz von Helicobacter pylori-Infektionen bei Patienten mit Gerinnungsstörungen. In: Scharrer I, Schramm W: 25. Hämophilie-Symposion Hamburg 1994. Berlin Heidelberg: Springer-Verlag, 1994:338

Endogenous Thrombin Potential and Thrombin Activatable Fibrinolysis Inhibitor in Patients with Hemophilia and von-Willebrand disease

U. Scholz, A. Siegemund, T. Siegemund, S. Petros, and L. Engelmann

Introduction

Hereditary hemophilia and von-Willebrand disease (vWD) represent the majority of the inherited bleeding disorders. The severity of bleeding symptoms is generally dependent on the degree of coagulation factor deficiency, although clinical experience shows that this is not the sole determinant.

Thrombin generation plays a central role in hemostasis. After initiation of coagulation by the factor VIIa-tissue factor complex, activated factor IX forms together with its cofactor, factor VIII, a tenase complex on the surface of activated platelets. This complex catalyzes the activation of factor X that is part of the prothrombinase complex involved in the generation of large amounts of thrombin. The ensuing thrombin burst is essential for the formation of a stable fibrin clot. Thrombin further amplifies its own generation by activating factor XI [1] and increasing the levels of activated factors V and VIII [2, 3]. The defect in hemophilia is thus mainly the deficiency in the tenase complex, which results in a deficiency in the intrinsic thrombin generation.

The von-Willebrand-factor (vWF) is known to have three functions: it serves as an adhesive ligand for platelets, thereby involved in their activation; it transports and stabilizes factor VIII; and it is also involved in the development of platelet procoagulant activity. Therefore, vWF is a factor that is also required for normal thrombin generation [4]. The influence of platelets on thrombin generation has been shown by studying the inhibitory effect of antiplatelet therapy on thrombin generation [5–7]. Reduced or inhibited thrombin production results in reduction in platelet contractile force, thus structurally weaker clot formation [8].

Besides formation of a fibrin clot, thrombin also prevents clot lysis via activation of the thrombin activatable fibrinolysis inhibitor (TAFI). TAFI is a carboxypeptidase B like proenzyme that is produced in the liver. Activation of TAFI is mediated via the factor XI dependent thrombin generation. After activation, TAFI inhibits fibrinolysis by removing carboxy-terminal lysine residues from fibrin that play a role in plasminogen binding and activation. The thrombin burst and TAFI activation protect the clot against premature lysis.

Plasma concentration of TAFI is stable and it does not show any circadian rhythm. Elevated levels are found in patients with venous thrombosis and in pregnancy, while disseminated intravascular coagulation is associated with reduced plasma concentrations of TAFI. In hemophilia, both normal and low levels of TAFI have

I. Scharrer/W. Schramm (Ed.)
33rd Hemophilia Symposion Hamburg 2002
© Springer-Verlag Berlin Heidelberg 2004

been reported [9–11]. In the present study, ETP in platelet poor plasma (ETP-PPP) and plasma TAFI concentrations were measured in patients with hemophilia A and B as well as vWD, and their interrelationship discussed.

Materials and Methods

74 adult patients with hemophilia A, 19 with hemophilia B, and 36 with vWD type 2 and 3 were included in the study. The control group comprised 232 healthy subjects.

In the patient population, blood samples were drawn under clinically stable condition (i.e. no current bleeding or any sign of acute infection). Repeated blood samples were also taken 30 minutes after a corresponding factor substitution that was necessary for elective procedures, which were mainly dental extractions or intraarticular injections. Thus, a total of 116, 49, and 42 samples were available in the group of hemophilia A and B, as well as vWD, respectively.

Factor VIII (FVIII) and factor IX (FIX) were measured with a one-stage assay. A turbidimetric assay (Dade Behring, Marburg) was used to measure the ristocetin cofactor (RCof) activity.

ETP-PPP was measured as described by Hemker and coworkers [12, 13] using an automated coagulation analyzer. In short, citrate blood was double centrifuged at 2860 g (each time for 20 minutes). 65 µl PPP was incubated with 15 µl clot inhibitor (Pefabloc FG, Pentapharm, Basel). The measurement lasted 20 minutes. Methyl sulfonylethyl oxycarbonyl-Val-Arg-pNA at a concentration of 860 µM was added as a substrate. ETP was given as arbitrary units (AU) and this corresponds to the area under the thrombin formation curve after subtracting the contribution by α2-macroglobulin.

Total TAFI antigen was measured with Coalize TAFI (Chromogenix), which is an ELISA technique. Coalize TAFI was used as a standard calibration substance.

The t test was applied for comparative parameters. Data are given as mean ± SD. A p value of < 0.05 was considered statistically significant.

Results

Table 1 shows ETP results at various concentrations of coagulation factors (RCof in vWD). A statistically significant difference was found only between controls and hemophilia B with a FIX activity < 10%.

When comparing ETP among the subgroups of patients, a significant difference was found in hemophilia B and vWD for FIX and RCof <10% vs. > 30%. No difference was found among subgroups of patients with hemophilia A.

Mean plasma TAFI concentration was significantly lower in hemophilia B for FIX concentrations <10% and 10–30% compared to controls, hemophilia A and vWD.

A positive correlation between ETP and TAFI was observed for hemophilia B (Fig. 1) but not for hemophilia A and vWD.

Fig. 2 shows that substitution with a FIX concentrate in a patient with hemophilia B resulted in an increase in ETP but no significant change in TAFI.

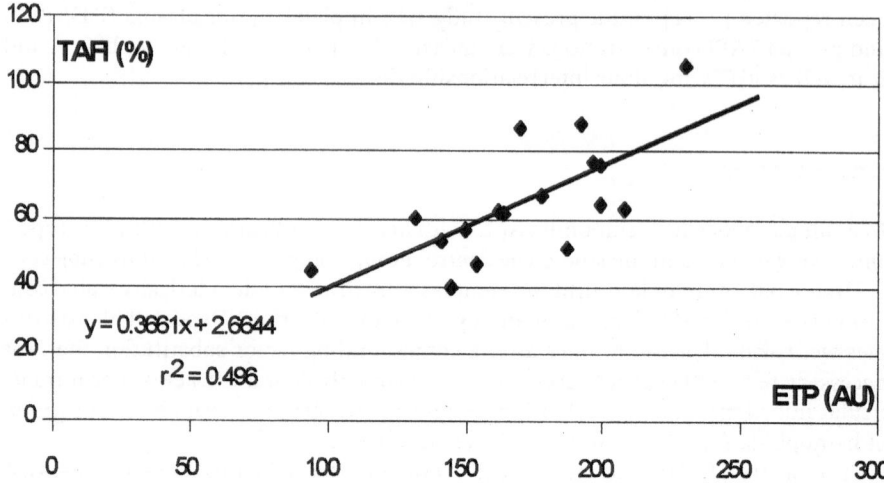

Fig. 1. Correlation between ETP and TAFI in hemophilia B.

Table 1. ETP-PPP and TAFI in hemophilia A and B and vWD at various concentrations of coagulation factors and in controls

Group	factor activity (%)	N	ETP (AU)	TAFI (%)
hemophilia A	<10	54	181.9 ± 39.9	71,5 ± 30,5
	10–30	24	178.9 ± 33.1	57,1 ± 16,1
	> 30	38	194.4 ± 56.8	61,3 ± 40,1
hemophilia B	< 10	20	166.8 ± 33.1	48,7 ± 21,3
	10–30	12	177.6 ± 35.9	52,6 ± 13,1
	> 30	17	206.7 ± 34.9	62,4 ± 27,1
vWd	< 10	8	180.2 ± 25.1	69,5 ± 17,8
	10–30	17	203.3 ± 36.8	74,1 ± 33,4
	> 30	17	206.7 ± 23.5	72,7 ± 26,1
controls		232	191.9 ± 28.8	85,6 ± 9,2

Discussion

Defective intrinsic thrombin generation as a result of deficiency in tenase complex is considered to be the main cause of bleeding in hemophilia A and B. Although the defect is complex, deficiency in thrombin generation also plays an important role in vWD.

Thrombin burst is essential for formation of a stable fibrin clot. Additionally, thrombin prevents premature clot lysis through activation of TAFI by the thrombin-dependent factor XI activation. Thrombin thus forms the fibrin clot and protects it as well.

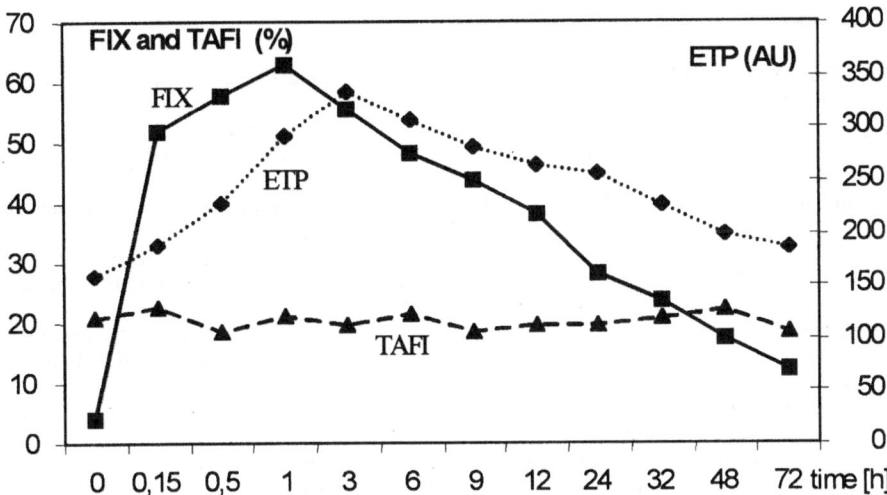

Fig. 2. Course of ETP and TAFI in a patient with hemophilia B after substitution with a factor IX concentrate.

In this study, a significant decrease in thrombin generation was found in patients with hemophilia B and vWD at <10% FIX and RCof, respectively. A clear difference at the concentrations investigated was not observed for hemophilia A. In general, patients with a residual factor activity of at least 10% seem to have normal thrombin generation.

Plasma concentration of TAFI antigen is reduced in patients with hemophilia and vWD; however, a significant reduction was found only in hemophilia B. Additionally, we have found a positive correlation between ETP and TAFI levels for hemophilia B in non-substituted state, but not for hemophilia A and vWD. The clinical significance of this finding is not clear. Mosnier et al. [11] reported that clot lysis time, which is a function of TAFI, is normal at FVIII concentrations >1%. They did not find any correlation between TAFI levels and bleeding complications in hemophilia A. As demonstrated in figure 2 we did not observe any significant change in plasma TAFI concentrations after substitution with a factor IX concentrate, although ETP was markedly increased. It could be argued that measurement of activated TAFI (TAFIa) may have been helpful in such a study. However, hitherto data did not clearly support this assumption, at least in hemophilia A [10].

In conclusion, we observed reduced thrombin generation in patients with hemophilia and vWD, and its extent varies depending on the type and degree of coagulation factor deficiency. Reduced ETP is associated with a reduction in TAFI. However, a defective inhibition of fibrinolysis could not be explained by plasma levels of TAFI antigen only.

References

1. Gilani D, Broze GJ Jr. Factor XI activation in a revised model of blood coagulation. Science 1991; 253: 909–12
2. Pieters J, Lindhout T, Hemker HC. In situ-generated thrombin is the only enzyme that effectively activates factor VIII and factor V in thromboplastin-activated plasma. Blood 1989; 74: 1021–4.
3. Butenas S, van`t Veer C, Mann KG. Evaluation of the initiation phase of blood coagulation using ultrasensitive assays for serine proteases. J Biol Chem 1997; 272: 21527–33
4. Keularts IM, Hamulyak K, Hemker HC, Béguin S. The effect of DDAVP infusion on thrombin generation in platelet-rich plasma of von-Willebrand type 1 and in mild haemophilia A patients. Thromb Haemost 2000; 84: 638–42
5. Keularts IM, Béguin S, de Zwaan C, Hemker HC. Treatment with GPIIb/IIIa antagonist inhibits thrombin generation in platelet rich plasma from patients. Thromb Haemost 1998; 80: 370–1
6. Hérault JP, Dol F, Gaich C, Bernat A, Herbert JM. Effect of clopidogrel on thrombin generation in platelet-rich plasma in the rat. Thromb Haemost 1999; 81: 957–60
7. Wegert W, Graff J, Kaiser D, Breddin HK, Klinkhardt U, Harder S. Effects of antiplatelet agents on platelet-induced thrombin generation. Int J Clin Pharmacol Ther 2002; 40: 135–41
8. Carr ME Jr, Martin EJ, Carr SL. Delayed, reduced or inhibited thrombin production reduces platelet contractile force and results in weaker clot formation. Blood Coagul Fibrinolysis 2002; 13: 193–7
9. Antovic J, Schulman S, Eelde A, Blomback M. Total thrombin-activatable fibrinolysis inhibitor (TAFI) antigen and pro-TAFI in patients with haemophilia A. Haemophilia 2001; 7: 557–560
10. Guo X, Okada N, Okada H. CPR – total (TAFI and activated TAFI) levels in plasma/serum of hemophiliacs. Microbiol Immunol 2000; 44: 77–78
11. Mosnier LO, Lisman T, van den Berg HM, Nieuwenhuis HK, Meijers JC, Bouma BN. The defective down regulation of fibrinolysis in hemophilia A can be restored by increasing the TAFI plasma concentration. Thromb Haemost 2001; 86: 1035–1039
12. Hemker HC, Wielders S, Kessels H, Béguin S. Continuous registration of thrombin generation in plasma, its use for the determination of the thrombin potential. Thromb Haemost 1993; 71: 617–24
13. Wielders S, Mukherjee M, Michiels J, Rijkers DT, Cambus JP, Knebel RW, Kakkar V, Hemker HC, Béguin S. The routine determination of the endogenous thrombin potential, first results in different forms of hyper- and hypocoagulability. Thromb Haemost 1997; 77: 629–636.

VIIc. Thrombophilic Disorders

Different Thrombotic Risk Factors – Contribution to the Endogenous Thrombin Potential

A. Siegemund, T. Siegemund, U. Scholz, S.Petros, and L. Engelmann

Background

Hemker [1] described the area under the thrombin generation curve as endogenous thrombin potential (ETP). He has shown that the ETP is suitable to express the hyper-coagulability of the plasma and an alternative way to control the therapy with anti-coagulants. The area under the thrombin generation curve is lowered under heparin, oral anticoagulants and also under hirudine. The well known prothrombin fragments F_{1+2} are parameters measuring the conversion from prothrombin to thrombin, but the ETP measures the development and the conversion of thrombin (capacity of the plasma to generate thrombin) and reflects direct the amount of circulating thrombin. Therefore measuring the ETP is a method for the global description of all components which are involved in the activation and inactivation of thrombin [2, 3]. Because of this underlying mechanism the ETP is increased in all cases of hyper-coagulability, in all cases of hypocoagulability this parameter is decreased.

Patients

In 563 patients from the University Hospital of Leipzig with objectively confirmed thrombosis we measured the following risk factors: PC-resistance (in cases of lowered ratio F V Leiden), prothrombin level and prothrombin mutation 20210 GA, the coagulation factors VIII:C, IX and XI, protein C and protein S and antithrombin (AT). Elevated levels of the coagulation factors were defined analogous to the Leiden Thrombophilia Study (LETS) [4, 5] with F II >115%, F VIII:C >150% [6], F IX >129% and F XI >123%. Protein C/S-deficiency was assumed if protein C-levels under 70% and protein S <60%. Hyperhomocysteinemia in our investigations are levels above 18 µmol/l. All patients with prothrombin time <70% were excluded and also patients with AT deficiency (because of the limited number of patients with hereditary defects).

Methods

The coagulation factors (II, VIII:C, IX, XI) were measured at the BCS (Dade Behring) with the corresponding deficient plasma, Thromborel R resp. Pathromtin SL, pro-

I. Scharrer/W. Schramm (Ed.)
33rd Hemophilia Symposion Hamburg 2002
© Springer-Verlag Berlin Heidelberg 2004

tein C as chromogenic method with Berichrom Protein C (all reagents from Dade Behring); protein S as free protein S and/or protein S clotting (Diagnostica Stago Asniere, France), homocysteine with HPLC (fluorometric detection, Spectra Physics); ETP as described by Hemker[2] with Pefabloc FG (Pentapharm Basel, Switzerland) as clot inhibitor, methyl-sulfonyl-ethyl-carbonyl-Val-Arg-pNA as substrate with a final concentration of 860 μmol/l. The ETP is expressed in AU (arbitrary units) and represents the area under the curve. The reference values were obtained from healthy blood donors. The vein punction was separately before blood donation.

Results

There exists a strong correlation between the number of thrombotic risk factors and the amount of generated thrombin (Fig.1). One risk factor alone is associated with a normal ETP, but two risk factors or more lead to an increase of ETP. This statistically significant difference was observed in all groups with more than one risk factor, whereby an additional risk factor contributes to an ETP-increase of about 5%. Four risk factors elevate the thrombin-forming capacity by nearly 20% (Table 1).

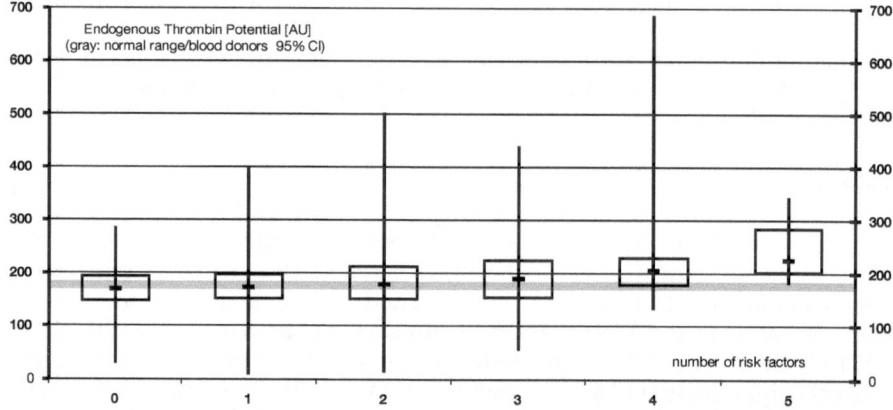

Fig. 1. Endogenous thrombin potential and the number of thrombotic risk factors

Table. 1. Endogenous thrombin potential [AU] and the number of thrombogenic risk factors

	number of thrombogenic risk factors				
	0	1	2	3	4
number of patients	271	250	184	79	42
mean	168,4	173,2	179,0	192,3	219,0
median	170,4	174,2	179,4	190,5	205,6
95% CI	163,6–173,0	167,0–179,6	170,5–187,3	178,5–206,1	193,4–244,8
p		0,037	<0,001	<0,001	0,002

Table 2. Endogenous thrombin potential [AU] and the different thrombotic risk factors

		mean	SD	N	95% CI
controls		176,9	29,4	98	171,1–182,7
factor II	<115%	163,2	49,2	930	160,0–166,4
	>115%	185,3	55,2	389	179,8–190,8
factor VIII:C	<159%	171,1	48,1	798	167,8–174,4
	>159%	171,0	57,0	473	165,9–176,1
factor IX	<129%	165,7	45,2	864	162,7–168,7
	>129%	177,8	58,4	508	172,7–182,6
factor XI	<123%	167,1	48,1	1060	164,2–170,0
	>123%	181,5	57,7	310	175,1–188,1

Our investigations have shown furthermore that not all thrombogenic risk factors contribute in the same manner to the ETP. We found out the following sequence (beginning with the highest contribution to the ETP): AT deficiency (not represented) and prothrombin allel 20210 GA, F II >115%, F IX >123%, F XI >129%. The differences between the investigated groups show a statistically significance (for example F II <115% vs. F II >115% p=0.002, F IX <129% vs F IX >129% p=0.002) or a borderline significance (F XI <123% vs. F XI >123% p=0.085, Table 2).

There is a simultaneous increase in ETP with higher levels of coagulation factors indicating a continuous dose-response relation between ETP (for instance F XI, Fig. 2). Elevated levels of F VIII: C and in contrast to other published data [7] F V-Leiden do not influence the ETP. On the contrary the simultaneous occurrence of F V-Leiden and prothrombin allel 20210 GA decrease the ETP. This is surprising, but with statistic significance (Fig. 3). The ETP-reduction is about 16%. Protein C/S-deficiency and hyperhomocysteinemia are also responsible for an ETP increase.

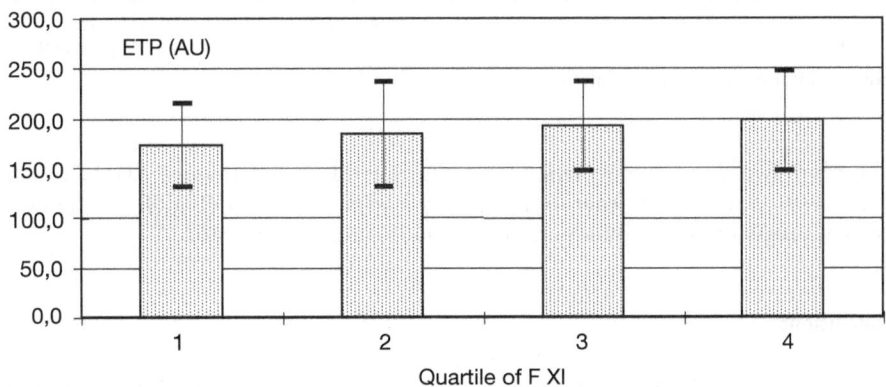

Fig. 2. ETP as function of F XI levels in patients with venous thrombosis (SD)

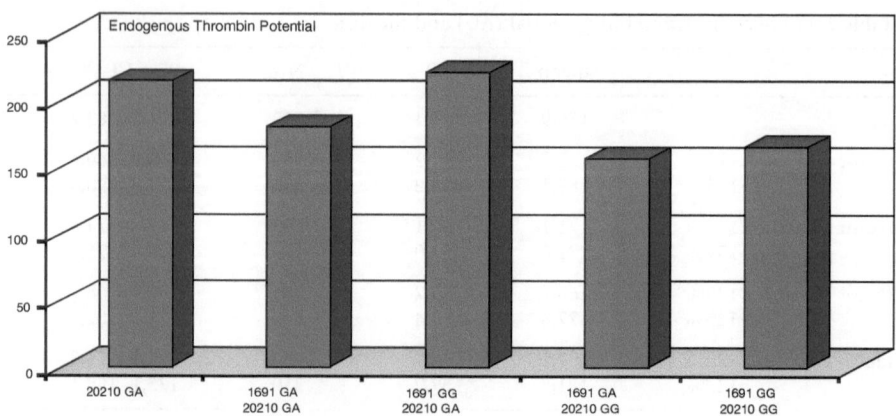

Fig. 3. ETP influenced by F V-Leiden and prothrombin allel 20210 GA

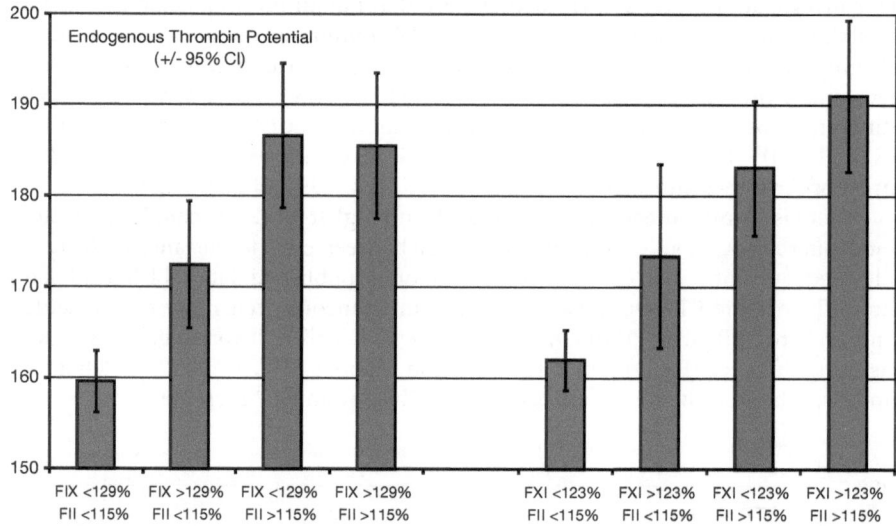

Fig. 4. ETP influenced by coagulation factor activity

In cases of two elevated coagulation factors (F II and F IX or F II and F XI) the rise in the measured thrombin generation capacity is especially clear (Fig.4). The highest value we register in the combination F II >115% and F XI >123%.

Conclusions

Several components of the coagulation cascade influence the thrombin generation capacity in different proportions. Patients with prothrombin allel 20210 GA and elevated levels of F II lie at the summit. In the same region the AT-deficiency is located. The proenzyme of the serine protease thrombin and the lack of its important inhibitor AT are responsible for the activation of the coagulation system. Because of the central role of the thrombin in the coagulation cascade this effect is clear. F IX and F XI also lead to a higher thrombin generation capacity. From the literature [8] and the now discussed cell-based model of blood coagulation [9] it is known that F XI gives a contribution to the secondary thrombin generation. The close relation between F XI levels and thrombin generation illustrates the renewed role of F XI in the coagulation cascade. Corresponding to the results of the LETS (Leiden Thrombophilia Study) elevated levels of this coagulation factors are thrombogenic. Our data emphasize these results and also the fact that only more than one risk factor are important for the thrombotic risk (LETS) [10].

There are further investigations necessary to explain the comparable thrombin generation capacity of patients with AT deficiency and prothrombin allel. The thrombin generation is in the same region, the thrombotic risk of such patients is different.

F V-Leiden does not influence the thrombin generation or reduce the thrombin generation of patients with prothrombin allel 20210 GA. Our thrombin generation test based on the combined activation (PT and aPTT based) of the coagulation cascade. A new aspect is changing concentration of activator substances in our test system.

Despite of all open questions the thrombin generation should be included in thrombophilia screening programs to recognize patients with hypercoagulability.

References

1. Hemker HC, Wielders S, Kessels H, Béguin S. Continuous registration of thrombin generation in plasma, its use for the determination of the thrombin potential. Thromb Haemost 193, 71: 617–24
2. Hemker HC, Béguin S: Thrombin generation in plasma: its assessment via the endogenous thrombin potential. Thromb Haemost 74: 134–38, 1995
3. Wielders S, Mukherjee M, Michiels M, Rijkers DTS, Cambus JP, Knebel RWC, Kakkar V, Hemker HC: The routine determination of the endogenous thrombin potential, first results in different forms of hyper- and hypocoagulability. Thromb Haemost 77: 629–36, 1997
4. Meijers JK, Tekelburg WL, Bouma BN, Bertina RM, Rosendaal FR. High levels of factor IX increase the risk of venous thrombosis. N Engl J Med 2000; 342: 696–701
5. van Hylckama Vileg A, van der Linden IK, Bertina RM, Rosendaal FR. High levels of factor IX increase the risk of venous thrombosis. Blood 2000, 95: 3678–82
6. Kraaijenhagen RA, in't Anker PS, Koopman MM et al. High plasma concentrations of factor VIII is a major risk factor for venous thromboembolism. Thromb Haemost 2000; 83: 5–9.
7. Butenas S, Mann KG. Blood coagulation. Biochemistry 2002; 67: 3–12
8. Gailani D, Broze GJ. Factor XI activation in a revised model of blood coagulation. Science 1991; 253: 909
9. Hoffman M, Monroe DM: A cell based model of hemostasis. Thromb Haemost 85: 958–65, 2001
10. Rosendaal FR: Venous thrombosis: a multicausal disease. Lancet 353: 1167–73,1999

Coagulation Parameters in Pregnancy: Low-Molecular-Weight Heparin Prophylaxis in Women with Thrombophilic Risk Factors

H.-H. Wolf, S. Seeger, A. Frühauf, O. Dorligschaw, and H.-J. Schmoll

Introduction

Thrombotic as well as fibrinolytic pathways of coagulation activation may be upregulated during pregnancy. Women with thrombophilic risk factors undergo a high risk for deep vein thrombosis and thromboembolism especially during the last trimenon and at term [1, 2].

Therefore, during pregnancy antithrombotic prophylaxis with low-molecular-weight (LMW) heparin could be indicated for some of those patients [3, 4]. Unfortunately, there are no randomized studies available to prove efficacy and adverse events of LMW heparin therapy according to the patients' prothrombotic risk factors.

As a pilot study we analyzed coagulation parameters in LMW heparin treated patients meanwhile pregnancy.

Patients' Characteristics

We report clinical data as well as laboratory profiles of 25 patients with at least one of the following thrombophilic risk factors: coagulation factor V Leiden (G1691A) or prothrombin (G20210A) mutations, low plasma concentrations of protein C or protein S, evidence of cardiolipin antibodies or lupus anticoagulant. 15 patients had a history of at least one deep vein thrombosis.

Therapy

Administration of dalteparin was adjusted to body weight. Dosage of LMW-heparin 4 hours after subcutaneous administration was efficacious to provide anti factor Xa plasma concentrations of 0,3 IU/ml.

Therapy was started within first and second trimester in 20 patients, within the third trimester in 5 patients, respectively, and was administered until day 14 post delivery. Acetylsalicylic acid has been administered additionally only in one patient presenting antiphospholipid antibody syndrome.

I. Scharrer/W. Schramm (Ed.)
33rd Hemophilia Symposion Hamburg 2002
© Springer-Verlag Berlin Heidelberg 2004

Changes in Coagulation System

From first to third trimester of pregnancy we saw a distinct rise in mean plasma concentrations of fibrinogen, F VII, F VIII, and vWF Collagen binding activity, to a lower amount of vWF Ristocetin Cofactor.

Table 1. Median plasma concentrations of coagulation factors

Parameter		median 1st Trimenon	2nd Trimenon	3rd Trimenon
F V	%	109,5	102	119
F VII	%	49	164	157
F VIII	%	122	141	173

Table 2. Median plasma concentrations of von-Willebrand-factor (vWF)

vW parameters		median 1st Trimenon	2nd Trimenon	3rd Trimenon
vWF CBA	%	58	111	ND
vWF Risto Co	%	116	132	113
vWF Ag	%	119	114	110

Significant increases were also seen in plasma concentrations of F1 + F2, PAI-1, TAT and PAP, not D-dimers from first to second trimester.

Table 3. Median plasma concentrations of fibrinolytic parameters

Parameter		median 1st Trimenon	2nd Trimenon	3rd Trimenon
Fibrinogen	g/l	2,1	4,4	4,5
F1 + F2	nmol/l	1,045	1,555	3,12
TAT	µg/l	2,4	4,4	4,5
D-dimer	mg/l	0,2	0,24	0,28

During pregnancy, there were low plasma concentrations of protein S (free) despite of continuous increase of total protein S (free and protein bound) resulting in protein S deficiency.

Table 4. Median plasma concentrations of coagulation parameters

Parameter		median 1st Trimenon	2nd Trimenon	3rd Trimenon
tissue factor	pg/ml	273	106	188
PAI-1	U/ml	1,5	3,4	6,25
F XIIa	ng/ml	2,01	2,34	3,11
F XII	%	80	100	97,5
PAP	µg/l	299,5	394,5	288,5

Different changes were seen in plasma concentrations of endogenous inhibitors of coagulation: median plasma concentrations of protein C were constantly low; median concentrations of activated factor XIIa, but not of factor XII concentration increased significantly.

Table 5. Median plasma concentrations of endogenous inhibitors of coagulation

Thrombophilic Parameters		median 1st Trimenon	2nd Trimenon	3rd Trimenon
Protein C	%	100	109	102
Protein S total	%	46	92	78
Protein S activity coag.	%	58	48	46
Protein S free	%	29	20	21

Fibrinolytic activity is impaired during normal pregnancy. We saw a 4-fold increase in endothelial-derived plasminogen-activator inhibitor (PAI-1).

D-dimer fragment of cross-linked fibrin slightly increased in dalteparin treated patients, mean F1 + F2 plasma concentrations increased significantly.

No thrombotic nor hemorrhagic complications were seen either in mothers or in children during pregnancy or labor. Diaplacental transmission of LMW-heparin has not been described yet.

The children presented normal gestational weight and were well at birth.

Conclusions

We conclude that antithrombotic prophylaxis with low-molecular heparin induced changes in activity of fibrinolytic as well as procoagulant parameters of coagulation [5].

Antithrombotic therapy with LMW-heparin seems to antagonize effectively pro-thrombotic coagulation parameters in pregnant risk patients and to inforce fibrinolytic activity.

During pregnancy dalteparin seems to be safe and useful in order to prevent deep vein thrombosis in patients with thrombophilic risk factors.

Studies on LMW heparin prophylaxis in subgroups according to the patients thrombophilic risk factors are requested to precise optimal onset, dosage and duration of LMW heparin administration.

References

1. Conrad J, Horellou M-H, Samana M-M. Inherited thrombophilia and gestational venous thromboembolism. Sem Thromb Hemostasis. 2003; 29: 121–142
2. Lockwood CJ. Inherited thrombophilias in pregnant patients: detection and treatment paradigm. Obstet Gyn. 2002; 99: 333–341
3. Bates SM, Ginsberg JS. Anticoagulation in pregnancy. Pharm Pract Manag Q. 1999; 19: 51–60
4. Ginsberg JS, Greer I, Hirsh J. Use of antithrombotic agents during pregnancy. Chest. 2001M 119; 122S–131S
5. Chan WS, Ginsberg JS. Diagnosis of deep vein thrombosis and pulmonary embolism in pregnancy. Thrombosis Research. 2002; 107; 85–91

VIId. Miscellaneous

Malignancy is not Associated with Decreased ADAMTS-13 Activity in Patients with Brain Tumors

M. Böhm, R. Gerlach, T. Scheuer, I. Stier-Brück, and I. Scharrer

Introduction

Von-Willebrand factor (vWF) mediates the adhesion of platelets to thrombogenic surfaces and platelet-to-platelet cohesion during thrombus growth. Upon secretion from vascular endothelium, vWF is degraded by the reducing activity of thrombospondin-1 [1] and the proteolytic activity of the vWF cleaving metalloprotease [2–3]. The metalloprotease shortens the vWF by cleaving the peptide bond Tyr^{1605}-Met^{1606} within domain A2. The enzyme has recently been identified as a new member of the ADAMTS (a disintegrin and metalloproteinase with thrombospondin type 1 motif) family and has been designated ADAMTS-13 [4–6]. Severe ADAMTS-13 deficiency is strongly associated with thrombotic thrombocytopenic purpura [6–13] and is caused by mutations in the ADAMTS-13 gene [6–8] or by inhibitory antibodies [9–10]. Oleksovicz et al. [14] first reported deficient activity of ADAMTS-13 in patients with disseminated malignancies. A total of 20 patients with metastatic tumors demonstrated significantly impaired ADAMTS-13 activity of $\leq 15\%$, whereas all patients with corresponding localized nonmetastatic tumors had ADAMTS-13 activities of $\geq 88\%$. The authors suggested, that low ADAMTS-13 activity could result in elevated levels of highly polymeric vWF, which might facilitate adhesive interactions with both circulating tumor cells and platelets, resulting in thrombus formation and the presumptive development of a metastatic colony. Fontana et al. [15] found mild ADAMTS-13 deficiency of 35% in 2 out of 4 patients with metastasizing neoplasia-associated microangiopathic hemolytic anemia (MAHA). Koo et al. [16] reported mild ADAMTS-13 deficiency (6–40%) in patients with various advanced stage-malignant tumors and in patients with colon cancer, grade IV, whereas all patients with limited stage-malignant tumors and colon cancer, stage II had ADAMTS-13 activities of >50%. To further investigate the role of ADAMTS-13 in tumor progression, we compared ADAMTS-13 activity and vWF:Ag in 30 patients with malignant brain tumors with 30 age-and sex-matched patients with benign brain tumors.

Materials and Methods

Study Population

60 patients with intracranial lesions as diagnosed by computerized tomography or magnetic resonance imaging were recruited for the study. Brain tumor classification

I. Scharrer/W. Schramm (Ed.)
33rd Hemophilia Symposion Hamburg 2002
© Springer-Verlag Berlin Heidelberg 2004

Table 1. Characteristics of the 60 patients included in the study. Brain tumors were classified according to the WHO grading system. There was no statistically significant age difference between patients with benign and malignant brain tumors (P>0.05, unpaired t-test).

Histological Diagnosis	Number of patients	Male/Female	Age (range; mean+/- SD)
Benign brain tumors	30	10/20	34-75; 55 +/-12
→ meningioma, WHO-GI	15	6/9	35-69; 56 +/-11
→ meningioma, WHO-GII	11	2/9	33-75; 55+/-16
→ pituitary tumors	3	2/1	44-66; 58+/-12
→ oligodendrogliom WHO-GII	1	0/1	39
Malignant brain tumors	30	10/20	41-74; 58 +/-8
→ glioblastoma-GIII-IV	14	4/10	44-74; 61+/-8
→ intracerebral metastasis	14	6/8	41-64; 55+/-8
→ meningioma-GIII	2	0/2	60-67; 64+/-5

was done according to the WHO grading system. Meningioma (WHO Grade I and II), pituitary tumors and oligodendroglioma (WHO grade II) were classified as benign tumors. Glioblastoma (WHO grade IV), intracerebral metastasis and meningioma (WHO grade III) were defined as malignant tumors.

Plasma Samples

Venous blood was drawn in citrated collection tubes from patients with brain tumors prior to surgery and centrifuged for 40 min at 4°C and 2500g. The platelet-poor plasma was subsequently stored at −20°C until tested. All individuals gave informed consent for blood sampling and research use.

ADAMTS-13 Activity

ADAMTS-13 activity was estimated by measuring the residual ristocetin cofactor activity of the degraded vWF substrate as described previously [13]. For assay calibration Imidazole buffer was replaced by heat-inactivated normal human plasma pool (30 min at 60°C and centrifuged for 15 min at 13000 rpm).

vWF Antigen

vWF:Ag was measured by enzyme immunoassay using rabbit anti-human vWF A0082 (DAKO, Denmark) for capture and peroxidase-conjugated rabbit anti-human vWF P0226 (DAKO, Denmark) for detection.

Data Analysis

Statistical analysis was performed using commercial software (Bias 7.01, Frankfurt, Germany). vWF:Ag, age and ADAMTS-13 activity were analyzed with Mann-Whitney-U-test. The relationship of ADAMTS-13 activity to vWF:Ag and age were examined using the Spearman correlation. Values of p lower 0.05 were considered statistically significant.

Results and Discussion

Mild ADAMTS-13 deficiency (normal range: 61–134%) was found in 2 patients with benign brain tumors (40%) and 7 patients with malignant brain tumors (42%), but there was no statistically significant difference in ADAMTS-13 activity for the age and sex matched patients with benign and malignant brain tumors (Fig. 1). Our results are in contrast to the findings of Oleksowicz et al. [14] and Koo et al. [16], who

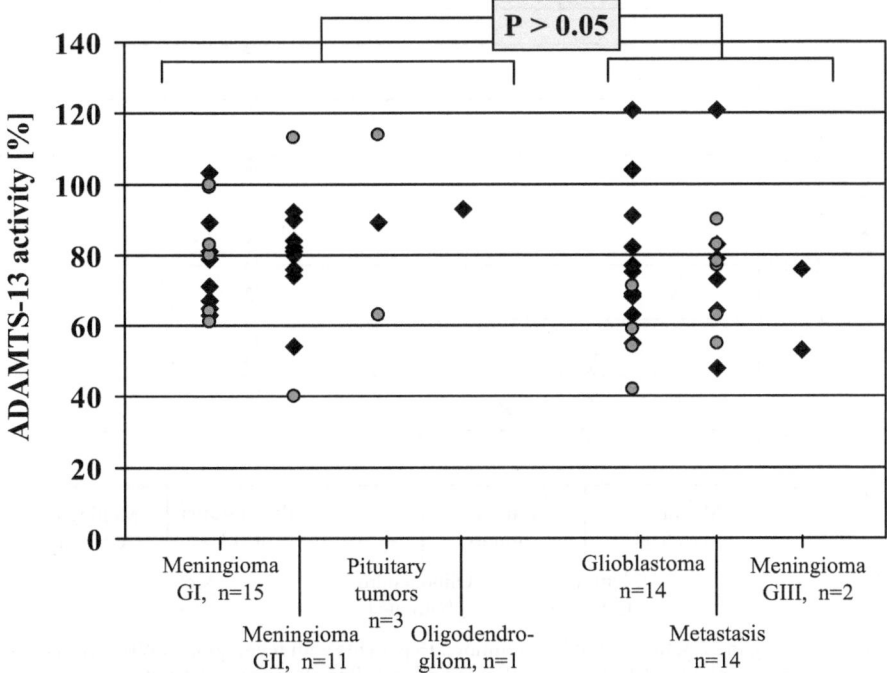

Fig. 1. ADAMTS-13 activity in 60 patients with brain tumors. 15 patients with meningioma, WHO-GI, 11 patients with meningioma, WHO-GII, 3 patients with pituitary tumors and 1 patient with oligodendrogliom, WHO-GII were classified as patients with benign tumors. 14 patients with glioblastoma, 14 patients with intracerebral metastasis and 2 patients with meningioma-GIII were classified as patients with malignant tumors. Benign tumors and malignant tumors were tested for statistical difference using the Mann-Whitney-U-Test (p > 0.05). Black diamonds and grey circles represent female (n=40) and male patients (n=20), respectively.

demonstrated an inverse correlation between ADAMTS-13 activity and metastasis and level of malignancy, respectively. Our data demonstrate, that advanced stage of malignancy and metastasis is not generally associated with decreased ADAMTS-13 activity. Mild ADAMTS-13 deficiency is found in a variety of clinical conditions like liver cirrhosis, uremia, acute inflammation [17], sepsis, heparin-induced thrombocytopenia, type 2 and myelodysplastic syndrome [18]. We found mild ADAMTS-13 deficiency in patients with acute ischemic stroke, disseminated intravascular coagulation, purpura rheumatica, lung fibroid and HELLP-syndrome (Böhm et al, Hemophilia Symposium 2002). The mechanism and the pathological relevance of low ADAMTS-13 activity in these conditions remain to be identified. However, these observations point to the necessity of stringent studies to establish a causal association between level of malignancy and/or metastasis and ADAMTS-13 deficiency. Since ADAMTS-13 is predominantly synthesized in the liver [6, 19], patients with liver failure should especially be excluded in such studies.

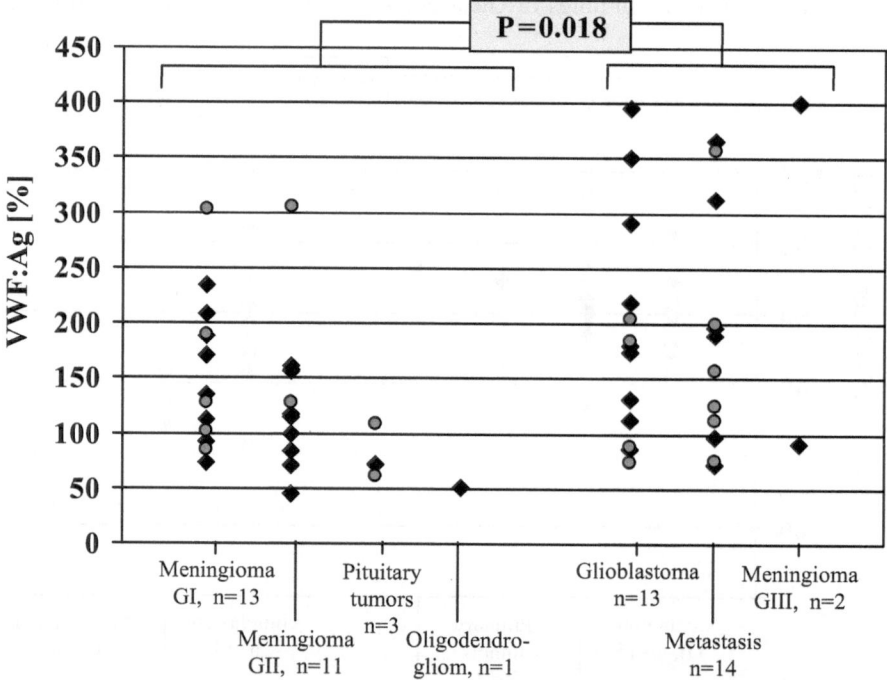

Fig. 2. vWF:Ag in 57 patients with brain tumors. 13 patients with meningioma, WHO-GI, 11 patients with meningioma, WHO-GII, 3 patients with pituitary tumors and 1 patient with oligodendrogliom, WHO-GII were classified as patients with benign tumors. 13 patients with glioblastoma, 14 patients with intracerebral metastasis and 2 patients with meningioma, WHO-GIII were classified as patients with malignant tumors. Benign tumors and malignant tumors were tested for statistical difference using the Mann-Whitney-U-Test (P=0.018). Black diamonds and grey circles represent female (n=38) and male patients (n=19), respectively. 2 patients with meningioma, WHO-GI and 1 patient with a glioblastom exhibited mild von-Willebrand Syndrome, type I and were subsequently excluded from this analysis.

Patients with malignant brain tumors could only be distinguished from patients with benign tumors by elevated levels of vWF:Ag (p=0.0062, unpaired t-test, Fig. 2). Our results are in concordance with data from several investigators, who found an association between impaired plasma vWF and stage of disease in patients with head and neck tumors [20], in patients with breast tumors [21] and in patients with colorectal tumors [22]. The mechanism of impaired plasma vWF:Ag is not fully understood, but might be a sign for the elevated tumor-dependent endothelial-cell proliferation.

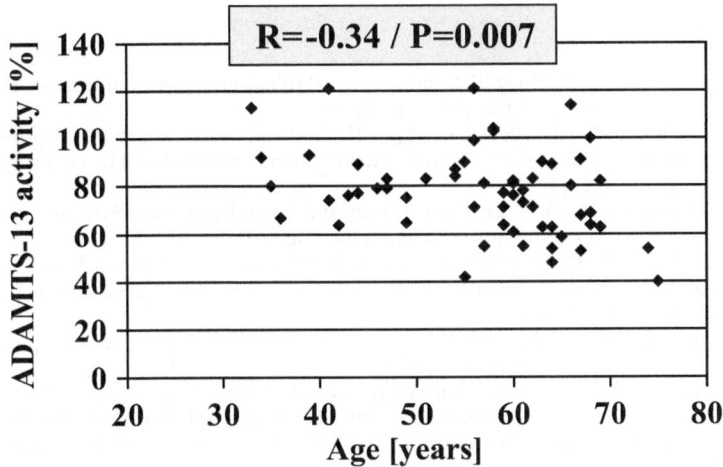

Fig. 3. Correlation between ADAMTS-13 activity and age of the investigated patients (n=60). The Spearman correlation coefficient was R = –0.34 (P=0.0071).

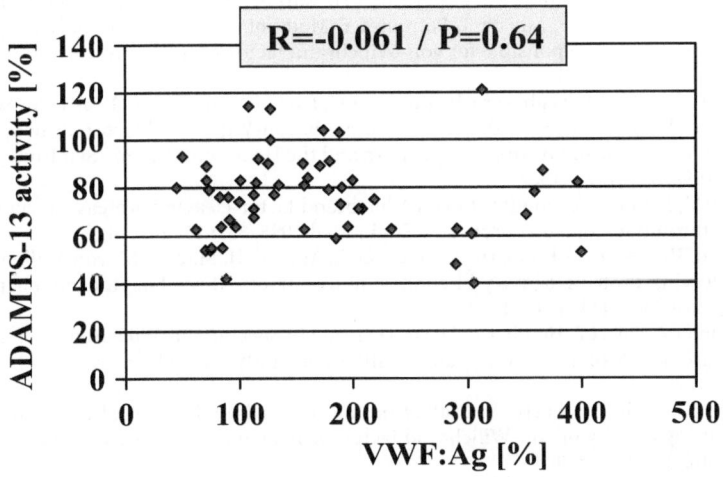

Fig. 4. Correlation between ADAMTS-13 activity and vWF:Ag for the investigated patients with the exception of 3 patients with mild von-Willebrand Syndrome, type I (n=57). The Spearman correlation coefficient was R= –0.061 (P=0.64).

ADAMTS-13 activity was influenced by the age of the patients (r=-0.34, p=0.0071, Pearson correlation, Fig. 4), as it was found by others [17, 23]. We did not detect a significant correlation between ADAMTS-13 activity and vWF:Ag (Fig. 5). At variance, Mannucci et al. [17] found an inverse correlation between vWF:Ag and ADAMTS-13 activity, which might be explained by differences in study population and/or the different laboratory method for assessment of ADAMTS-13 activity.

References

1. Xie L, Chesterman CN, Hogg PJ. Control of von-Willebrand factor multimer size by throm-bospondin-1. J Exp Med 2001; 193: 1341–1349
2. Furlan M, Robles R, Lämmle B. Partial purification and characterisation of a protease from human plasma cleaving von-Willebrand factor to fragments produced by in vivo proteolysis. Blood 1996; 10: 4223–4234
3. Tsai HM. Physiologic Cleavage of von-Willebrand Factor by a Plasma Protease is Dependent on its conformation and requires Calcium ion. Blood 1996; 10: 4235–4244
4. Fujikawa K, Suzuki H, McMullen B, Chung D. Purification of human von-Willebrand factor-cleaving protease and its identification as a new member of the metalloproteinase family. Blood 2001; 98: 1662–1666
5. Gerritsen HE, Robles R, Lämmle B, Furlan M. Partial amino acid sequence of purified von-Willebrand factor-cleaving protease Blood 2001; 98: 1654–1661
6. Levy GG, Nichols WC, Lian EC, Foroud T, McClintick JN, McGee BM, Yang AY, Siemieniak DR, Stark KR, Gruppo R, Sarode R, Shurin SB, Chandrasekaran V, Stabler SP, Sabio H, Bouhassira EE, Upshaw JD, Ginsburg D, Tsai HM. Mutations in a member of the ADAMTS gene family cause thrombotic thrombocytopenic purpura. Nature 2001; 413: 488–494
7. Schneppenheim R, Budde U, Oyen F, Angerhaus D, Aumann V, Drewke E, Hasenpflug W, Häberle J, Kentouche K, Kohne E, Kurnik K, Mueller-Wiefel D, Obser T, Santer R, Sykora KW. Blood 2002; prepublished online October 17, 2002
8. Kokame K, Matsumoto M, Soejima K, Yagi H, Ishizashi H, Funato M, Tamai H, Konno M, Kamide K, Kawano Y, Miyata T, Fujimura Y. Mutations and common polymorphisms in ADAMTS13 gene responsible for von-Willebrand factor-cleaving protease activity. PNAS 2002; 99: 11902–11907
9. Furlan M, Robles R, Galbusera M, Remuzzi G, Kyrle PA, Brenner B, Krause M, Scharrer I, Aumann V, Mittler U, Solenthaler M, Lämmle B. von-Willebrand factor-cleaving protease in thrombotic thrombocytopenic purpura and the Hemolytic-Uremic Syndrome. N Engl J Med 1998, 339: 1578–1584
10. Tsai HM, Lian EC. Antibodies to von-Willebrand factor-cleaving protease in acute throm-botic thrombocytopenic Purpura. N Engl J Med 1998, 339: 1585–1594
11. Allford SL, Harrison P, Lawrie AS, Liesner R, Mackie IJ, Machin SJ. von-Willebrand fac-tor-cleaving protease activity in congenital thrombotic thrombocytopenic purpura. Br J Haematol 2000; 111: 1215–1222
12. Veyradier A, Obert B, Houllier A, Meyer D, Girma JP. Specific von-Willebrand factor-cleaving protease in thrombotic microangiopathies: a study of 111 cases. Blood 2001; 98: 1765–1772
13. Böhm M, Vigh T, Scharrer I. Evaluation and clinical application of a new method for measuring activity of von-Willebrand factor-cleaving metalloprotease (ADAMTS13). Ann Hematol 2002; 81: 430–435
14. Oleksowicz L, Bhagwati N, DeLeon-Fernandez M. Deficient activity of von-Willebrand's factor cleaving protease in patients with disseminated malignancies. Cancer Res 1999; 59: 2244–2250

15. Fontana S, Gerritsen HE, Kremer Hovinga J, Furlan M, Lämmle B. Microangiopathic hae-molytic anaemia in metastasizing malignant tumours is not associated with a severe defi-ciency of the von-Willebrand factor-cleaving protease. Br J Haematol 2001; 113:100–102

16. Koo BH, Oh D, Chung SY, Kim NK, Park S, Jang Y, Chung KH. Deficiency of von-Willebrand factor-cleaving protease activity in the plasma of malignant patients. Thromb Res 2002; 105: 471–476

17. Mannucci PM, Canciani MT, Forza I, Lussana F, Lattuada A, Rossi E. Changes in health and disease of the metalloprotease that cleaves von-Willebrand factor. Blood 2001; 98: 2730–2735

18. Bianchi V, Robles R, Alberio L, Furlan M, Lämmle B. von-Willebrandfactor-cleaving pro-tease (ADAMTS13) in thrombocytopenic disorders: a severely deficient activity is specific for thrombotic thrombocytopenic purpura. Blood 2002; 100: 710–713

19. Zheng X, Chung D, Takayama TK, Majerus EM, Sadler JE, Fujikawa K. Structur of von-Willebrand factor-cleaving protease (ADAMTS13), a metalloprotease involved in thrombotic thrombocytopenic purpura. J Biol Chem 2001; 276: 41059–41063

20. Sweeney JD, Killion KM, Pruet CF, Spaulding MB. von-Willebrand factor in head and neck cancer. Cancer 1990; 66 (11): 2387–2389

21. Rohsig LM, Damin DC, Stefani SD, Castro CG Jr, Roisenberg I, Schwartsmann G. von-Willebrand factor antigen levels in plasma of patients with malignant breast disease. Braz Jmed Biol Res 2001; 34 (9): 1125–1129

22. Damin DC, Rosito MA, Gus P, Roisemberg I, Bandinelli E, Schwartsmann G. von-Willebrand factor in colorectal cancer. Int J Colorectal Dis 2002; 17 (1): 42–45

23. He S, Cao H, Magnusson CGM, Eriksson-Berg M, Mehrkash M, Schenck-Gustafsson K, Blombäck M. Are increased levels of von-Willebrand factor in Chronic Coronary Heart Disease caused by decrease in von-Willebrand factor cleaving protease activity? A study by an Immunoassay with antibody against intact bond 842Tyr-843Met of the von-Willebrand factor protein. Thromb Res 2001; 103: 241–248

Analysis of Factor VIII RNA from Hemophilia A Patients with no Detectable Mutation in the Coding Regions

O. El-Maarri, U. Herbiniaux, M. Watzka, J. Graw, C. Uen,
J. Schröder, H.H. Brackmann, W. Schramm, R. Schwaab,
C. Müller-Reible, E. Seifried, and J. Oldenburg

Summary

Here on we report on the detailed RNA analysis of the factor VIII cDNA from patients that have either putative splicing site mutations or patients with no previously detected DNA mutations by mutation screening and also sequencing of the complete factor VIII cDNA. This protocol proofs to be effective, simple and able to detect splicing errors, thus showing evidence for the causality of splicing defects for the hemophilia A disease in those individuals. Patients that were negative for mutation detection protocols and also show a normal mRNA might be potential candidates for the discovery of novel allelic or non allelic mutations leading to a hemophilia A phenotype.

Introduction

Hemophilia A is caused by absence or deficiency of factor VIII (FVIII) coagulation activity due to a great variety of mutations in the FVIII gene. These include the common intron 22 and intron 1 inversions, point mutations, deletions and insertions (Oldenburg, 2001). However, in spite of applying all available techniques for mutation analysis (Oldenburg et al., 2001), no mutation can be identified in a small subpopulation of about 2% of patients in either the exons, the splice sites or the promoter region (Klopp et al., 2002). These findings point to other still unknown mutation mechanisms that might be related to the FVIII gene or other genes interacting with it. In the present study we addressed this subject by analyzing the FVIII RNA in those patients where no mutation has been identified. FVIII mRNA analysis is hampered by the very small amounts of ectopic mRNA that can be obtained from the patients lymphocytes. The protocol presented herein represents a robust procedure suitable for routine mRNA studies.

Materials and Methods

RNA was extracted from 2.5 ml peripheral blood samples. We performed 4 different reverse transcriptions with the primers indicated in the Figure (horizontal arrows). Later on we performed two rounds of RT PCRs for each region resulting in a total of eight templates covering the complete F VIII cDNA. We then cloned all products with abnormal size in a TA cloning vector and sequenced the inserts.

I. Scharrer/W. Schramm (Ed.)
33rd Hemophilia Symposion Hamburg 2002
© Springer-Verlag Berlin Heidelberg 2004

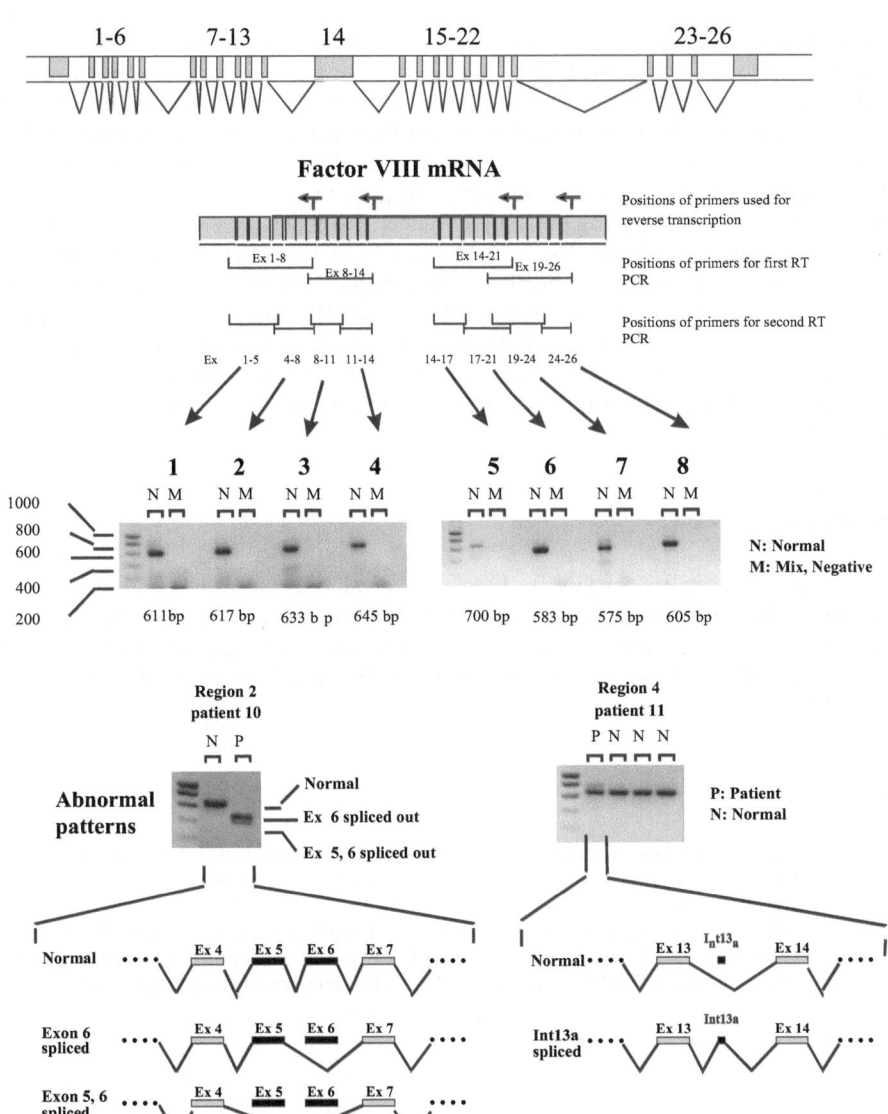

Fig. 1. Flowchart of the RNA analysis in the factor VIII gene; the amplified regions are shown under the factor VIII mRNA; Horizontal arrows represent the positions of the primers used for the reverse transcription.

Results and Discussions

So far we analyzed 4 patients. We found two abnormal bands in two of them, patient number 10 has splicing errors (IVS 6+3 A>G) involving exons 5 and 6 that were revealed by skipping either exon 6 or both, exons 5 and 6. In patient 11 a 136 bp insert from intron 13 was spliced in additionally to a causative intron 1 inversion mutation. Our approach proved to be useful in detecting abnormal splicing mutations that are not located within the coding region of the F VIII gene but are lying in the introns and results in an unusual splicing pattern. Moreover, the absence of any mutation in the factor VIII gene on both the DNA and RNA levels, in a number of patients indicates that some other factor(s) or control region(s) may be involved. These could be proteins needed specifically for secretion of the factor VIII molecule or involved in post transactional modification. Alternatively, unknown factors that affect the expression rate or the stability of the mRNA could be involved; to address this, a detailed mapping and characterization of the factor VIII promoter and expression control is needed.

Conclusions

The protocol presented in this study enables a reliable extraction and analysis of ectopic FVIII mRNA from the patients blood lymphocytes. The technique allows to clearly assign the causality of splice site mutations and furthermore will represent an important tool for the elucidation of novel mutation mechanisms leading to hemophilia A.

References

1. Oldenburg J, Ivaskevicius V, Rost S, Fregin A, White K, Holinski-Feder E, Muller CR, Weber BH. Evaluation of DHPLC in the analysis of hemophilia A. J Biochem Biophys Methods. 2001, 47 (1–2): 39–51
2. Oldenburg J, Mutation profiling in Hemophilia A. Thromb Haemost. 2001. 85: 577–9
3. Klopp N, Oldenburg J, Uen C, Schneppenheim R, Graw J. 11 hemophilia A patients without mutations in the factor VIII encoding gene. Thromb Haemost. 2002, 88 (2): 357–60

FISH for Carrier Detection of large Deletions in the Factor VIII Gene

T. Förster, M. Guttenbach, C.R. Müller, and J. Oldenburg

Introduction

Hemophilia A is a common congenital bleeding disorder caused by a deficiency of coagulation factor VIII. The disease is inherited in a X-linked recessive pattern with an estimated incidence of 1 per 5000–10000 males. The gene encoding factor VIII is large (186 kb) and is located about 1 MB from the telomere in Xq28. Female carriers which are usually asymptomatic transmit hemophilia A to 50% of their male descendants.

Large deletions represent 3% of the molecular defects in severe hemophilia A. While they can easily be detected in males by PCR and Southern Blot it is more demanding to determine the presence of a large deletion in a female. The second intact X-chromosome complicates the results of PCR based methods and at a best semi-quantitative results e.g. by Southern Blotting can be obtained.

In order to unequivocally assign the status of a potential female carrier of a large deletion we have established FISH (fluorescence in situ hybridization) for individual F-VIII exons.

Methods

PCR products containing individual exons and part of their adjacent introns were amplified from BAC clones carrying parts of the FVIII gene to generate probes of about 5 kb each. After labeling with fluorescent nucleotides the probes were hybridized to metaphase chromosomes of four mothers of patients with known deletions. An X-chromosomal probe of the centromeric region was used as an internal control (Fig. 1, 3).

Results and Discussion

All four women turned out to be carriers of the familial deletion (Fig. 2). With probes of the deleted exon only one of the two X-chromosomes was labeled (Fig. 1). In contrast probes of flanking exons showed signals on both X-chromosomes (Fig. 3). The extend of the deletion (as known from PCR analysis in the patient) could be confirmed by FISH in all cases.

I. Scharrer/W. Schramm (Ed.)
33rd Hemophilia Symposion Hamburg 2002
© Springer-Verlag Berlin Heidelberg 2004

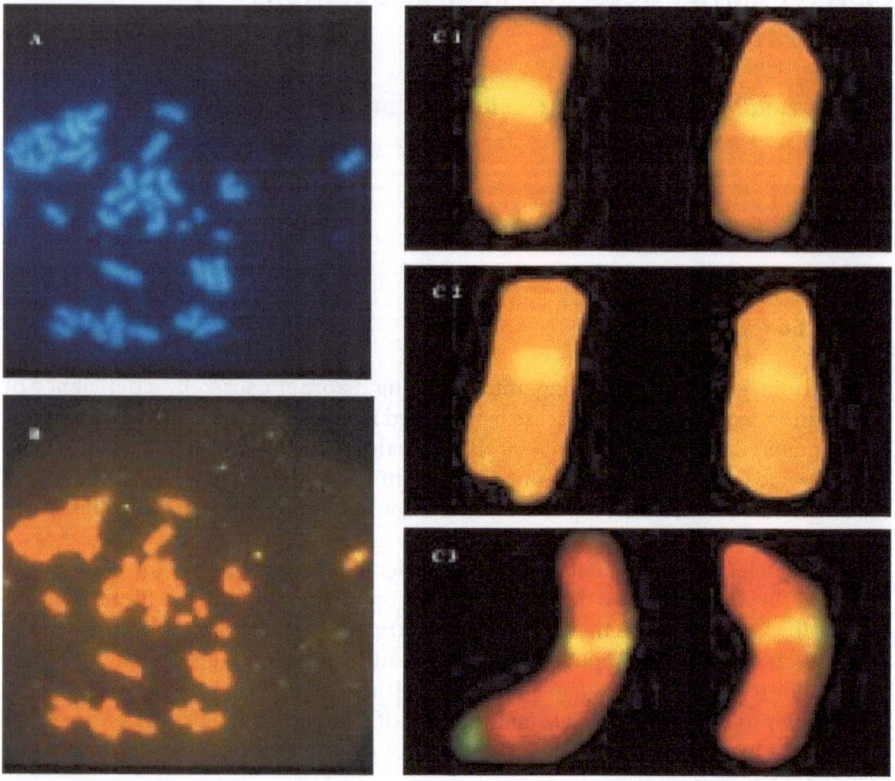

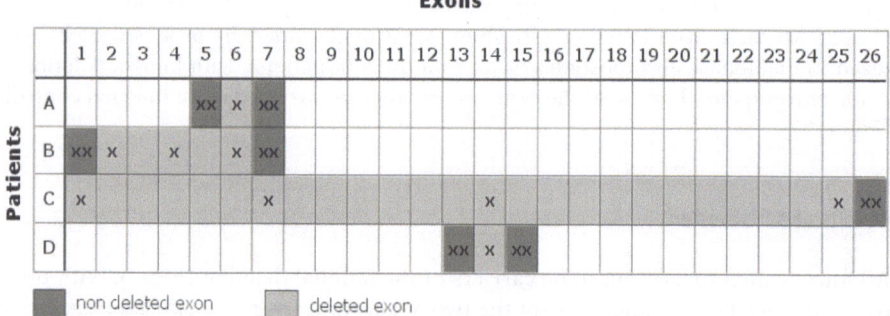

Fig. 1. Hybridization with a probe of a deleted exon. Only one of the two X chromosomes is labeled. X-chromosomes are additionally labeled by a centromeric probe for easy recognition.
A, B: Whole metaphases of one female patient in DAPI and FITC
C1 – C3: Enlargement of the two X-Chromosomes of three different metaphases of the same female patient

Exons

Patients	1	2	3	4	5	6	7	8	9	10	11	12	13	14	15	16	17	18	19	20	21	22	23	24	25	26
A					xx	x	xx																			
B	xx	x		x		x	xx																			
C	x				x									x											x	xx
D													xx	x	xx											

■ non deleted exon   ▢ deleted exon

Fig 2. Overview of the deletions in the four female patients A-D. The colored boxes indicate the extend of deletions known from PCR analysis in the male index patient. FISH results are shown as x or xx. x stands for one signal in the metaphase and xx stands for one signal each on both X-chromosomes.

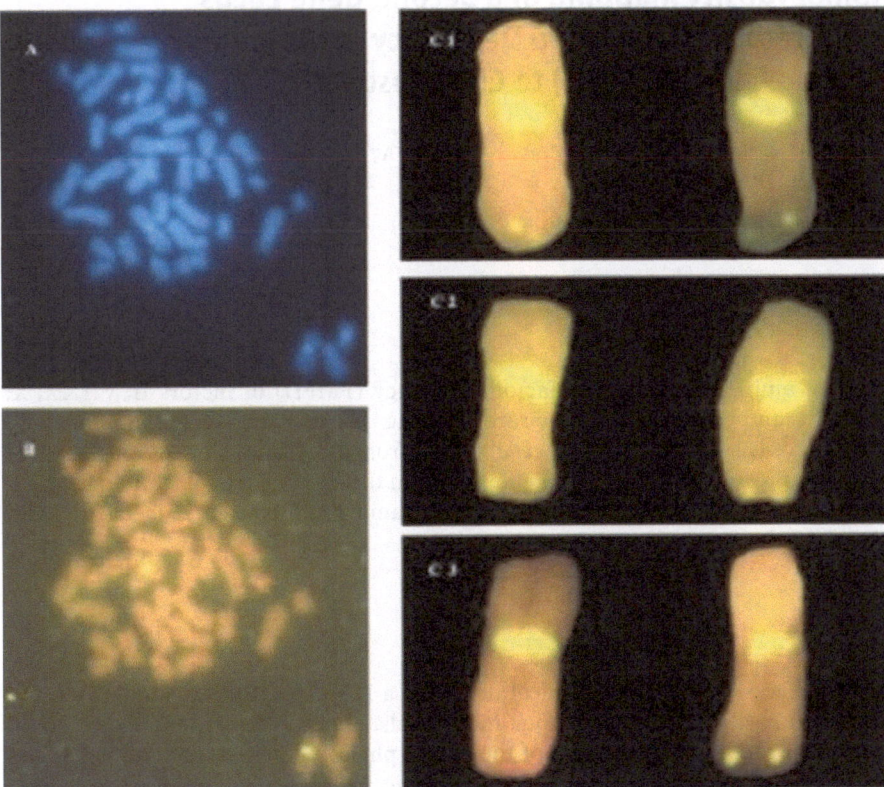

Fig. 3. Hybridization with a probe of a non-deleted exon. Both X- chromosomes are labeled. X-chromosomes are additionally labeled by a centromeric probe for easy recognition.
A, B: Whole metaphases of one female patient in DAPI and FITC; C1 – C3: Enlargement of the two X-Chromosomes of three different metaphases of the same female patient

Conclusion

FISH-technique is well suited for direct visualization and unequivocally assignment of a large deletion in a female carrier.

References

1. Oldenburg J (2001) Mutation profiling in hemophilia A. Thromb Haemost 85: 577–579
2. Oranwiroon S, Akkarapatumwong V, Pung-Amritt P, Treesucon A, Veerakul G, Mahasandana C, Panyim S, Yenchitsomanus P (2001). Determination of hemophilia A carrier status by mutation analysis. Haemophilia; 7: 20–5

Homozygosity Mapping of a Second Gene Locus for Hereditary Combined Deficiency of Vitamin K-Dependent Clotting Factors (FMFD) to Chromosome 16

A. Fregin, S. Rost, W. Wolz, A. Krebsova, C.R. Muller, and J. Oldenburg

Introduction

Familial multiple coagulation factor deficiency (FMFD) of factors II, VII, IX, X, protein C and protein S is a very rare bleeding disorder with autosomal recessive inheritance [1]. The disease may result either from a defective resorption/transport of vitamin K to the liver, or from a mutation in one of the genes encoding gamma-carboxylase (GGCX) or other proteins of the Vitamin K 2, 3-epoxide reductase (VKOR, Fig. 1) [2, 3].

Patients

We have recently presented clinical details of a Lebanese (Fam. A) and a German family (Fam. B) with ten and four individuals, respectively, where we proposed autosomal recessive inheritance of the FMFD phenotype [1]. Direct sequencing of gamma-carboxylase and microsomal epoxide hydrolase revealed no mutation. Biochemical investigations of vitamin K metabolites in patients' serum showed a significantly increased level of vitamin K epoxide, thus, suggesting a defect in one of the subunits of the vitamin K 2, 3-epoxidase reductase (VKOR) complex.

Results and Discussion

We have assigned a second gene for hereditary combined multiple coagulation factor deficiency (FMFD) to chromosome 16p12-q21 by homozygosity mapping (Fig. 2). A phenotype related to human coagulation factor deficiency has been described in rats and mice as resistance to the anticoagulant drug warfarin (Fig. 1). Alterations in the warfarin binding site of the VKOR could lead to a phenotype of warfarin resistance, while alterations in another part of the enzyme would result in the FMFD phenotype with bleeding tendency due to a lack of recycled vitamin K1H2. The genes responsible for warfarin resistance have been mapped in mice (*war*) to chromosome 7 at a position of 62.5 cM and in rats (*Rw*) to chromosome 1q35-42 (5, 6). Chromosomes 7 of mouse and 1 of rat share extensive areas of synteny (Fig. 3). Several anchor loci flanking the locus for warfarin resistance, both in mouse and rat, are located on the short arm of human chromosome 16. Colocalization

I. Scharrer/W. Schramm (Ed.)
33rd Hemophilia Symposion Hamburg 2002
© Springer-Verlag Berlin Heidelberg 2004

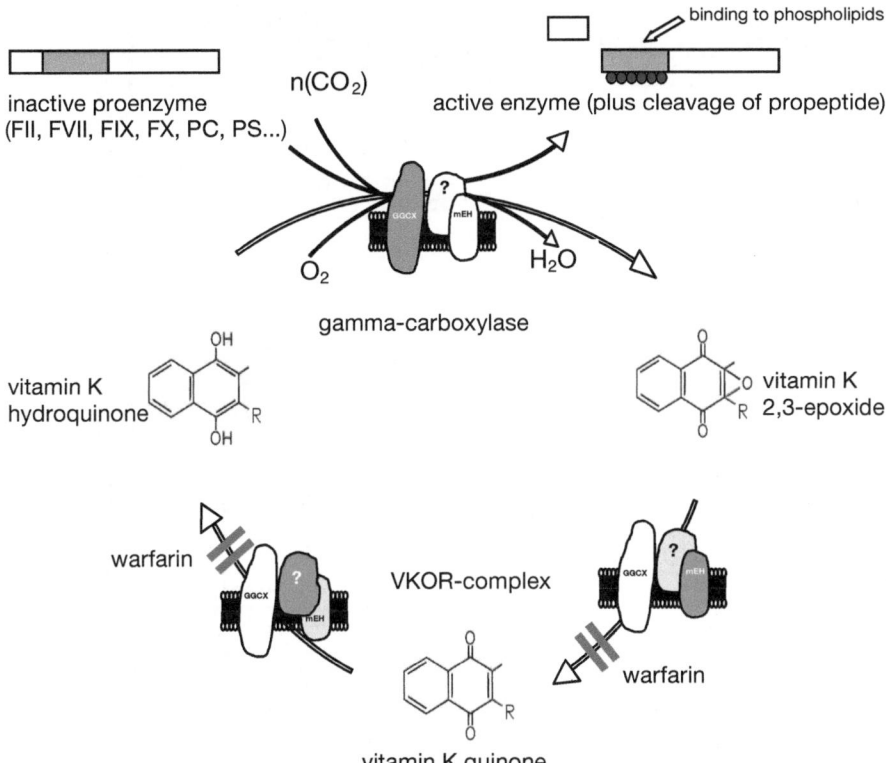

Fig. 1. A model of the Vitamin K cycle. Vitamin K dependent coagulation factors attain their ability to attach to phospholipids via modification by gamma-carboxylase. Vitamin K hydroquinone is oxidized to its 2, 3-epoxide by this process. The epoxide is reduced to the active cofactor by the vitamin K 2, 3-epoxide reductase. This multienzyme-complex is inhibited by the anticoagulant warfarin, which leads to a phenotype similar to FMFD.

Table 1. Two point LOD score values (MLINK) for linkage between FMFD and selected chromosome 16 markers based on the two families, obtained at different recombination fractions.

Order	Comp.	McM	FcM	q = 0	q =.01	q =.05	q =.1	q =.2	q =.3	q =.4
D16S420	31130	51.65	43.44	-infini	1.32	1.75	1.71	1.31	0.77	0.25
D16S3093	36625	52.51	52.12	-infini	-0.74	-0.11	0.09	0.18	0.13	0.04
D16S3131	37256	52.61	53.17	-infini	-0.15	0.40	0.52	0.45	0.26	0.08
D16S261	40460	53.69	64.17	3.39	3.32	3.03	2.67	1.91	1.13	0.38
D16S690	52906	53.69	65.97	3.39	3.32	3.03	2.67	1.91	1.13	0.38
D16S3080	55810	53.69	66.39	1.88	1.84	1.68	1.48	1.05	0.61	0.20
D16S409	62310	53.69	67.33	3.08	3.02	2.77	2.45	1.78	1.06	0.36
D16S419	63668	56.83	78.35	-infini	1.32	1.75	1.71	1.31	0.77	0.25
D16S3039	65124	56.83	92.29	-infini	1.32	1.73	1.68	1.26	0.72	0.23
D16S3096	91611	69.66	120.05	-infini	-1.39	-0.17	0.20	0.34	0.24	0.08

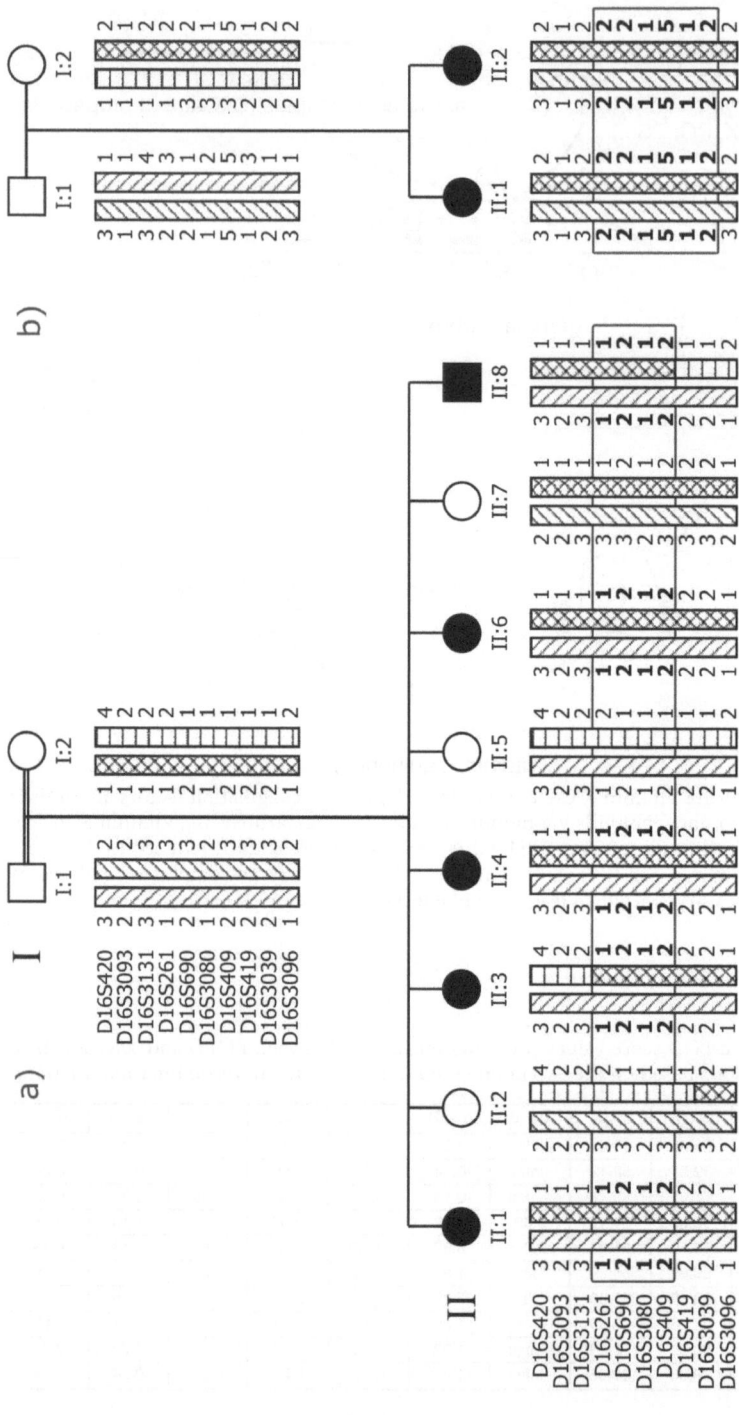

Fig. 2. Pedigrees of FMFD families with informative haplotypes from selected markers. The open rectangle demarcates the candidate gene region, which comprises only homozygous markers. Markers in the rectangle, presumably inherited IBD (identical-by-descent), are denoted in bold.

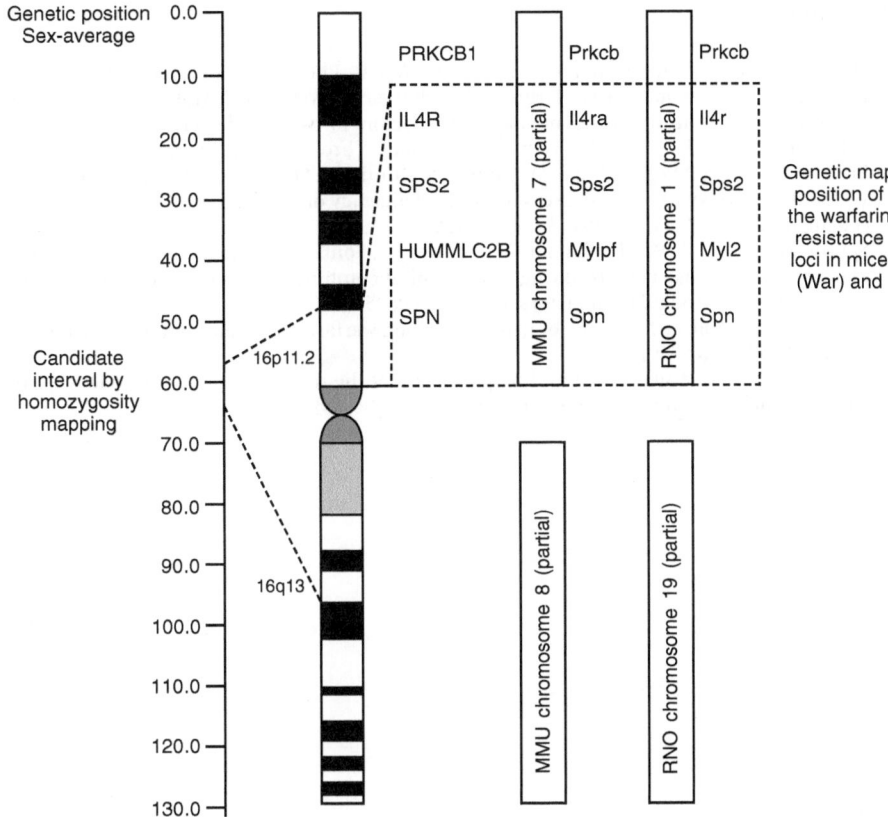

Fig. 3. Position of the candidate inter-val by homozygosity on chromosome 16. The small bar on the left resembles the candidate interval in the genetic map. The projection on the idiogram of chromosome 16 shows the physical dimension of this area. The human to mouse/rat homology regions present genes surrounding the locus for resistance to warfarin. By comparing chromosomal maps of these species, the candidate interval could be confined to 16p12-p11.

of FMFD in humans and warfarin resistance in mouse and rat on homologous chromosomal segments implies that both phenotypes may be allelic.

Assuming a single gene for both phenotypes, mouse-human homology maps would restrict the candidate gene region to the proximal short arm of chromosome 16.

Supported by grants of the DFG (OI 100/3-1) and Baxter Germany

References

1. Oldenburg J, von Brederlow B, Fregin A, Rost S, Wolz W, Eberl W, Eber S, Lenz E, Schwaab R, Brackmann HH, Effenberger W, Harbrecht U, Schurgers LJ, Vermeer C, Müller CR. Congenital deficiency of vitamin K dependent coagulation factors in two families presents as a genetic defect of the vitamin K-epoxide-reductase-complex. Thromb Haemost. 2000; 84: 937–941
2. Brenner B, Sanchez-Vega B, Wu S-M, Lanir N, Stafford DW, Solera J. A missense mutation in γ-glutamyl carboxylase gene causes combined deficiency of all vitamin K-dependent blood coagulation factors. Blood. 1998; 92: 4554–4559
3. Spronk HMH, Farah RA, Buchanan GR, Vermeer C, Soute BAM. Novel mutation in the γ-glutamyl carboxylase gene resulting in congenital combined deficiency of all vitamin K-dependent blood coagulation factors. Blood. 2000; 96: 3650–3652
4. MacSwiney FJ, Wallace ME. A major gene controlling warfarin-resistance in the house mouse. J Hyg. 1976; (Lond) 76: 173–181
5. Kohn HK, Pelz HJ. A gene anchored map position of the rat warfarin-resistance locus, RW, and ist orthologs in mice and humans. Blood. 2000; 96: 1996–1998

First Case of Compound Heterozygosity in the Gamma-Glutamyl Carboxylase Gene Causing Combined Deficiency of all Vitamin K-Dependent Blood Coagulation Factors

S. Rost, A. Fregin, D. Koch, M. Compes, W. Wolz, C.R. Müller, and J. Oldenburg

Introduction

Hereditary combined deficiency of all vitamin K-dependent coagulation factors (FMFD, Familial Multiple Coagulation Factor Deficiency) is a very rare bleeding disorder, with only 14 cases described as yet [1]. The clinical presentation is variable with respect to the residual activities of the affected proteins, the response to oral substitution of vitamin K and to the involvement of skeletal abnormalities. The phenotype may result either from a mutation within the gamma-glutamyl carboxylase gene or a mutation affecting the vitamin K 2, 3-epoxid reductase (VKOR) complex. While the responsible gene(s) of the VKOR complex are still unknown, two different mutations have been reported in the gamma-glutamyl carboxylase gene in two consanguineous families [2, 3].

Patient

In the present study we report on a third family in which the index patient, an one year old boy, showed a mild deficiency of all vitamin K dependent coagulation factors with activities ranging from 20 to 30% of normal (Table 1). High doses of intravenously administered vitamin K led to an increase of the factor activities to 50–60%, however the factor activities could not be restored to normal and decreased again when vitamin K substitution was stopped.

Table 1. Vitamin K dependent factor levels in the index patient. (before and after Vitamin K substitution; in percentage of normal range)

	Quick	Factor II	Factor VII	Factor X
Before Vitamin K	18–25	21	42	36
After Vitamin K	53	40	62	65

Results and Discussion

Sequence analysis of all exons and flanking intron regions of the gamma-glutamyl carboxylase gene in the index patient revealed a splice site mutation of exon 3 (IVS2-1 G>T; Fig. 1) and a missense mutation in exon 11 (R485P; Fig. 2). Both mutations were

I. Scharrer/W. Schramm (Ed.)
33rd Hemophilia Symposion Hamburg 2002
© Springer-Verlag Berlin Heidelberg 2004

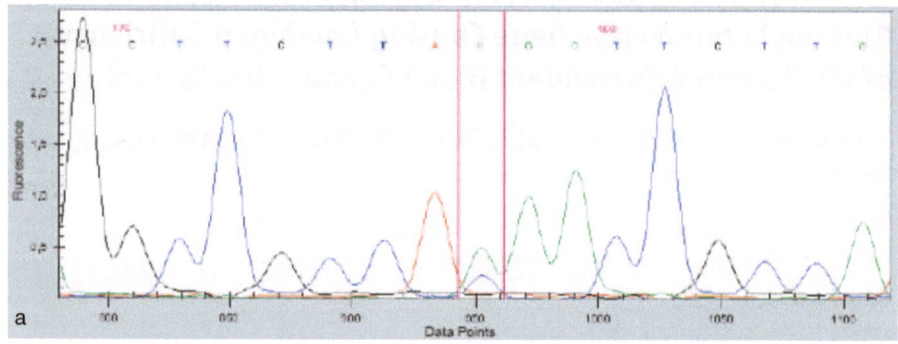

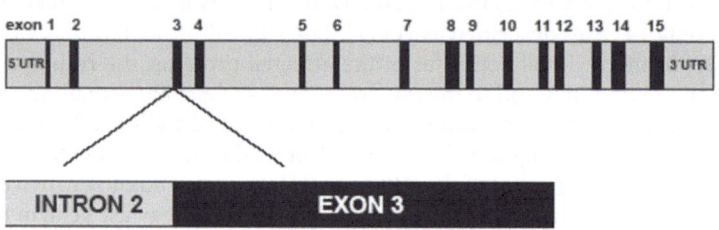

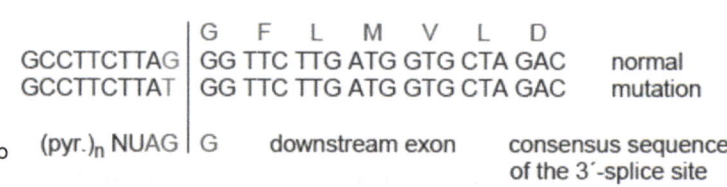

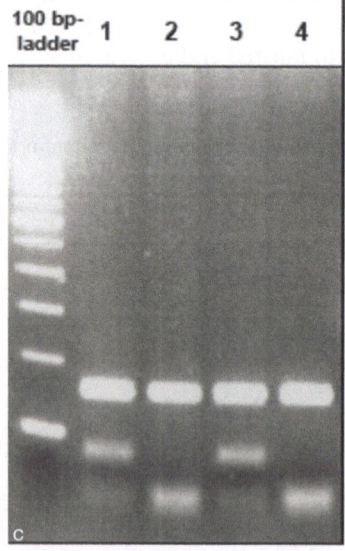

Fig. 1 a–c. Identification of the splice site mutation. (a) Sequence analysis of exon 3 of the gamma-glutamyl carboxylase gene in the index patient. A heterozygous G to T mutation in the last nucleotide of intron 2 was detected in both strands. This splice site mutation is predicted to result in a loss of the whole exon 3 during splicing process leading to a truncated protein. (b) Schematic representation of the gamma-glutamyl carboxylase gene. The intronexon-border of exon 3 and the sequence containing the mutation is shown in detail. (c) RFLP-analysis of exon 3 using the restriction enzyme Dde I. This digestion leads either to 79 bp- and 153 bp-fragments in case of mutation (1 = father and 3 = patient) or to 36 bp-, 43 bp- and 153 bp-fragments in the wildtype (2 = mother, 4 = negative control). 100 unrelated blood donors were examined by this method, thus excluding a frequent polymorphism at this restriction site.

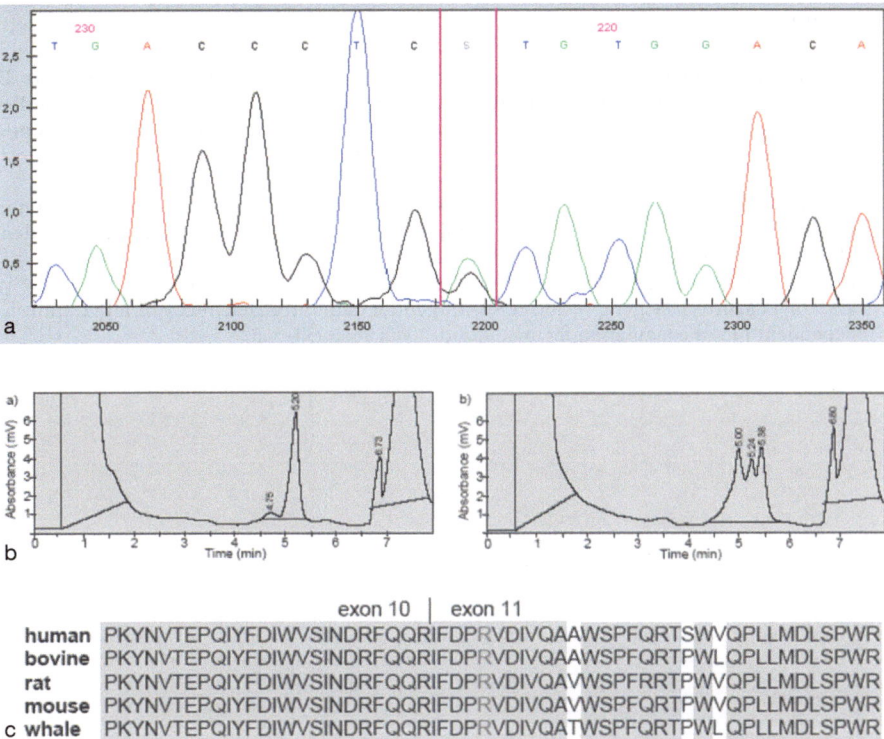

Fig. 2 a–c. Identification of the R485P missense mutation. **(a)** Sequence analysis of exon 11 of the gamma-glutamyl carboxylase gene in the index patient. This revealed a heterozygous G to C transversion in both strands resulting in the conversion of an arginine codon (CGT) to a proline codon (CCT) at residue 485 in the protein. **(b)** DHPLC analysis of exon 11 of the gamma-glutamyl carboxylase gene in a negative control (a) and the index patient (b). In this way, 100 healthy blood donors were screened for the missense mutation and all showed the pattern of the negative control. **(c)** Comparison of the aminoacid sequence similarity of a part of exon 10 and 11 in five different species. The mutated arginine 485 lies in a highly conserved region indicating an important role of this protein domain.

not found in 200 unrelated chromosomes of healthy blood donors, thus excluding the presence of frequent polymorphisms at these sites.

The present patient is the first case of a compound heterozygote for mutations in the gamma-glutamyl carboxylase gene. Both mutations are likely to be causative: The first changes the conserved consensus sequence of the 3'-splice site of intron 2, while the second introduces a novel proline, which is known to have significant impact on the secondary structure of proteins. Both mutations have not been published before and represent the third and the fourth mutations described so far within the gamma-glutamyl carboxylase gene.

Supported by grants of the DFG (OI 100/3-1) and Baxter Germany

References

1. Oldenburg J, von Brederlow B, Fregin A, Rost S, Wolz W, Eberl W, Eber S, Lenz E, Schwaab R, Brackmann HH, Effenberger W, Harbrecht U, Schurgers LJ, Vermeer C, Müller CR. Congenital deficiency of vitamin K dependent coagulation factors in two families presents as a genetic defect of the vitamin K-epoxide-reductase-complex. Thromb Haemost. 2000; 84: 937–941
2. Brenner B, Sanchez-Vega B, Wu S-M, Lanir N, Stafford DW, Solera J. A missense mutation in γ-glutamyl carboxylase gene causes combined deficiency of all vitamin K-dependent blood coagulation factors. Blood. 1998; 92: 4554–4559
3. Spronk HMH, Farah RA, Buchanan GR, Vermeer C, Soute BAM. Novel mutation in the γ-glutamyl carboxylase gene resulting in congenital combined deficiency of all vitamin K-dependent blood coagulation factors. Blood. 2000; 96: 3650–3652

Phosphatidylserine in the Neonatal and Adult Platelet Membrane: A Comparison

T. Rehak, G. Cvirn, M. Petritsch, H. Köfeler, and W. Muntean

Introduction

Neonatal platelets are described as hyporeactive [1, 2]. Hypothesized to be immature, they differ in many aspects from adult platelets: morphologically they have a similar size, but markedly less α-granules, less pseudopods, smaller glycogen deposits and less microtubular structures [3]. In function tests aggregation response particularly to epinephrine and collagen is reduced, and markers of platelet activation, analyzed by flow cytometry, show lower expression after activation with physiological agonists [4]. Realizing these facts neonatal platelets are mainly characterized by a low reserve capacity [5].

Negatively charged phospholipids, i.e. phosphatidylserine (PS), are localized in the inner cell membrane-leaflet of resting platelets. After activation they are immediately exposed in the outer leaflet [6, 7], generating a procoagulant surface for plasmatic clotting factors to assemble on the platelet surface as coagulation complexes, i.e., tenase and prothrombinase complexes [8]. Platelets also express protein binding sites for several clotting factors [9, 10, 11], which seem to play an important role in coordinating assembly of the coagulation complexes. The procoagulant effect of PS is estimated high, since an inherited disorder called Scott Syndrome [12] is known, which is characterized by a lack of membrane expression of procoagulant phospholipids leading to hemorrhagic complications.

The aim of our study was to investigate whether phosphatidylserine in neonatal platelets differs from that in adult platelets in its total amount, its exposure on the platelet surface and its effect on the thrombin generation.

We, therefore, used mass spectrometry to determine the amount of total PS, flow cytometry for detecting the exposure of PS, and a recently described subsampling method to monitor the time-course of thrombin generation in plasma [13].

Methods

Blood Preparation

Blood was taken from umbilical cord of term neonates immediately after vaginal delivery. For normal adult controls blood was collected by cubital venipuncture from healthy volunteers who had not taken aspirin or other drugs for at least 10 days. In both cases blood was collected into tubes containing 0.1M citrate.

I. Scharrer/W. Schramm (Ed.)
33rd Hemophilia Symposion Hamburg 2002
© Springer-Verlag Berlin Heidelberg 2004

Platelet Isolation

1 ml of citrated blood was centrifuged at 2300 rpm for 20 min at room temperature, subsequently the plasma was removed. Blood cells were resuspended in 2 ml of phosphate buffered saline and centrifuged at 1500 rpm for 15 min at room temperature. Washing procedures were repeated three times. After resuspension and centrifugation at 400 rpm for 15 min the supernatant platelet suspension was taken for further analysis. Platelet counts were determined on a Sysmex counter and suspensions were adjusted.

Mass Spectrometry

Lipid extracts of platelets were dried under stream of nitrogen and redissolved in 250 μl of chloroform/methanol 2:1 containing either 10 mM ammonium acetate for positive ion analysis or no additive for negative ion measurements. A set of internal standards for intensity correction and quantification was added directly before performing lipid extracts.

Mass spectrometric analysis was performed with a triple quadruple instrument model TSQ 7000 (Finnigan, San Jose, CA) equipped with a nano-electrospray source (Protana, Odense, Denmark) operating at a typical flow rate of 20–80 nl/min. The instrument was used either in single stage MS mode for detection of total positive or negative ions or in tandem MS mode for product ion, precursor ion or neutral loss scan analysis as previously described [14]. The relative intensity of each $[M+H]^+$ and $[M+H]^-$ was determined from phospholipid specific scan analysis as described [14]. This corrected intensities were used to calculate phospholipid concentration via a set of internal standards [15].

To identify the fatty acid composition of each molecular species, product ion scan analysis of the different molecular species and parent ion scans for all major fatty acids were performed.

Aliquots of 10–20 μl were transferred into the nano-electrospray capillary, and the spray was started by applying 800 V to the capillary. For each spectrum 60 repetitive scans of 2s duration were averaged. All tandem MS experiments were performed with argon as collision gas at a nominal pressure of 2.3 mTorr. Collision energy settings were employed as described [14].

Flow Cytometry

Platelet Activation

For negative controls 100 μl of platelet suspension ($20*10^3$ cells/μl) were incubated with PBS and GPRP (1 mg/ml final concentration). For thrombin-stimulated samples 100 μl of platelet suspension were incubated with 100 μl Thrombin (Sigma, USA, 1U/ml final concentration), PBS and GPRP. For Ionophor-stimulated samples 100 μl of platelet suspension were incubated with 10 μl Calcium Ionophor A23187 (Calbiochem, USA, 20 μM final concentration), PBS and GPRP. Samples were incubated for 15 min at room temperature.

Antibodies

For annexin V measurements 12 x 75 mm polypropylene tubes were prepared to a total volume of 400 μl containing: 300 μl of either stimulated or resting platelet suspension as described above and 100 μl of 1X Binding Buffer containing 0.25 μg/ml FITC-annexin V. After gentle mixing, the samples were incubated for 15 min at room temperature in the dark and subsequently diluted with 500 μl 1X binding buffer.

All tubes were analyzed within one hour after preparation using a FACScan flow cytometer (Becton-Dickinson).

Thrombin Generation

To either resting platelet suspension ($2.5*10^6$ cells/μl) or Ionophor-stimulated platelet suspension (final concentration of Ionophor: 20 μM) the components of prothrombinase complex were added: FXa (final concentration: 1.5 pM), FVa (final concentration: 3 pM). After adding FII (final concentration: 4 nM) and calcium chloride (final concentration: 5 μM) a subsampling method was used to monitor the time course of thrombin generation:

At timed intervals 10 μl aliquots were withdrawn from the tube and subsampled into 490 μl PBS containing 225 μM S2238. The reaction was stopped after 6 min by addition of 250 μl 50% acetic acid. The amount of generated thrombin was quantitated by measuring the absorbency by double wavelength (405–690 nm) in the Anthos microplate reader 2001 (Anthos Labtec Instruments GmbH, Austria).

Results

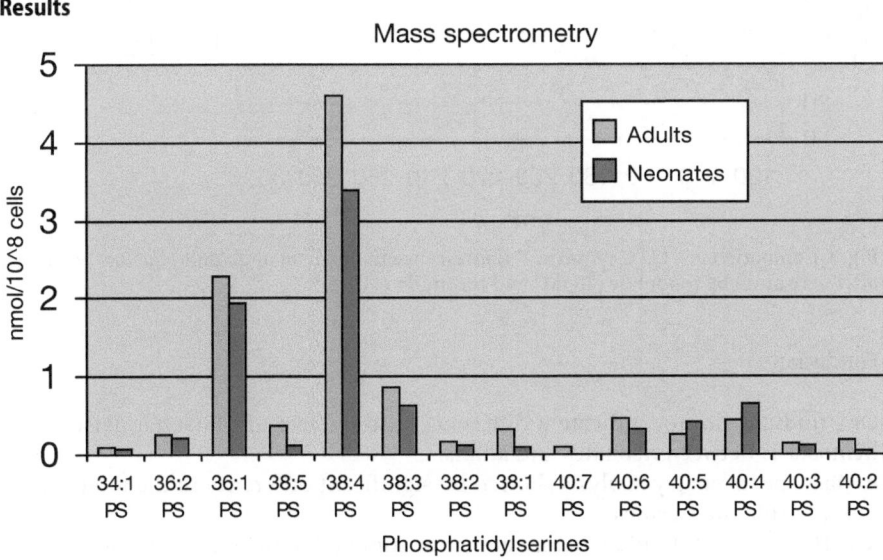

Fig. 1. Categorization of phosphatidylserines into length and number of double bonds of their fatty acids.

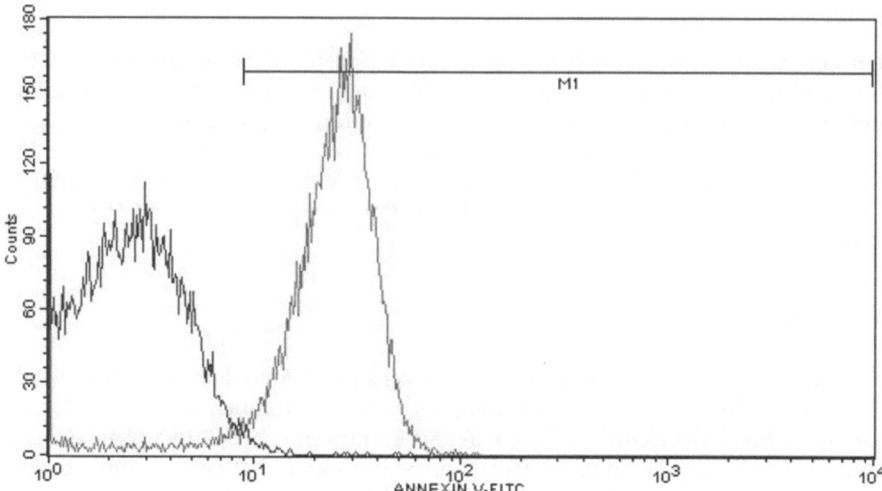

Fig. 2. Flow cytometry histogram showing the g1-control (blue) and the FITC-annexin labeled platelets (red) after Ionophor stimulation. A marker was set including ~1% of g1-control-events and the percentage of FITC-annexin V labeled events in the marker region was taken for statistical analysis.

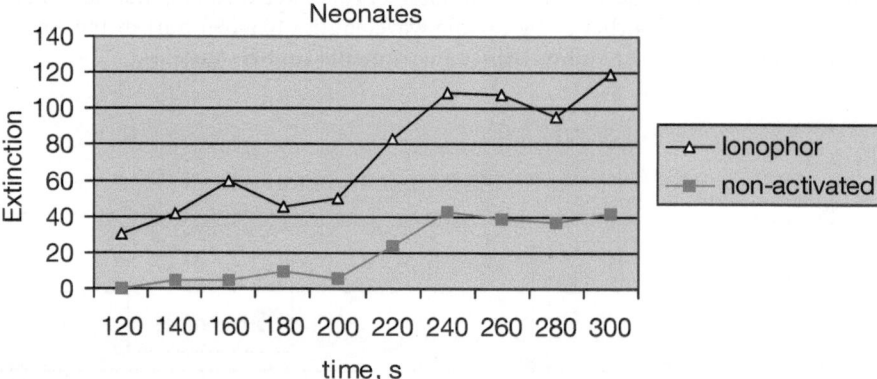

Fig. 3. Comparison of FITC-annexin V fluorescence in neonatal and adult platelets before and after activation by Ionophor (20μM) and thrombin (1U/ml)

Conclusion

Our findings do not indicate a difference in the effect of phosphatidylserine on hemostasis between neonates and adults:
- Mass spectrometry analysis showed no significant difference in the total amount of phosphatidylserines.
- FITC-annexin V binding before and after stimulation by Ionophor was similar.
- No significant difference was detected in the supporting effect of phosphatidylserine on thrombin generation.

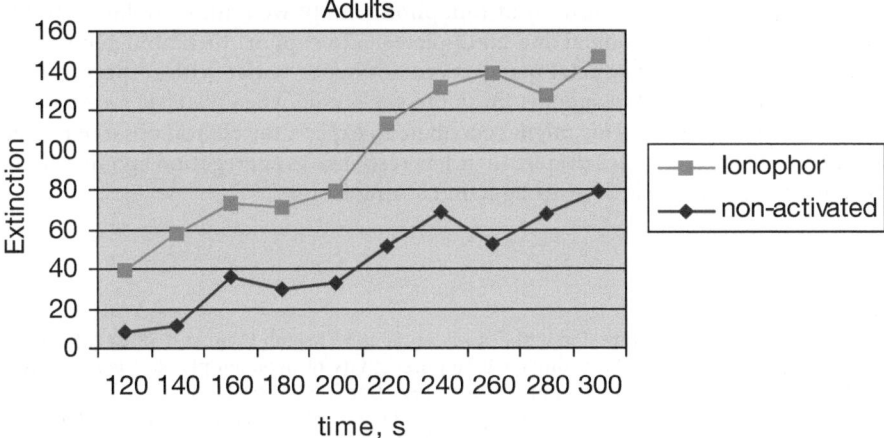

Fig. 4. Thrombin generation in the presence or absence of Ionophor

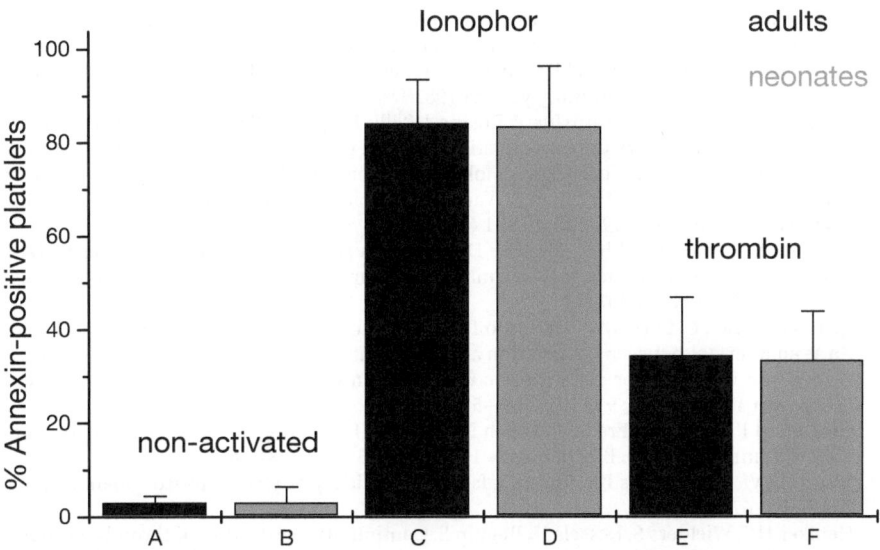

Fig. 5. Thrombin generation before and after stimulation of neonatal platelets by Ionophor

Discussion

Platelets play an important role in primary hemostasis and are closely linked to plasmatic coagulation. Phosphatidylserine as a part of cell membrane is a procoagulant factor enabling coagulation factors to assemble to coagulation complexes and thus to generate large amounts of thrombin. In our study we did not detect significant differences in the total amount of PS. Furthermore, same amounts of PS were exposed to the outer leaflet after addition of Ionophor. Finally, we found similar ability of Ionophor-stimulated neonatal and adult platelets to support thrombin generation. Our data indicate that neonatal platelets are not hyporeactive with respect to their ability to expose PS and to support thrombin generation when platelets are activated by addition of Ionophor. This might contribute to explain the clinical observed excellent hemostasis of neonates despite their low response to aggregation agonists in in-vitro tests and low levels of procoagulant clotting factors.

References

1. Michelson AD. Platelet function in the newborn. Semin Thromb Hemost 1998; 24 (6): 507–12
2. Grosshaupt B, Muntean W, Sedlmayr P. Hyporeactivity of neonatal platelets is not caused by preactivation during birth. Eur J Pediatr 1997 Dec; 156 (12): 944–8
3. Saving KL, Jennings DE, Aldag JC, Caughey RC. Platelet ultrastructure of high-risk premature infants. Thromb Res 1994 Mar 15; 73 (6): 371–84
4. Rajasekhar D, Kestin AS, Bednarek FJ, Ellis PA, Barnard MR, Michelson AD. Neonatal platelets are less reactive than adult platelets to physiological agonists in whole blood. Thromb Haemost 1994 Dec; 72 (6): 957–63
5. Andrew M. Developmental hemostasis: relevance to thromboembolic complications in pediatric patients. Thromb Haemost 1995 Jul; 74 (1): 415–25
6. Bevers EM, Comfurius P, Zwaal RF. Changes in membrane phospholipid distribution during platelet activation. Biochim Biophys Acta 1983 Dec 7; 736 (1): 57–66
7. Zwaal RF, Bevers EM, Comfurius P, Rosing J, Tilly RH, Verhallen PF. Loss of membrane phospholipid asymmetry during activation of blood platelets and sickled red cells; mechanisms and physiological significance. Mol Cell Biochem 1989 Nov 23-Dec 19; 91 (1–2): 23–31
8. Sumner WT, Monroe DM, Hoffman M. Variability in platelet procoagulant activity in healthy volunteers. Thromb Res 1996 Mar 1; 81 (5): 533–43
9. Ahmad SS, Rawala-Sheikh R, Monroe DM, Roberts HR, Walsh PN. Comparative platelet binding and kinetic studies with normal and variant factor IXa molecules. J Biol Chem 1990 Dec 5; 265 (34): 20907–11
10. Cirino G, Cicala C, Bucci M, Sorrentino L, Ambrosini G, DeDominicis G, Altieri DC. Factor Xa as an interface between coagulation and inflammation. Molecular mimicry of factor Xa association with effector cell protease receptor-1 induces acute inflammation in vivo. J Clin Invest 1997 May 15; 99 (10): 2446–51
11. Greengard JS, Heeb MJ, Ersdal E, Walsh PN, Griffin JH. Binding of coagulation factor XI to washed human platelets. Biochemistry 1986 Jul 1; 25 (13): 3884–90
12. Weiss HJ, Vicic WJ, Lages BA, Rogers J. Isolated deficiency of platelet procoagulant activity. Am J Med 67: 206, 1979
13. Hemker HC, Wielders S, Kessels H, Beguin S. Continuous registration of thrombin generation in plasma, its use for the determination of the thrombin potential.: Thromb Haemost 1993 Oct 18; 70 (4): 617–24
14. B. Brügger, G. Erben, R. Sandhoff, F. T. Wieland, W.-D. Lehmann. Quantitative analysis of biological membrane lipids at the low picomole level by nano-electrospray ionization tandem mass spectrometry. Proc. Natl. Acad. Sci. U.S.A. 94: 2339–2344. 1997
15. Koivusalo M, Haimi P, Heikinheimo L, Kostiainen R, Somerharju P. Quantitative determination of phospholipid compositions by ESI-MS: effects of acyl chain length, unsaturation, and lipid concentration on instrument response. J Lipid Res 2001 Apr; 42 (4): 663–72

Low Protein C, Tissue Factor Pathway Inhibitor, and Antithrombin allow Sufficient Thrombin Generation in Neonatal Plasma

G. Cvirn, S. Gallistl, T. Rehak, G. Jürgens, and W. Muntean

Introduction

Despite physiological low levels of contact and vitamin K dependent factors, [1, 2] neonates show no easy bruising, no increased bleeding during surgery, and good wound healing.

Therefore, we investigated whether physiological low concentrations of the inhibitors activated protein C (APC), tissue factor pathway inhibitor (TFPI), and antithrombin (AT) possibly compensate for the low levels of procoagulant factors and allow efficient thrombin generation. In contrast to conventional in-vitro clotting assays, where high amounts of thromboplastin reagents are applied to initiate clotting, we used low amounts of relipidated tissue factor (rTF). It has been shown that coagulation activation via the extrinsic pathway with low amounts of rTF is probably more physiological than the activation commonly used in standard assay systems [3]. Activation of protein C was induced by endogenously generated thrombin in the presence of added soluble thrombomodulin (TM) [4].

Material and Methods

Collection and Preparation of Plasma

Cord blood was obtained immediately following the delivery of 28 full term infants (38–42 weeks gestational age). Newborns with Apgar scores of 9 or less five minutes after delivery were excluded from the study. Blood was collected into 0.1 M citrate using a two syringe technique, centrifuged at room temperature for 15 min at 2800 x g, pooled and stored at -70°C in propylene tubes until assayed. FV and FVIII activities were elevated over the respective adult values, other pro- and anticoagulant factors were in the normal range for neonates. In the same way plasma from 18 healthy adults was collected from the antecubital vein, prepared, and checked.

Activation of Plasma

Three hundred µl plasma with different TFPI and/or AT levels were incubated with 100 µl of PBS containing lipidated recombinant human TF (1.25-10 pM final concen-

I. Scharrer/W. Schramm (Ed.)
33rd Hemophilia Symposion Hamburg 2002
© Springer-Verlag Berlin Heidelberg 2004

tration) and soluble TM (2–10 nM final concentration) for 1 minute at 37°C. After subsequent incubation with 20 μl PBS containing H-Gly-Pro-Arg-Pro-OH (Pefabloc FG, 1.0 mg/ml final concentration) to inhibit fibrin polymerization, [5] plasma samples were activated by addition of 12 μl 0.5 M CaCl$_2$.

Determination of Clotting Time

Clotting times were determined by means of the optomechanical coagulation analyzer Behring Fibrintimer II from Dade Behring Marburg GmbH, Marburg, Germany, which applies the turbodensitometric measuring principle.

Determination of Thrombin Generation

We used a subsampling method derived from a recently described technique. [5] Plasmas were prepared and activated as described above. At timed intervals 10 μl aliquots were withdrawn from the activated plasma and subsampled into 490 μl PBS containing 255 μM S-2238. Amidolysis of S-2238 was stopped after 6 min by addition of 250 μl 50% acetic acid. The amount of thrombin generated was quantitated by measuring the absorbency by double wave length (405–690 nm) in the Anthos microplate-reader 2001, from Anthos Labtec Instruments GmbH, Salzburg, Austria. The total amidolytic activity measured is caused by the simultaneous activity of free thrombin and the alpha 2-macroglobulin (α2-M)/thrombin complex. Free thrombin generation curves were calculated by mathematical treatment of total amidolytic activity curves using a method developed by Hemker et al.

The area under the free thrombin generation curve has been called »thrombin potential (TP)«. The TP has been shown to be a suitable parameter to reflect the thrombogenic potency in a given plasma sample.

Determination of APC Generation

Plasmas were prepared and activated as described above. At timed intervals 20 μl aliquots were withdrawn from the activated plasma and subsampled into 280 μl PBS containing 3 mM S 2366 and 0.1 mM I-2581 to block thrombin activity. After 15 min, 100 μl of 50 % actetic acid was added to terminate the chromogenic substrate conversion. After each reaction was stopped, 250 μl of the reaction mixture was transferred to an ELISA plate, and the absorbency was measured at 405 nm in the Anthos microplate reader. The molar concentrations of the generated APC were calculated from reference curves constructed by measuring the activity of purified human APC (0–20 nM) with S 2366 [6].

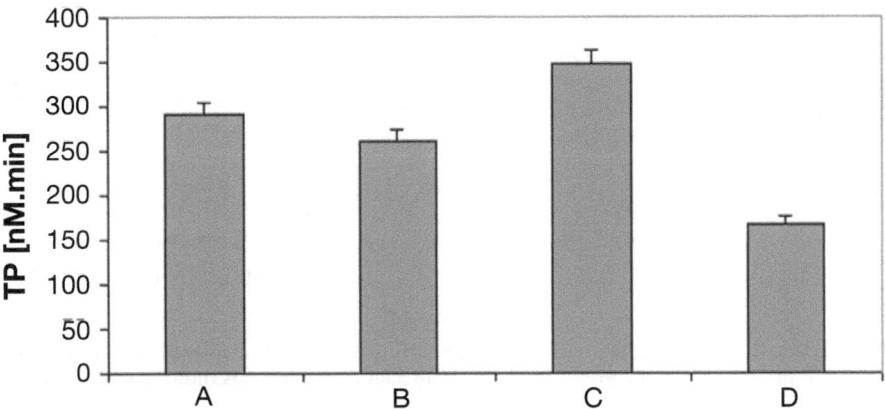

Fig. 1. Effect of addition of TM on TF-initiated thrombin generation. Thrombin potential (TP) is displayed in reactions initiated by 5 pM TF in cord plasma in the absence of TM (A), in the presence of 4 nM TM (B), and in adult plasma in the absence of TM (C), and in the presence of 4 nM TM (D).

Results

Effects of the Addition of 4 nM of Thrombomodulin (TM) on Thrombin Potential (TP) in Cord and Adult Plasma

Suppression of the TP due to addition of 4 nM of TM was significantly less pronounced in cord plasma (291 to 261 nM.min) than in adult plasma (347 to 167 nM.min, p of differences <0.001), shown in Figure 1. Accordingly, the clotting time (the time that elapses until a level of 10–20 nM of thrombin is formed in the reaction mixture) was significantly less prolonged in cord plasma (204 to 233 s) than in adult plasma (219 to 311s, p of differences <0.001).

Effects of the Addition of TM on APC Generation in Cord and Adult Plasma

Formation of APC dose-dependently increased in the presence of increasing amounts of TM in both cord and adult plasma (data not shown). APC generation started simultaneously with thrombin formation, and, therefore, occurred significantly earlier in cord plasma. Approximately same amounts of APC were generated in cord and adult plasma (Fig. 2).

Effect of TFPI and AT on the Anticoagulant Action of TM in Cord Plasma

The capability of 4 nM of TM to suppress thrombin formation and to prolong clotting time is significantly less pronounced in cord plasma containing TFPI and AT at physiological levels (the TP was decreased from 291 to 261 nM.min, the clotting time

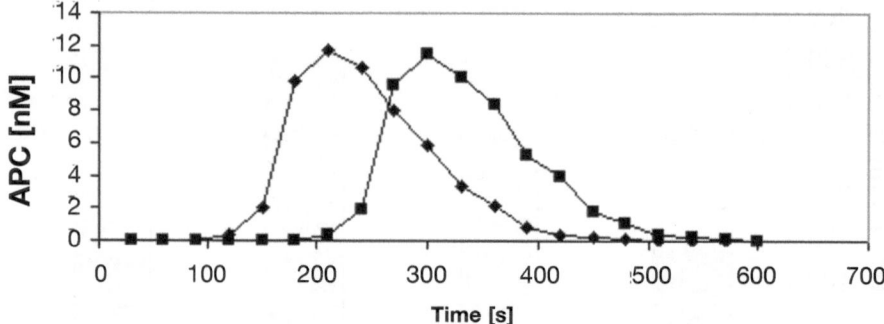

Fig. 2. Effect of TM on APC generation. APC generation over time is displayed in both cord (◆) and adult plasma (■) in the presence of 4 nM TM, clot formation was induced by addition of 2.5 pM of TF.

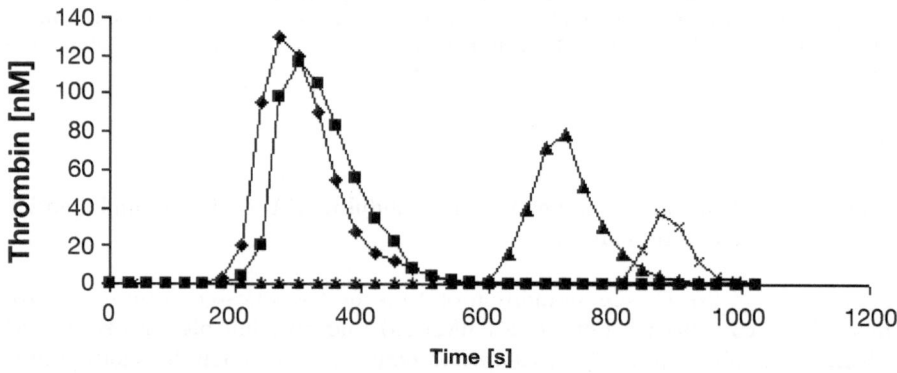

Fig. 3. Effect of TFPI and AT on the anticoagulant action of 4 nM TM in cord plasma. Free thrombin generation over time is displayed in reactions initiated by 5 pM TF in cord plasma containing physiological levels of TFPI and AT in the absence of TM (◆), in the presence of 4 nM TM (■), and in cord plasma containing TFPI and AT at adult levels in the absence of TM (▲), and in the presence of 4 nM TM (✖).

was prolonged from 204 to 233 s) compared to that in cord plasma containing TFPI and AT at adult levels (the TP was decreased from 182 to 81 nM.min, the clotting time was prolonged from 617 to 815 s, p of differences <0.001), shown in Fig. 3.

Conclusions

The low anticoagulant capacity of the three inhibitors APC, TFPI, and AT in cord plasma allows enhanced thrombin formation associated with shorter clotting times compared to adult plasma when low amounts of rTF are applied to initiate clot formation.

Our results might contribute to explain the clinical observed excellent hemostasis in neonates despite low levels of procoagulant factors, i.e. prothrombin.

References

1. Andrew M, Paes B, Milner R, Johnston M, Mitchell L, Tollefsen DM, Powers P. Development of the human coagulation system in the full-term infant. Blood 1987; 70: 165–72
2. Nardi M, Karpatkin M. Prothrombin and protein C in early childhood: normal adult levels are not achieved until the fourth year of life. J Pediatr 1986; 109: 843–5
3. Davie EW, Fujikawa K, Kisiel W. The coagulation cascade: Initiation, maintenance and regulation. Biochemistry 1991; 30: 10363–70
4. Dittman WA. Thrombomodulin: biology and potential cardiovascular applications. Trends Cardiovasc Med 1991; 8: 331–6
5. Wielders S, Mukherjee M, Michiels J, Rijkers DT, Cambus JP, Knebel RW, Kakkar V, Hemker HC, Beguin S. The routine determination of the endogenous thrombin potential, first results in different forms of hyper- and hypocoagulability. Thromb Haemost 1997; 77: 629–36
6. Varadi K, Siekmann J, Turecek PL, Schwarz HP. Phospholipid-bound tissue factor modulates both thrombin generation and APC-mediated factor a inactivation. Thromb Haemost 1999; 82: 1673–9

Subject Index